Aaron M. Fischman • Rahul S.Patel
Robert A. Lookstein
Editors

Transradial Access in Interventional Radiology

Background, Applications and Techniques

Springer

Editors
Aaron M. Fischman
Department of Diagnostic
Molecular and Interventional Radiology
Icahn School of Medicine at Mount Sinai
New York, NY
USA

Rahul S. Patel
Department of Diagnostic
Molecular and Interventional Radiology
Icahn School of Medicine at Mount Sinai
New York, NY
USA

Robert A. Lookstein
Department of Diagnostic
Molecular and Interventional Radiology
Icahn School of Medicine at Mount Sinai
New York, NY
USA

ISBN 978-3-030-81677-3 ISBN 978-3-030-81678-0 (eBook)
https://doi.org/10.1007/978-3-030-81678-0

This Springer imprint is published by the registered company Springer Nature Switzerland AG
The registered company address is: Gewerbestrasse 11, 6330 Cham, Switzerland

This book is dedicated to Harold A. Mitty, MD, FSIR, the father of interventional radiology at Mount Sinai. He is a dedicated mentor, innovator, and pioneer. His life's work will always be remembered and cherished by countless generations of IRs.

Preface

> The secret of change is to focus all of your energy, not on fighting the old, but building on the new. – Socrates (470–399BC)

> If I had asked the public what they wanted, they would have said a faster horse. – Henry Ford

When I think about the evolution of transradial access in interventional radiology, I often remind myself how long it took for the cardiology community to fully adopt this technique and the many obstacles along the way. Since we performed our first chemoembolization from the radial artery in 2012, the hope was that we could learn from prior successes and failures and move forward rapidly in a thoughtful and energetic way. Since then, the technique has rapidly evolved and improved, and has become the preferred arterial access point in our center and many other centers around the world. In many ways, we have learned a lot from the pioneers before us in this space like Lucien Campeau and Ferdinand Kiemeneji. In other ways, much of our knowledge was gained via diligence, creativity, trial and error, and a constant desire to innovate. As we did this, our medical device industry partners watched and listened. New devices were developed. We tried new things together. We had some failures but many more successes. The true beneficiaries of these collaborative efforts are our patients. Transradial access has been shown to be safe, cost effective, technically feasible even in dire circumstances, and more comfortable for patients. There are many among us that are satisfied with the status quo and don't see any need to change or deviate from the current path (see Henry Ford's quote above). That's OK to a point, but then we need to remember who we are and where we came from. We trained to think outside the box. We trained to innovate. We trained to advance minimally invasive intervention to improve the lives of our patients. This book represents almost a decade of experience in the world of transradial access in interventional radiology. It is our hope that you use what is written in this book as a guide in your career-long exploration of what is possible.

New York, NY, USA — Aaron M. Fischman

Contents

1 **The Advent of Transradial Interventions: An Overview** 1
Chidubem Ugwueze and Aaron M. Fischman

2 **Anatomy and Physical Exam** 11
Matthew Tangel and Joseph J. Titano

3 **Nursing Assessment** 19
Aaron M. Fischman, Adie Friedman, and Jacxelyn Moran

4 **Procedure Suite Setup** 25
Kristina Prachanronarong and Vivian Bishay

5 **Recovery Room and Post-procedure Care** 31
Kristina Prachanronarong and Vivian Bishay

6 **Access Complications and Management** 37
Naveen Galla and Rajesh I. Patel

7 **Transradial Access for Renal and Mesenteric Artery Disease** 51
Nicholas Voutsinas and Robert A. Lookstein

8 **Transradial Access for Interventional Oncology: Chemoembolization and Radioembolization Applications** 57
Samuel Z. Maron, Nickolas Dreher, Joseph J. Titano, and Edward Kim

9 **Transradial Access for Peripheral Arterial Disease: Aortoiliac Applications** 63
Alex Sher, Raghuram Posham, Samuel Z. Maron, and Rami O. Tadros

10 **Transradial Access for Peripheral Arterial Disease: Infrainguinal Applications** 75
Raghuram Posham, Alex Sher, Samuel Z. Maron, and Rami O. Tadros

11 Aortic Endoleak Following Endovascular Aortic Repair 87
Wayne Martin Bauknight and Rahul S. Patel

12 Transradial Access for Peripheral Arterial Disease: Subclavian and Upper Arm Interventions 113
Shashidhara Murthy, Rahul S. Patel, and Aaron M. Fischman

13 Transradial Access in Uterine Artery Embolization 123
Ricki Korff, Shaun Honig, and Scott Nowakowski

14 Prostate Artery Embolization 133
Jason Gruener and Ardeshir R. Rastinehad

15 Hemodialysis Access Interventions 147
Timothy Carlon and Joseph J. Titano

16 Carotid and Vertebral Intervention 163
Reade De Leacy, Devin V. Bageac, Brett Marinelli, Sayan Manna, and J. Mocco

17 Endovascular Neurosurgery and Stroke Intervention 177
Reade De Leacy, Devin V. Bageac, Jennifer M. Watchmaker, Sayan Manna, and J. Mocco

18 Acute Hemorrhage and Trauma 195
David Kestenbaum and Robert Blue

19 Transulnar Arterial Access 211
Daryl Goldman, Jun Yeop Lee, and Mona Ranade

20 Distal Transradial Arterial Access 221
Daryl Goldman, Raghuram Posham, and Mona Ranade

21 Transradial Access for Bariatric Embolization 233
Mario A. Cedillo, Kirema Garcia-Reyes, and Aaron M. Fischman

Index 243

Contributors

Devin V. Bageac Departments of Neurosurgery and Diagnostic, Molecular and Interventional Radiology, Icahn School of Medicine at Mount Sinai, New York, NY, USA

Wayne Martin Bauknight Northwestern Medicine, Chicago, IL, USA

Vivian Bishay Department of Diagnostic, Molecular and Interventional Radiology, Icahn School of Medicine at Mount Sinai, New York, NY, USA

Robert Blue Department of Diagnostic, Molecular and Interventional Radiology, Icahn School of Medicine at Mount Sinai, New York, NY, USA

Timothy Carlon Department of Diagnostic, Molecular and Interventional Radiology, Icahn School of Medicine at Mount Sinai, New York, NY, USA

Mario A. Cedillo Department of Diagnostic, Molecular and Interventional Radiology, Icahn School of Medicine at Mount Sinai, New York, NY, USA

Reade De Leacy Departments of Neurosurgery and Diagnostic, Molecular and Interventional Radiology, Icahn School of Medicine at Mount Sinai, New York, NY, USA

Nickolas Dreher Department of Diagnostic, Molecular and Interventional Radiology, Icahn School of Medicine at Mount Sinai, New York, NY, USA

Aaron M. Fischman Department of Diagnostic, Molecular and Interventional Radiology, Icahn School of Medicine at Mount Sinai, New York, NY, USA

Adie Friedman Department of Radiology, Memorial Sloan Kettering Cancer Center, New York City, NY, USA

Naveen Galla Department of Diagnostic, Molecular and Interventional Radiology, Icahn School of Medicine at Mount Sinai, New York, NY, USA

Kirema Garcia-Reyes Department of Diagnostic, Molecular and Interventional Radiology, Icahn School of Medicine at Mount Sinai, New York, NY, USA

Daryl Goldman Department of Diagnostic, Molecular and Interventional Radiology, Icahn School of Medicine at Mount Sinai, New York, NY, USA

Jason Gruener Department of Diagnostic, Molecular and Interventional Radiology, Icahn School of Medicine at Mount Sinai, New York, NY, USA

Shaun Honig Department of Diagnostic, Molecular and Interventional Radiology, Icahn School of Medicine at Mount Sinai, New York, NY, USA

David Kestenbaum Department of Diagnostic, Molecular and Interventional Radiology, Icahn School of Medicine at Mount Sinai, New York, NY, USA

Edward Kim Department of Diagnostic, Molecular and Interventional Radiology, Icahn School of Medicine at Mount Sinai, New York, NY, USA

Ricki Korff Department of Diagnostic, Molecular and Interventional Radiology, Icahn School of Medicine at Mount Sinai, New York, NY, USA

Jun Yeop Lee Department of Diagnostic, Molecular and Interventional Radiology, Icahn School of Medicine at Mount Sinai, New York, NY, USA

Robert A. Lookstein Department of Diagnostic, Molecular and Interventional Radiology, Icahn School of Medicine at Mount Sinai, New York, NY, USA

Sayan Manna Departments of Neurosurgery and Diagnostic, Molecular and Interventional Radiology, Icahn School of Medicine at Mount Sinai, New York, NY, USA

Brett Marinelli Departments of Neurosurgery and Diagnostic, Molecular and Interventional Radiology, Icahn School of Medicine at Mount Sinai, New York, NY, USA

Samuel Z. Maron Department of Diagnostic, Molecular and Interventional Radiology, Icahn School of Medicine at Mount Sinai, New York, NY, USA

J. Mocco Departments of Neurosurgery and Diagnostic, Molecular and Interventional Radiology, Icahn School of Medicine at Mount Sinai, New York, NY, USA

Jacxelyn Moran Department of Diagnostic, Molecular and Interventional Radiology, Icahn School of Medicine at Mount Sinai, New York, NY, USA

Shashidhara Murthy Department of Diagnostic, Molecular and Interventional Radiology, Icahn School of Medicine at Mount Sinai, New York, NY, USA

Scott Nowakowski Department of Diagnostic, Molecular and Interventional Radiology, Icahn School of Medicine at Mount Sinai, New York, NY, USA

Rahul S. Patel Department of Diagnostic, Molecular and Interventional Radiology, Icahn School of Medicine at Mount Sinai, New York, NY, USA

Rajesh I. Patel Department of Diagnostic, Molecular and Interventional Radiology, Icahn School of Medicine at Mount Sinai, New York, NY, USA

Raghuram Posham Department of Diagnostic, Molecular and Interventional Radiology, Icahn School of Medicine at Mount Sinai, New York, NY, USA

Kristina Prachanronarong Department of Diagnostic, Molecular and Interventional Radiology, Icahn School of Medicine at Mount Sinai, New York, NY, USA

Mona Ranade Department of Radiology, University of California, Los Angeles, Los Angeles, CA, USA

Ardeshir R. Rastinehad Department of Urology, Lenox Hill Hospital, Northwell Health, New York, NY, USA

Alex Sher Department of Diagnostic, Molecular and Interventional Radiology, Icahn School of Medicine at Mount Sinai, New York, NY, USA

Rami O. Tadros Department of Surgery, Division of Vascular Surgery, Icahn School of Medicine at Mount Sinai, New York, NY, USA

Matthew Tangel Department of Diagnostic, Molecular and Interventional Radiology, Icahn School of Medicine at Mount Sinai, New York, NY, USA

Joseph J. Titano Department of Diagnostic, Molecular and Interventional Radiology, Icahn School of Medicine at Mount Sinai, New York, NY, USA

Chidubem Ugwueze Department of Diagnostic, Molecular and Interventional Radiology, Icahn School of Medicine at Mount Sinai, New York, NY, USA

Nicholas Voutsinas Department of Diagnostic, Molecular and Interventional Radiology, Icahn School of Medicine at Mount Sinai, New York, NY, USA

Jennifer M. Watchmaker Departments of Neurosurgery and Diagnostic, Molecular and Interventional Radiology, Icahn School of Medicine at Mount Sinai, New York, NY, USA

Chapter 1
The Advent of Transradial Interventions: An Overview

Chidubem Ugwueze and Aaron M. Fischman

Abbreviations

CABG	Coronary arterial bypass graft
CAD	Coronary arterial disease
ESC	European Society of Cardiology
PCI	Percutaneous coronary interventions
PTCA	Percutaneous transluminal coronary angioplasty
TCT	Transcatheter Cardiovascular Therapeutics
TRA	Transradial
TREAT	TransRadial Endovascular Advanced Therapies
TRI	Percutaneous transradial interventions

Historical Highlights of Transradial Artery Catheterization

- 1947: Dr. Radner performs first transradial artery catheterization by surgical exposure and ligation of the artery for thoracic aortography.
- 1964: Campeau and Bourassa began using distal radial arteriotomy to perform coronary angiography.
- 1989: Campeau publishes his series of 100 coronary angiograms using a percutaneous access of the distal radial artery using a 5F sheath.

C. Ugwueze (✉) · A. M. Fischman
Department of Diagnostic, Molecular and Interventional Radiology,
Icahn School of Medicine at Mount Sinai, New York, NY, USA
e-mail: chidubem.ugwueze@mountsinai.org; aaron.fischman@mountsinai.org

A. M. Fischman et al. (eds.), *Transradial Access in Interventional Radiology*,
https://doi.org/10.1007/978-3-030-81678-0_1

- 1992: Masaki Otaki applies percutaneous transradial coronary angiography in Japanese patients.
- 1992: Kiemeneij performs first percutaneous transradial coronary balloon angioplasty.
- 1994: Fajadet performs first transradial intervention live streaming from Toulouse to the Transcatheter Cardiovascular Therapeutics conference in Washington.
- 1999: First noncoronary transradial cases performed in Japan.
- 2013 and 2015 ESC consensus statement making the transradial approach the standard of care for percutaneous coronary interventions.
- 2014: First Annual TransRadial Endovascular Advanced Therapies (TREAT) Conference.
- 2016: A review of 1500 transradial noncoronary cases performed at the Mount Sinai Hospital is published.

Preamble

The history of intravascular access is a story of persistent endeavor by clinicians to apply the newest techniques in improving the lives of their patients. These applications of new techniques have meant safer and more minimally invasive routes for entering the arterial system to perform diagnostic and interventional procedures. Over the course of the last quarter century, percutaneous vascular access via the radial artery has emerged as a standard for arterial access proliferating and contributing enormously to improvements in quality of life and decreased procedural complication and mortality rates. These advancements are a result of nonlinear incremental technical and clinical refinements that made percutaneous transradial access the standard for percutaneous coronary interventions in many countries. Interest in a transradial approach was present early in the development of the fields of interventional radiology and cardiology. For instance, in 1947, Stig Radner performed an intracranial angiography via the radial artery at Lund University, Sweden. Dr. Charles Dotter's method for nonselective coronary angiography published in 1958 was performed via radial access. The next documented successful applications of transradial access in clinical practice were in 1989 by Lucien Campeau at the Montreal Heart Institute. Prior to Campeau's 1989 report, this technique was obscure and underutilized. This chapter attempts to delineate the steps that led from early enthusiasm during the founding of Interventional Cardiology and Interventional Radiology to the eventual increasing prevalence of transradial interventions in both fields.

Origins of Transradial Approach

In March 1947, Stig Radner performed the first radial artery access procedure, via surgical exposure, for intracranial angiography by injecting contrast into the vertebral artery [1]. He repeated this technique in a series of patients for thoracic aortography in 1948 [2]. It is striking that Radner's first intracranial angiography attempt was reportedly performed on himself [3]. He was definitely a pioneer way ahead of his time. However, because of the technical difficulties, risks, and time consumption inherent in performing arterial catheterization by surgical exposure (Fig. 1.1) followed by surgical ligation or suturing of the vessel, other innovators sought percutaneous catheterization, introducing a catheter into the blood vessel through the skin via needle stick, as an alternative to surgical cutdowns. In 1949, Gunnar Jonsson, a Swedish radiologist, performed the first percutaneous thoracic aortography when he cannulated the common carotid artery using trocar technique, entering the artery with a blunt cannula and a sharp inner needle. The procedure was prematurely aborted because the operator feared that the blunt and inflexible cannula would damage the aortic wall [4]. A year later the availability of flexible thin-walled polyethylene tubes made percutaneous access more feasible [5]. In 1951, two groups performed percutaneous arterial catheterization using these more flexible tubes, Peirce into the femoral artery for aortography and Donald, Kesmodel, Rollins, and Paddison into the common carotid artery for cerebral angiography [6, 7]. These subsequent percutaneous catheterizations were performed by passing the polyethylene tube through large bore needles. Despite the breakthrough, this method was unreliable and carried a significant risk of access site hemorrhage given that the needle puncture was larger than the polyethylene tube caliber. Thus, in 1953, Sven Seldinger, then a second year radiology resident, solved this problem by replacing the needle with the same size catheter using a metal leader, now referred to as guidewires [8].

Despite the introduction of the Seldinger technique, use of a percutaneous transradial approach (Fig. 1.2) remained limited because vascular catheters at the time were still relatively too large and inflexible to be accommodated in the smaller

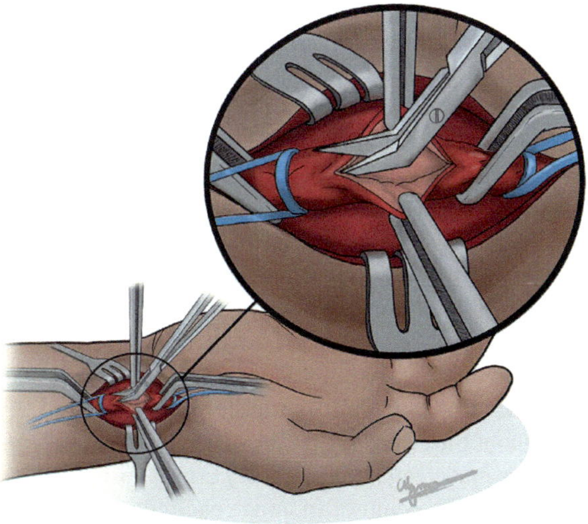

Fig. 1.1 Representation of surgical exposure of the radial artery. Encircled is the arteriotomy that allows for vascular access. (Illustration by Chidubem Ugwueze)

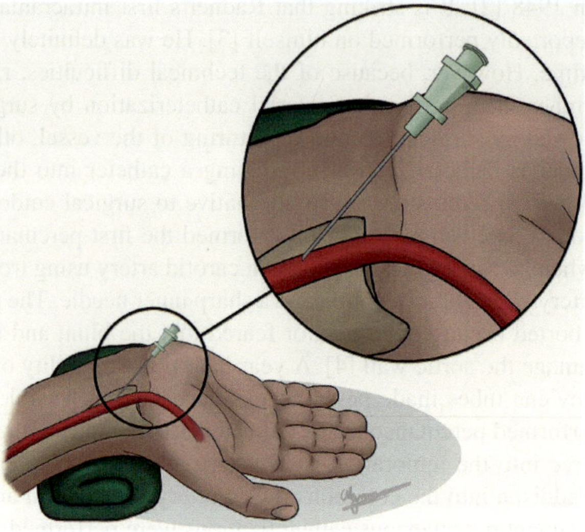

Fig. 1.2 Representation of percutaneous needle access of the radial artery (Illustration by Dr. Chidubem Ugwueze)

caliber of the artery. In 1964 Campeau and Bourassa, at the Montreal Heart Institute, began accessing the distal radial artery, inserting 7F catheters via surgical exposure for coronary angiography [9]. Besides this, 1947 through 1989 was otherwise void of documented advances or increased prevalence of transradial procedures. During this same time frame, the more accommodating caliber of the femoral arteries facilitated a proliferation in percutaneous transfemoral coronary angiography and interventions.

Coronary angiography was first performed in 1958 when F Mason Sones, a cardiologist at the Cleveland Clinic, fortuitously cannulated the ostia of the right coronary artery and selectively opacified the vessel via a distal brachial arteriotomy [10]. At the time of Sones' serendipitous discovery, there were multiple other investigators attempting different non-selective methods of aortic root injections to opacify the coronary arteries. One of these investigators was Dr. Charles Dotter, the father of interventional radiology. He published his occlusive aortography method for coronary arteriography in 1958. Dotter's aortic root injection method, and those of Lehman et al. and Richard and Thal, was deemed to carry additional risks without the optimal visualization achieved by Sones' selective cannulation. Hence, Sones' selective method became the standard [11–14, 15].

Ricketts and Abrams performed the first percutaneous transfemoral coronary angiography in 1961 [16]. However, it was the independent and parallel work done by radiologists Dr. Judkins and Dr. Amplatz on preshaped catheters that truly facilitated the dissemination of the coronary angiography as a diagnostic technique throughout the radiology and cardiology world [17, 18]. This is because preshaped catheters made engaging coronary arterial ostia much easier, reducing the technical difficulty and amount of training required to achieve proficiency in the procedure.

The diagnostic prowess of coronary angiography had a transformative impact on the evaluation and treatment of coronary arterial disease (CAD). It served as an effective roadmap and stimulus for significant innovation in the surgical and percutaneous treatment of CAD. Sones' early coronary angiographic studies demonstrated that the internal mammary implant used in the Vineberg procedure, the surgical procedure at the time aimed at alleviating the symptoms of CAD, was grossly inadequate. A series of postoperative coronary arteriography performed 1 year after the procedure demonstrated collateral flow to the ischemic myocardium in only 54% of the cases studied [14, 19]. This discovery played a role in motivating the subsequent development of the Coronary Arterial Bypass Graft (CABG) surgery by Dr. Rene Favaloro, also at the Cleveland Clinic [20]. Sones visualized the first patent aorto-coronary vein graft in 1967. The clinical success of Favaloro's saphenous vein bypass graft (CABG) was so dramatic that by the early 1970s it had become the most common surgical procedure in the USA [14].

The 1970s was also very notable for the birth of percutaneous transluminal coronary angioplasty (1977). Inspired by Dotter's 1964 transluminal angioplasty for the treatment of atherosclerotic obstruction of the femoral artery, Dr. Andreas Gruentzig, a German radiologist and father of interventional cardiology, performed the first percutaneous transluminal coronary angioplasty (PTCA) in 1977 [21–23]. This was the spark that created the field of interventional cardiology and later made percutaneous coronary interventions (PCIs) a standard intervention for CAD. It began by establishing coronary angioplasty as a credible alternative to coronary arterial bypass grafting. The evolution of percutaneous coronary stenting and resultant improvement in long-term efficacy allowed for PCI to make this big leap.

Development and Acceptance of Transradial Approach in Interventional Cardiology

Transfemoral coronary artery stent placement raised the question of how to safely remove the large bore catheter from the groin access site without significant hemorrhage. This dilemma was notably more complicated than coronary angiography or angioplasty because of the need for anticoagulation/antiplatelet therapy to prevent the newly deployed coronary arterial stent from thrombosing. Despite valiant efforts by both the patient (prolonged immobilization and hospital stays) and physician (dosing medications, monitoring INR and aPTT, and timing access sheath removal), there was a significant high rate of femoral bleeding complications [24]. Hence, when Dr. Lucien Campeau published his series of 100 percutaneous coronary angiography using the distal radial artery in 1989, a fellow cardiologist, Dr. Kiemeneij, saw transradial's value; the shallow path of the radial artery made it easily compressible and the dual blood supply to the hand, for potentially reducing bleeding risk and post procedural complications. In the early 1990s, when catheters small enough to facilitate a radial approach became available, Dr. Kiemeneij began using a 6F radial access system for PCI at his hospital, the Onze Lieve Vrouwe Gasthuis (OLVG) in Amsterdam.

In August 1992, Dr. Kiemeneij performed the first transradial PCI, a coronary balloon angioplasty, shortly followed by a percutaneous transradial coronary stent placement in 1993 [25]. He first presented his work on transradial PCI as a poster presentation at the American Heart Association (AHA) conference in 1993. Conference attendees were intrigued. Nevertheless, the perceived technical difficulty and novelty of the approach proved to be too much of a barrier for a significant number of early enthusiastic adopters at the time. One early adopter made a huge difference. With Dr. Kiemeneij's permission and guidance, Dr. Fajadet live-streamed a percutaneous transradial coronary intervention from his hospital in Toulouse to the 1994 Transcatheter Cardiovascular Therapeutics (TCT) conference in Washington [24]. When thousands of interventional cardiologists in the audience witnessed the patient walk out of the Cath lab immediately after the procedure, there was thunderous applause. This live-streamed demonstration provided international exposure that caused practitioners in several countries to adopt the transradial approach. Percutaneous transradial interventions then transitioned from being championed by one center, Dr. Kiemeneij's OLVG, to multiple centers all around the world.

Increasing adoption of percutaneous transradial interventions (TRI) provided ample data demonstrating that TRI was delivering on its promise. Papers published from 1992 to 1997 showed reduced rates of major access site bleeding resulting in less mortality, increased patient comfort, and decreased costs [24]. The ACCESS study was the first randomized clinical trial showing the equivalence in clinical outcomes between radial, brachial, and femoral access with less transradial access site complications [26]. The mounting evidence helped to overcome the reluctance many clinicians had to learn the newer radial approach. With increasing international adoption and cooperation with medical device companies, dedicated radial access puncture sets, sheaths, catheters, and hemostasis devices were created resulting in even better outcomes and lower threshold for clinicians to start a radial program.

With the turn of the millennium came a series of randomized clinical trials further solidifying the superiority of the transradial approach in reducing bleeding risk and mortality rates; the MORTAL, RIVAL, RIFLE STEACS, and MATRIX studies [27–30]. This accumulation of evidence led the European Society of Cardiology (ESC) to declare the radial access the method of choice for coronary interventions first in 2013 and then affirmed as Class I Level B in 2015 [31]. The transradial approach had gone from obscure experiment to standard of care.

The Evolution of Interventional Radiology and Its Adoption of the Transradial Approach

As alluded to above, the field of interventional radiology stemmed from Charles Dotter's 1964 angioplasty of a stenosed femoral artery. Concurrent to Dotter's breakthrough, Stanley Baum (a radiologist) and Moreye Nusbaum (a surgeon), at the University of Pennsylvania, Philadelphia, pioneered catheter directed embolization for treating acute gastrointestinal bleeding [32]. In 1970, Charles Dotter also reported controlling an acute upper gastrointestinal bleed by selective embolization using autologous clot as the embolic material [33]. Work by Dr. Tetsuro Kato, a Japanese urologist, further demonstrated the importance of embolic material. In 1981, Kato's work showed that delivering microcapsules containing chemotherapeutic agents into tumor supplying arteries was superior to local intra-arterial injection of antitumor agents [34].

A partnership between Juan Parodi, a vascular surgeon, and Julio Palmaz, a radiologist, which began at the 1988 TCT meeting in Washington DC eventually led to the first successful endovascular repair of an abdominal aortic aneurysm in September 1990 [33]. The Palmaz stent, a metal stent, was shortly approved for use in peripheral vessels in 1991. These embolic methods, stents, and stent-grafts, pioneered by Dotter, Kato, Parodi, and Palmaz, allowed for the proliferation of endovascular diagnostic and therapeutic procedures to tamponade bleeds, deliver chemotherapy locally into tumors, restore the lumen of stenosed and dissected vessels, exclude aneurysms, and close arteriovenous fistulas all throughout the body. Percutaneous transfemoral access was utilized for all these early noncoronary arterial interventions.

The first noncoronary percutaneous TRAs were performed in Japan in 1999 [35, 36]. However, uptake into interventional radiology practice was sluggish. By 2011, high volume cardiology clinics in Canada, Europe, and Asia were performing 95% of PCIs via the radial approach. In the USA, this number among interventional cardiologists was a little more than 10% [37]. In the early 2000s, TRA was shown to be feasible and safe for treating peripheral arterial disease [38]. However, at that time, TRA was effectively absent in interventional radiology practices.

Utilizing the technique described in Japan, Dr. Aaron Fischman, an interventional radiologist, performed the first chemoembolization in the USA using the transradial technique on April 19, 2012, at the Mount Sinai Hospital in New York [39]. Shortly thereafter, Dr. Marcelo Guimaraes also performed a TRA chemoembolization in 2013 at the Medical University of South Carolina. Recognizing the significant impact TRA could have on IR practice, in 2013, Dr. Fischman and Dr. Rahul Patel, and other Interventional Radiologists at the Mount Sinai Hospital, published a series of papers demonstrating the feasibility for TRA for uterine artery embolization, prostate artery embolization, hepatic radioembolization, renal artery interventions, peripheral vascular disease, and a call to action for other IRs to start utilizing the transradial access [40–43]. This was the beginning of the development of the largest TRA program in the USA for noncoronary interventions. It was felt at the time that education and training for TRA was severely lacking in the USA outside of major training programs performing TRA. Teaching courses and workshops began popping up across the country as well as at national meetings such as Society of Interventional Radiology (SIR) in 2013. This was shortly followed by the inaugural annual TransRadial Endovascular Advanced Therapies (TREAT) conference in New York in 2014 dedicated specifically to noncoronary TRA interventions and live teaching cases. The largest single-center review of the feasibility of TRA for noncoronary interventions was published in 2016 with 1500 cases performed at the

Mount Sinai Hospital [44]. There is an accumulation of evidence at multiple centers demonstrating that the transradial approach is feasible and safe for noncoronary interventions with patients having a preference for TRA [45–48]. Similar to Kiemeneij's experience at OLVG, TRA in Interventional Radiology is currently transitioning from a single center endeavor to being widely adopted in multiple centers in the USA.

References

1. Radner S. Intracranial angiography via the vertebral artery: preliminary report of a new technique. Acta Radiol. 1947;28:838–42.
2. Radner S. Thoracal aortography by catheterization from the radial artery. Acta Radiol. 1948;29:178–80.
3. Bertrand O, Rao S. Best practices for transradial approach. Philadelphia: Lippincott Williams & Wilkins; 2014.
4. Jonsson G. Thoracic aortography by means of a cannula inserted percutaneously into the common carotid artery. Acta Radiol. 1949;31:376–86.
5. Helmsworth JA, McGUIRE J, Felson B. Arteriography of the aorta and its branches by means of the polyethylene catheter. Am J Roentgenol Radium Ther. 1950;64:196–213.
6. Peirce EC 2nd. Percutaneous femoral artery catheterization in man with special reference to aortography. Surg Gynecol Obstet. 1951;93:56–74.
7. Donald DC. An improved technic for percutaneous cerebral angiography. AMA Arch Neurol Psychiatry. 1951;65:508.
8. Seldinger SI. Catheter replacement of the needle in percutaneous arteriography. A new technique. Acta Radiol Suppl. 1953;434:47–52.
9. Campeau L. Entry sites for coronary angiography and therapeutic interventions: from the proximal to the distal radial artery. Can J Cardiol. 2001;17:319–25.
10. Sones FM Jr, Shirey EK. Cine coronary arteriography. Mod Concepts Cardiovasc Dis. 1962;31:735–8.
11. Dotter CT, Frische LH. Visualization of the coronary circulation by occlusion aortography: a practical method. Radiology. 1958;71:502–24.
12. Lehman JS, Novack P, Kasparian H, Likoff W, Perlmutter HI. Selective coronary arteriography. Radiology. 1964;83:846–53.
13. Lemmon WM, Stauffer Lehman J, Boyer RA. Suprasternal transaortic coronary arteriography. Circulation. 1959;19:47–54.
14. Ryan TJ. The coronary angiogram and its seminal contributions to cardiovascular medicine over five decades. Circulation. 2002;106:752–6.
15. Payne MM. Charles Theodore Dotter. The father of intervention. Tex Heart Inst J. 2001;28:28–38.
16. Ricketts HJ, Abrams HL. Percutaneous selective coronary cine arteriography. JAMA. 1962;181:620–4.
17. Judkins MP. Selective coronary arteriography. I. A percutaneous transfemoral technic. Radiology. 1967;89:815–24.
18. Amplatz K, Formanek G, Stanger P, Wilson W. Mechanics of selective coronary artery catheterization via femoral approach. Radiology. 1967;89:1040–7.
19. Gorlin R, Taylor WJ. Selective revascularization of the myocardium by internal-mammary-artery implant. N Engl J Med. 1966;275:283–90.
20. Favaloro RG. Bilateral internal mammary artery implants. Operative technic--a preliminary report. Cleve Clin Q. 1967;34:61–6.

21. Dotter CT, Judkins MP. Transluminal treatment of arteriosclerotic obstruction. Description of a new technic and a preliminary report of its application. Circulation. 1964;30:654–70.
22. Meier B. The first patient to undergo coronary angioplasty — 23-year follow-up. N Engl J Med. 2001;344:144–5.
23. Grüntzig A. Transluminal dilatation of coronary-artery stenosis. Lancet. 1978;311:263.
24. Kiemeneij F. The history and evolution of transradial coronary interventions. In: Transradial approach for percutaneous interventions; 2017. p. 3–7. https://doi.org/10.1007/978-94-017-7350-8_1.
25. Kiemeneij F, Laarman GJ. Percutaneous transradial artery approach for coronary stent implantation. Catheter Cardiovasc Diagn. 1993;30:173–8.
26. Kiemeneij F, Laarman GJ, Odekerken D, Slagboom T, van der Wieken RA. Randomized comparison of percutaneous transluminal coronary angioplasty by the radial, brachial and femoral approaches: the access study. J Am Coll Cardiol. 1997;29:1269–75.
27. Chase AJ, et al. Association of the arterial access site at angioplasty with transfusion and mortality: the M.O.R.T.A.L study (Mortality benefit Of Reduced Transfusion after percutaneous coronary intervention via the Arm or Leg). Heart. 2008;94:1019–25.
28. Jolly SS, et al. Radial versus femoral access for coronary angiography and intervention in patients with acute coronary syndromes (RIVAL): a randomised, parallel group, multicentre trial. Lancet 2011;377:1409–20.
29. Romagnoli E, et al. Radial versus femoral randomized investigation in ST-segment elevation acute coronary syndrome: the RIFLE-STEACS (Radial Versus Femoral Randomized Investigation in ST-Elevation Acute Coronary Syndrome) study. J Am Coll Cardiol. 2012;60:2481–9.
30. Valgimigli M, et al. Radial versus femoral access in patients with acute coronary syndromes undergoing invasive management: a randomised multicentre trial. Lancet. 2015;385:2465–76.
31. Hamon M, et al. Consensus document on the radial approach in percutaneous cardiovascular interventions: position paper by the European Association of Percutaneous Cardiovascular Interventions and Working Groups on Acute Cardiac Care** and Thrombosis of the European Society of Cardiology. EuroIntervention. 2013;8:1242–51.
32. Nusbaum M, Baum S, Blakemore WS. Clinical experience with the diagnosis and management of gastrointestinal hemorrhage by selective mesenteric catheterization. Ann Surg. 1969;170:506–14.
33. Mauro MA, Murphy KPJ, Thomson KR, Venbrux AC, Morgan RA. Image-guided interventions e-book: expert radiology series. Philadelphia: Elsevier Health Sciences; 2020.
34. Kato T, et al. Magnetic microcapsules for targeted delivery of anticancer drugs. Appl Biochem Biotechnol. 1984;10:199–211.
35. Yamashita T, et al. Transradial approach for noncoronary angiography and interventions. Catheter Cardiovasc Interv. 2007;70:303–8.
36. Shiozawa S, et al. Transradial approach for transcatheter arterial chemoembolization in patients with hepatocellular carcinoma: comparison with conventional transfemoral approach. J Clin Gastroenterol. 2003;37:412–7.
37. Frangos C, Noble S. How to transform you into a radialist: literature review. Cardiovasc Med. 2011;14:277–82.
38. Sanghvi K, Kurian D, Coppola J. Transradial intervention of iliac and superficial femoral artery disease is feasible. J Interv Cardiol. 2008;21:385–7.
39. Shiozawa S, Tsuchiya A, Endo S, Kumazawa K, Ogawa K. Transradial approach for transcatheter arterial chemoembolization in patients with hepatocellular carcinoma. Nihon Shokakibyo Gakkai Zasshi. 2002;99:1450–4.
40. Resnick NJ, et al. Uterine artery embolization using a transradial approach: initial experience and technique. J Vasc Interv Radiol. 2014;25:443–7.
41. Bishay V, et al. Transradial approach for hepatic radioembolization: initial results and technique. J Vasc Interv Radiol. 2014;25:S88.

42. Isaacson AJ, Fischman AM, Burke CT. Technical feasibility of prostatic artery embolization from a transradial approach. AJR Am J Roentgenol. 2016;206:442–4.
43. Sher A, et al. Safety and feasibility of transradial infrainguinal peripheral arterial disease interventions. J Vasc Surg. 2020. https://doi.org/10.1016/j.jvs.2020.02.016.
44. Posham R, et al. Transradial approach for noncoronary interventions: a single-center review of safety and feasibility in the first 1,500 cases. J Vasc Interv Radiol. 2016;27:159–66.
45. Thakor AS, et al. Transradial access for interventional radiology: single-centre procedural and clinical outcome analysis. Can Assoc Radiol J. 2017;68:318–27.
46. Styczen H, et al. Initial experience with transradial access for cerebrovascular procedures: is it feasible and safe? World Neurosurg. 2020;136:e593–600.
47. Liu LB, et al. Patient experience and preference in transradial versus transfemoral access during transarterial radioembolization: a randomized single-center trial. J Vasc Interv Radiol. 2019;30:414–20.
48. Yamada R, et al. Transradial versus transfemoral arterial access in liver cancer embolization: randomized trial to assess patient satisfaction. J Vasc Interv Radiol. 2018;29:38–43.

Chapter 2
Anatomy and Physical Exam

Matthew Tangel and Joseph J. Titano

Brachial Artery Anatomy

The brachial artery is a continuation of the axillary artery, beginning at the lateral margin of the teres major muscle and coursing in the anteromedial aspect of the arm. Once it reaches the antecubital fossa, the brachial artery divides into the radial and ulnar arteries (Fig. 2.1).

It is helpful to be aware of some of the anatomic variants of the brachial artery in order to safely navigate a catheter to the thoracic aorta. The most common variant is a high origin of the radial artery from the brachial artery above the humeral

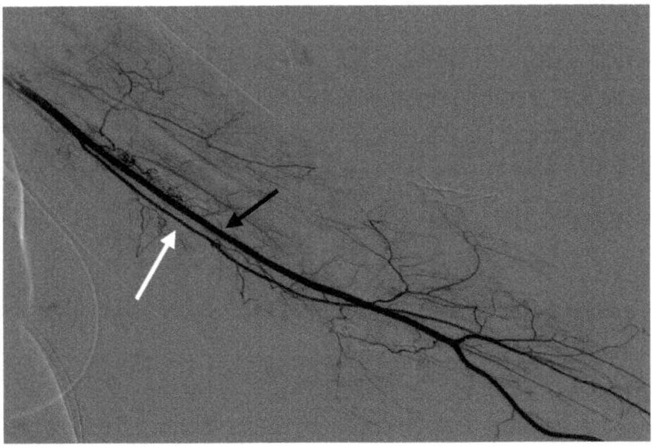

Fig. 2.1 Left upper extremity angiogram demonstrating normal brachial artery anatomy. The black arrow denotes the brachial artery. The white arrow denotes the profunda brachial artery

M. Tangel (✉) · J. J. Titano
Department of Diagnostic, Molecular and Interventional Radiology,
Icahn School of Medicine at Mount Sinai, New York, NY, USA
e-mail: matthew.tangel@mountsinai.org; joseph.titano@mountsinai.org

A. M. Fischman et al. (eds.), *Transradial Access in Interventional Radiology*,
https://doi.org/10.1007/978-3-030-81678-0_2

Table 2.1 Brachial artery variants and their frequency [1]

Brachial artery variants	Frequency (%)
Radial artery origin from proximal brachial artery	12
Persistent superficial brachial artery	1–2
Ulnar artery origin from proximal radial artery	1–2
Accessory brachial artery	0.1
Common interosseous artery origin from proximal brachial artery	<0.1

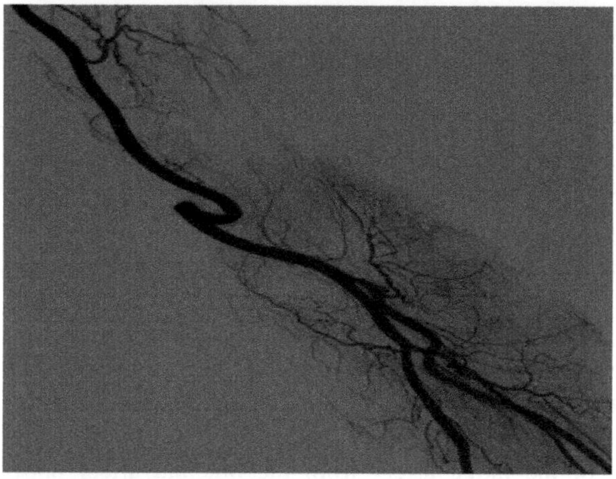

Fig. 2.2 Brachial artery loop

intercondylar line, with an incidence of approximately 12%. Other, less common variants include a persistent superficial brachial artery, accessory brachial artery where there is duplication and it rejoins the distal brachial artery in the antecubital fossa, and brachial artery loops [1]. Variant arterial anatomy arising from the brachial artery is listed in Table 2.1 (Fig. 2.2).

Radial Artery Anatomy

The radial artery originates deep in the cubital fossa at the level of the radial tuberosity and continues along the lateral, volar aspect of the forearm. Only the fascia and skin overlie the radial artery in the lower third of the forearm, where it resides between the tendons of the brachioradialis and the flexor carpi radialis and is situated superficial to the pronator quadratus and radius. The inherent anatomy of the radial artery in the lower third of the forearm renders it an excellent access point for catheter-guided procedures: it is easy to palpate, superficial, and the underlying radius acts as a backdrop for effective compression to achieve hemostasis. Once the radial artery reaches the radial styloid process, it takes a turn dorsally and passes deep to the tendons of the extensor pollicis brevis and abductor pollicis longus in the anatomic snuff box [2]. This can also serve as a site for radial artery access.

There are several well-known anatomic variants of the radial artery, including aplasia or hypoplasia, partial duplication, and complete duplication; however, the most commonly encountered anatomic variant that alters the approach to navigating a catheter centrally is a radial artery loop [3]. Anatomic variants of the radial artery, excluding radial artery loops, are listed in Table 2.2 (Fig. 2.3).

Table 2.2 Radial artery variants and their frequency [1]

Radial artery variants	Frequency (%)
High origin (both axillary and brachial)	14–17
Dorsal continuation	1
Partial duplication	0.8
Complete duplication	0.1
Aplasia or hypoplasia	0.1

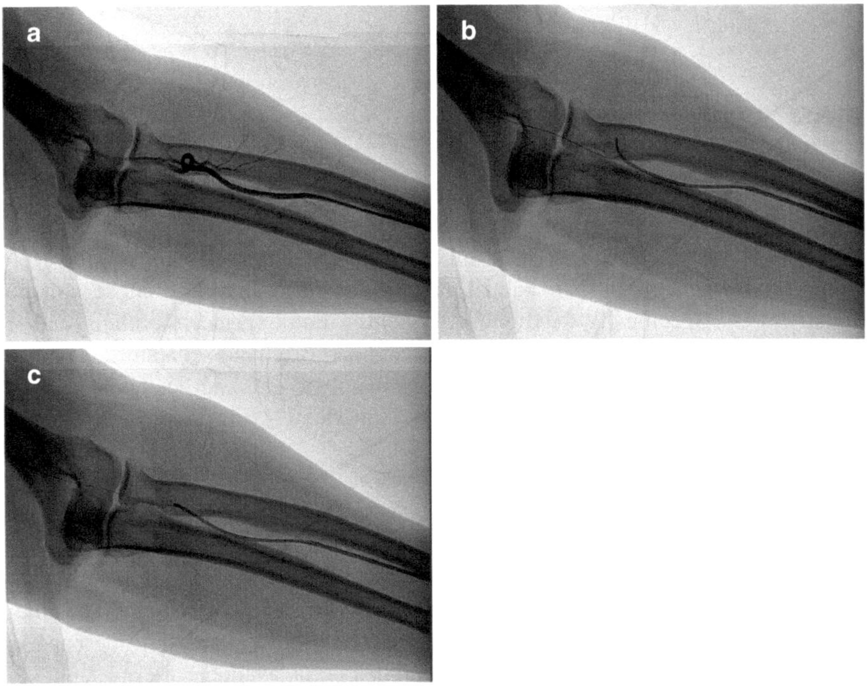

Fig. 2.3 (**a**) Radial artery loop. (**b**) This was successfully crossed with a 0.016″ wire. (**c**) Successful reduction of the loop once the catheter was advanced and back tension was applied

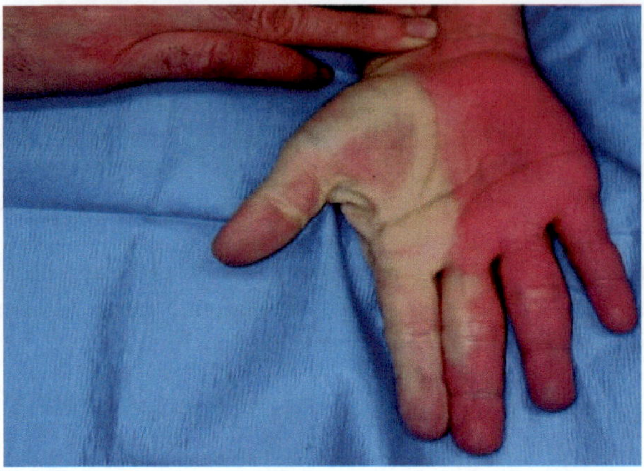

Fig. 2.4 Case where occlusion pressure applied to the radial artery resulted in poor flow to the radial aspect of the hand, specifically the thumb, index finger, and medial aspect of the third digit. This finding implies that the ulnar artery does not supply sufficient collateral flow to the deep palmar arch. Radial artery access in this patient may render them at risk for ischemia of the thumb and index finger

Blood Supply to the Hand

Blood supply to the hand arises from dual perfusion via the radial and ulnar arteries. These arteries form a complete anastomotic arcade via the deep and superficial palmar arches to supply the hand. The radial artery is the dominant supply to the deep palmar arch, which gives rise to palmar metacarpal arteries that anastomose with the digital vessels. Specifically, the digital artery of the thumb (princeps pollicis) and of the radial side of the index finger (radialis indicis) originate separately from the deep palmar arch. The ulnar artery is the main supply to the superficial palmar arch, which gives rise to the common palmar digital arteries [2] (Fig. 2.4).

Physical Exam

Perhaps the most important factor in determining whether a patient would be amenable to radial artery access is assessing if the dual blood supply to the hand is intact. In some patients, the dominant or potentially only available arterial supply to the hand is via the radial artery. If the radial artery were to be accessed in these patients, they could be at risk for hand ischemia not only perioperatively, but in the postoperative period as well.

Modified Allen Test

Traditionally, a modified Allen test was performed to ensure adequate perfusion to the hand. This test consists of simultaneously applying pressure to the radial and ulnar arteries until the hand turns a bluish hue. The ulnar artery compression is then released, and if the hand achieves a normal tone after several seconds, it implies that the ulnar artery is patent and the anastomotic arcade of the hand is intact; therefore, cannulation of the radial artery would not render the patient at risk for hand ischemia. One significant caveat of the modified Allen test is it is very subjective in nature and is prone to false positive and false negative results [4]. It is because of these shortcomings that the Barbeau test is preferred to assess patients prior to radial artery cannulation [5].

Barbeau Test

The Barbeau test constitutes placing a pulse oximeter to the ipsilateral thumb to get a baseline waveform, and subsequently applying occlusion pressure to the radial artery. The operator then observes the waveform for any changes in its amplitude. The changes in the waveform are assigned to a grading system that ranges from A to D. Each of these grades and their corresponding waveforms supply a wealth of information regarding the integrity of the anastomotic arcade of the hand and feasibility for safe radial artery access [6] (Fig. 2.5).

Barbeau Grade	Waveform		Interpretation
	Compression start	After 2 minutes	
A	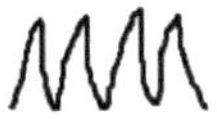	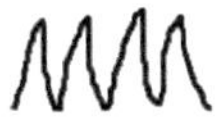	collaterals
B	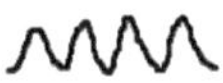	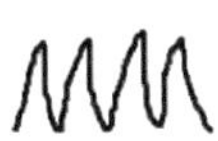	Dampening of the waveform with return to normal within 2 minutes. Indicates a good collateral network
C	—	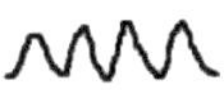	Complete loss of the waveform initially, with return to a Indicates poor collateralization, but still a candidate for radial artery access
D	—	—	No waveform, even after 2 minutes. No collateral network is present. Radial artery access iscontraindicated

Fig. 2.5 Barbeau waveforms and their significance

Sonographic Assessment of the Radial Artery

After the Barbeau test is completed, the radial artery should be investigated sonographically. This is best performed using a linear array, high frequency transducer that will provide excellent resolution of superficial structures, such as the radial artery in the wrist [7]. The radial artery will appear as a structure with a round, thin echogenic wall that surrounds an anechoic center, has pulsatile vascular flow on color Doppler, and will produce a "triphasic" waveform on pulse Doppler related to rapid antegrade flow during systole, transient reversal of flow during early diastole, and return of slow antegrade flow during late diastole [8] (Fig. 2.6).

Many studies have been performed to assess the average diameter of the radial artery, and the consensus is in the vicinity of 2.3 ± 0.4 mm [9–11]. Ideally, the radial artery should measure greater than 2 mm to be able to accommodate many of the sheaths that are placed via radial artery access and reduce risk of stretching injury [12]. One way to help increase the diameter of the radial artery prior to access is to place a paste consisting of nitroglycerin and local anesthetic to the wrist to both maximally dilate the artery and also minimize pain. One study has demonstrated the effectiveness of this paste, where patients who had it applied had an increase in their radial artery cross-sectional diameter by on average 16.5 ± 4.2% [13].

Once the radial artery is identified, the ultrasound settings should be adjusted to achieve optimal visualization. The field depth should be adjusted so that only the radial artery and adjacent, relevant structures are visualized. Gain can be increased or decreased to help with differentiating fine anatomic details. The focal point should be adjusted to be at the level, or just deep to the radial artery. Optimizing these settings not only aids in assessing the radial artery, but also will make needle visualization during access much easier.

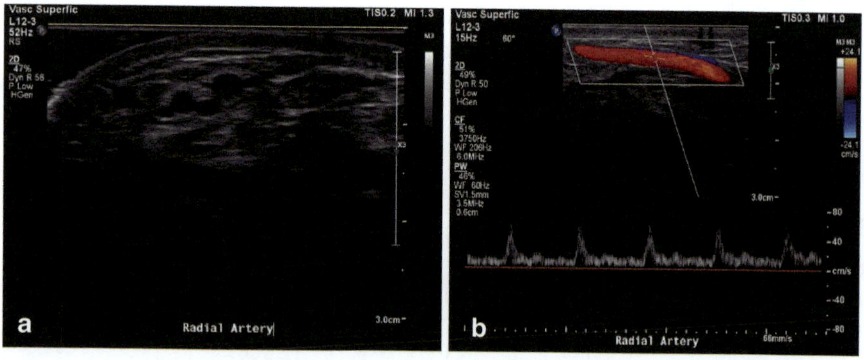

Fig. 2.6 (**a**) Gray scale visualization of the radial artery. Incidentally, this patient was found to have partial duplication of the radial artery. (**b**) Long-axis view of the radial artery with color Doppler and pulse Doppler demonstrating the triphasic waveform

References

1. Kadir S, Brothers MF. Atlas of normal and variant angiographic anatomy. Philadelphia: W.B. Saunders Company; 1991.
2. Rosse C, Gaddum-Rosse P, Hollinshead WH. Hollinsheads textbook of anatomy. Philadelphia: Lippincott-Raven Publishers; 1997.
3. Lo TS, Nolan J, Fountzopoulos E, et al. Radial artery anomaly and its influence on transradial coronary procedural outcome. Heart. 2008;95:410–5.
4. Hirai M, Kawai S. False positive and negative results in Allen test. J Cardiovasc Surg (Torino) [Internet]. 1980; [cited 2019 Oct 29]. Available from: https://www.ncbi.nlm.nih.gov/pubmed/7391126.
5. Barbeau GR, Arsenault F, Dugas L, Simard S, Larivière MM. Evaluation of the ulnopalmar arterial arches with pulse oximetry and plethysmography: comparison with the Allen's test in 1010 patients. Am Heart J. 2004;147(3):489–93.
6. Barbeau GR, Arsenault F, Dugas L, Simard S, Larivière MM. Evaluation of the ulnopalmar arterial arches with pulse oximetry and plethysmography: comparison with the Allens test in 1010 patients. Am Heart J. 2004;147:489–93.
7. Weiner MM, Geldard P, Mittnacht AJ. Ultrasound-guided vascular access: a comprehensive review. J Cardiothorac Vasc Anesth. 2013;27:345–60.
8. Hinwood D, Donnelly R, London NJM. ABC of arterial and venous disease: non-invasive methods of arterial and venous assessment. BMJ. 2000;321:0008270.
9. Okuyan H, Hızal F, Taçoy G, Timurkaynak T. Angiographic evalution of the radial artery diameter in patients who underwent coronary angiography or coronary intervention. J Am Coll Cardiol. 2013. https://doi.org/10.1016/j.jacc.2013.08.666.
10. Beniwal S, Bhargava K, Kausik SK. Size of distal radial and distal ulnar arteries in adults of southern Rajasthan and their implications for percutaneous coronary interventions. Indian Heart J. 2014;66:506–9.
11. Ashraf T, Panhwar Z, Habib S. Size of radial and ulnar artery in local population. J Pak Med Assoc. 2010;60:817–9.
12. Yoo B-S, Yoon J, Ko J-Y, Kim J-Y, Lee S-H, Hwang S-O, et al. Anatomical consideration of the radial artery for transradial coronary procedures: arterial diameter, branching anomaly and vessel tortuosity. Int J Cardiol. 2005;101(3):421–7.
13. Beyer AT, Ng R, Singh A, Zimmet J, Shunk K, Yeghiazarians Y, Ports TA, Boyle AJ. Topical nitroglycerin and lidocaine to dilate the radial artery prior to transradial cardiac catheterization: a randomized, placebo-controlled, double-blind clinical trial. Int J Cardiol. 2013;168:2575–8.

Chapter 3
Nursing Assessment

Aaron M. Fischman, Adie Friedman, and Jacxelyn Moran

Introduction

As the specialty of Interventional Radiology (IR) has evolved, there has been an effort to establish IR as both a clinical and technical practice, rather than solely a procedural one. This helps provide longitudinal care and a reliable referral service [1]. For this reason, it is crucial that IR health professionals stay up to date on the fundamentals that help ensure optimal patient care. Specifically, this chapter reviews the preprocedural management for vascular cases performed via radial artery access.

A comprehensive preprocedural patient evaluation is imperative to reduce the risk of adverse events in transradial (TR) access cases. The role of the IR nurse is to collect and record data pertaining the status of the patient and to communicate this information to members of the health-care team [2]. Guidance on preprocedural patient management can be obtained from use of modern assessment tools which aim to reduce costs and optimize patient care [3]. One study showed that such standardized implementation in TR access procedures reduced the door-to-procedure time, decreased the number of post-procedure complications, quickened rehabilitation and reduced hospital stay length, reduced hospital costs, and improved patient satisfaction [4]. Important topics that should be considered during preoperative evaluation will be described.

A. M. Fischman · J. Moran (✉)
Department of Diagnostic, Molecular and Interventional Radiology,
Icahn School of Medicine at Mount Sinai, New York, NY, USA
e-mail: aaron.fischman@mountsinai.org; Jacxelyn.moran@mountsinai.org

A. Friedman
Department of Radiology, Memorial Sloan Kettering Cancer Center, New York City, NY, USA

A. M. Fischman et al. (eds.), *Transradial Access in Interventional Radiology*,
https://doi.org/10.1007/978-3-030-81678-0_3

Orienting the Patient

Patient education and orientation is crucial for guaranteeing patient satisfaction, comfort, and reduced anxiety. Studies have demonstrated that causes for malpractice suits in radiology departments often include procedural complications and poor physician-patient rapport [5]. Welcoming staff-patient encounters as well as comprehensive procedure information and updates help patients feel less anxious and better prepared prior to their IR procedure [6]. Patient procedure information can be provided in form of pamphlets, information sheets, or online resources and videos. In regard to TR access cases, one study showed that increased anxiety was a risk factor for radial artery vasospasm [7]. Patients with less anxiety will tend to be more cooperative during the procedure and may require less sedation.

Informed Consent

The informed consent gives the patient the opportunity to comprehend the intervention that they are about to undergo and to decide whether they wish to pursue treatment. The health professional must take responsibility to thoroughly explain the procedure in terms of preparation, expectations, risks, benefits, success rate, and alternative treatment options. In one survey, 61% of IR clinic responders reported providing patients with information sheets about the procedure during the consent process [8]. One study suggests that patient anxiety decreases and patient satisfaction increases when they are able to discuss procedure details in advance [6].

Patients should be told what to anticipate during the procedure, such as their level of awareness, the amount of pain to be felt, the type of medications to be administered, the duration of the procedure, and their positioning on the procedure table. Patients should be informed that access of the radial artery is typically painless and improves patient comfort and post procedural independence, removing the need for an uncomfortable groin compression for hemostasis [9, 10]. The expected probability of success for the procedure should be disclosed. Especially relevant to TR access cases is informing the patient about the possibility of needing a different access site, since this may affect discharge plans [11]. Anatomical variation between patients can make maneuvering through the arterial tree more time consuming. There is a learning curve for proceduralists utilizing TR access, initially causing longer procedure times and greater radiation and contrast exposure to the patient [3]. Because of the increased technical demand for TR cases, a case may need to be converted to a transfemoral (TF) access case. Prior studies have shown that the access site crossover rate for TR procedures is 1.8% [12]. Risk factors for TR access failure or crossover to a different access site include female sex, older age, and obesity [13]. A decrease in TR access failures is correlated with greater procedural cases performed [14].

In addition to discussing risk factors for the procedure itself, potential side effects from undergoing TR access should be specifically addressed during the consent process. In terms of TR access complications, a small risk of hematoma, compartment syndrome, arteriovenous fistula, pseudoaneurysm, and bleeding exists, albeit less so than in TF access cases [11, 15]. Patients can be informed that TR access has a reduced rate of complications when compared to TF access with many studies showing that TF access has a higher rate of major bleeding, pseudoaneurysms, arteriovenous fistula, and hematomas which typically lead to longer hospital stays and greater costs as well as worsened morbidity and mortality [11, 13, 15]. The superficial location, away from any major anatomical landmarks, and smaller size of the radial artery reduces the chance for these complications [11]. Additionally, access of the radial artery requires smaller catheters, and its location allows for easy compressibility for hemostasis purposes.

Radial artery spasm can cause pain and procedure delay and occurs more often with smaller radial artery size and longer procedure duration [16, 17]. There is also a very rare risk of post procedural radial artery occlusion and hand ischemia. Reduced risk of radial artery occlusion has been identified with use of smaller catheters, intra-arterial heparin administration, immediately catheter removal following the procedure, and less than 4-hour post procedural compression [16]. Unlike TF access, the dual arterial supply of the hand reduces the chance of limb ischemia. A few studies have demonstrated that there is endothelial damage to the radial artery following TR access, and rarely, changes in hand function and physiology can be identified, such as change in temperature or strength [18]. Bruising is one of the most common post procedural findings after TR access, and patients should be prepared for this [19].

During the consenting process, it is also important to review post-procedure expectations with the patient. Post procedural hemostasis at the radial artery access site can be achieved by compression with the use of a pressure device, usually for 1–2 hours [11]. The patient must understand that the amount of time for use of the compression device will vary and that premature removal of the device may increase the risk of hematoma [10]. In terms of activity level following the procedure, patients are not required to stay bed-bound after the procedure as is required after TF access [14]. This in turn decreases the workload on the staff as the patient is able to ambulate on their own with decreased need for supervision. One study showed that TR access, in comparison to TF access, correlated with reduced nurse workload in standardized, systematic vascular procedures, reducing the number of resources needed for patient care, as well as improving costs of care and efficiency of IR procedures [20]. Post-procedure wrist pain can be managed with over-the-counter medication as needed, elevating the arm, and applying ice [13].

History, Physical Exam, and Medications

During the preprocedural period there should be a review of pertinent patient medical history and physical exam that may impact transradial access [13]. Obesity, elderly patients, and female sex have been linked to an increased occurrence of TR access complications [16]. In older patients with tortuous thoracic aortas, it can be more challenging to direct the catheter into the descending thoracic aorta. Patients with advanced vascular disease or small-vessel vasculitis are at greater risk for failed TR access procedure [11]. History of prior radial access may reduce the chance of successful TR access due to altered anatomy. Patients should be asked if they have ever had any hand or arm trauma or surgery such as axillary lymph node dissection. TR access should be reconsidered in patients with chronic renal disease who may require hemodialysis access in the future [11]. In certain patient populations, risk of bleeding complication is higher due to medical conditions such as chronic kidney disease and thrombocytopenia [15]. The patient should be educated about possible adverse effects of bleeding while receiving anticoagulation therapy [13].

Peripheral intravenous access and identification bands should be placed in the contralateral arm of TR access, commonly the right arm [9, 15]. Any jewelry should be removed from the arm that is to be accessed. Baseline vital signs should include height since patients of short stature tend to have smaller and shorter ascending aortas, which may increase the difficulty of TR access [11].

Baseline radial and ulnar pulses should be documented, as well as the color and temperature of the extremities. The extent and baseline of hand functionality and pain level should be noted. If the area to be imaged involves the descending thoracic aorta or below the diaphragm, left arm access is generally preferred so that the catheter does not lay across the origins of the carotid arteries. Any existing hemodialysis fistula or shunt deters ipsilateral TR access [13]. Ultrasound examination can be obtained to measure the size of the radial artery preoperatively.

A common test used to examine the blood supply to the hand is the Allen test. The Allen test starts by occluding the radial and ulnar arteries for 1 minute while the patient makes a fist followed by observing return of blood flow in the patient's unclenched hand as soon as compression of the ulnar artery is released [9, 11]. Return of blood flow to the hand within 10 seconds is normal [9].Alternative exams include the modified Allen test and the Barbeau test which incorporate pulse oximetry and plethysmography. These tests use a pulse oximeter on second digit which evaluates the waveform while altering the blood supply to the hand [14]. In patients who have had previous TR access, a reverse Allen test, which tests radial artery flow, can be performed to check for radial artery occlusion [14]. If the patient has an abnormal result from any of these tests, then an alternative access site should be considered [13].

The IR nurse is typically responsible for providing medications preprocedurally and for monitoring the patient's physiologic and hemodynamic state following administration [21]. Prior to TR access, prolonged preprocedural application of topical medications, such as EMLA, can help reduce radial artery spasm [22, 23]. In our department, the nurses apply Lidocaine and Prilocaine Cream USP, 2.5%/2.5%, as well as Nitroglycerin Ointment USP, 2%, mixed together and applied over the radial artery access site at least 30 min prior to the procedure. Depending on the type of vascular procedure, varying levels of sedation may be utilized. Low dose fentanyl and midazolam has been shown to reduce patient discomfort and in turn the incidence of radial artery spasm [15].

References

1. Soares GM. The value of clinical interventional radiology. J Am Coll Radiol. 2011;8(5):318–24.
2. Chan D, Downing D, Keough CE, Saad WA, Annamalai G, d'Othee BJ, Ganguli S, Itkin M, Kalva SP, Khan AA, Krishnamurthy V. Joint practice guideline for sterile technique during vascular and interventional radiology procedures: from the society of interventional radiology, association of perioperative registered nurses, and association for radiologic and imaging nursing, for the society of interventional radiology (Wael Saad, MD, Chair), standards of practice committee, and endorsed by the cardiovascular interventional radiological society of Europe and the Canadian interventional radiology association. J Vasc Interv Radiol. 2012;23(12):1603–12.
3. Zhu L, Xu J, Wang Q, Xu F, Chen J. Nursing care of transradial angiography and intervention in a tertiary hospital in shanghai: a best practice implementation project. JBI Database System Rev Implement Rep. 2016;14(5):286–94.
4. Li M, Liu H. Implementation of a clinical nursing pathway for percutaneous coronary intervention: a prospective study. Geriatr Nurs. 2018;39(5):593–6.
5. Craciun H, Mankad K, Lynch J. Risk management in radiology departments. World J Radiol. 2015;7(6):134.
6. Lundén M, Lundgren SM, Persson LO, Lepp M. Patients' experiences and feelings before undergoing peripheral percutaneous transluminal angioplasty. J Vasc Nurs. 2013;31(4):158–64.
7. Ercan S, Unal A, Altunbas G, Kaya H, Davutoglu V, Yuce M, Ozer O. Anxiety score as a risk factor for radial artery vasospasm during radial interventions: a pilot study. J Am Coll Cardiol. 2013;62(18 Supplement 2):C3.
8. O'Dwyer HM, Lyon SM, Fotheringham T, Lee MJ. Informed consent for interventional radiology procedures: a survey detailing current European practice. Cardiovasc Intervent Radiol. 2003;26(5):428–33.
9. Nickolaus MJ, Gilchrist IC, Ettinger SM. The way to the heart is all in the. AACN Clin Issues. 2001;12(1):62–71.
10. Shah S, Gindi R, Basir MB, Khandelwal A, Alqarqaz M, Zaidan M, Voeltz M, Koenig G, Kim HE, O'Neill WW, Alaswad K. Optimal TR-band weaning strategy while minimizing vascular access site complications. Cardiovasc Revasc Med. 2019;20(2):133–6.
11. Dunne ML, Phillips E. Transradial vascular access: a growing trend. Nurse Pract. 2014;39(8):50–4.
12. Posham R, Biederman DM, Patel RS, Kim E, Tabori NE, Nowakowski FS, Lookstein RA, Fischman AM. Transradial approach for noncoronary interventions: a single-center review of safety and feasibility in the first 1,500 cases. J Vasc Interv Radiol. 2016;27(2):159–66.
13. Mullin MK. Transradial approach versus transfemoral approach for coronary angiography and coronary angioplasty. Crit Care Nurs Q. 2014;37(2):159–69.
14. Cale L, Constantino RE. Transitioning to transradials: a collaborative process in the cardiac catheterization laboratory. Dimens Crit Care Nurs. 2013;32(1):1–5.
15. Mason PJ, Shah B, Tamis-Holland JE, Bittl JA, Cohen MG, Safirstein J, Drachman DE, Valle JA, Rhodes D, Gilchrist IC. American Heart Association Interventional Cardiovascular Care Committee of the Council on Clinical Cardiology; Council on Cardiovascular and Stroke Nursing; Council on Peripheral Vascular Disease; and Council on Genomic and Precision Medicine. An update on radial artery access and best practices for transradial coronary angiography and intervention in acute coronary syndrome: a scientific statement from the American Heart Association. Circ Cardiovasc Interv. 2018;11(9):e000035.
16. Amoroso G, Laarman GJ, Kiemeneij F. Overview of the transradial approach in percutaneous coronary intervention. J Cardiovasc Med. 2007;8(4):230–7.
17. Steffenino G, Fabrizi MD, Baralis G, Tomatis M, Mogna A, Dutto M, Dutto MS, Conte L, Lice G, Cavallo S, Porcedda B. Implementation of radial arterial access for cardiac interventions: a strong case for quality assurance protocols by the nursing staff. J Cardiovasc Med. 2011;12(2):116–21.

18. Maki KA, Griza DS, Phillips SA, Wolska BM, Vidovich MI. Altered hand temperatures following transradial cardiac catheterization: a thermography study. Cardiovasc Revasc Med. 2019;20(6):496–502.
19. Cosman TL, Arthur HM, Natarajan MK. Prevalence of bruising at the vascular access site one week after elective cardiac catheterisation or percutaneous coronary intervention. J Clin Nurs. 2011;20(9-10):1349–56.
20. Amoroso G, Sarti M, Bellucci R, Puma FL, D'Alessandro S, Limbruno U, Canova A, Petronio AS. Clinical and procedural predictors of nurse workload during and after invasive coronary procedures: the potential benefit of a systematic radial access. Eur J Cardiovasc Nurs. 2005;4(3):234–41.
21. Goodhart J, Page J. Radiology nursing. Orthop Nurs. 2007;26(1):36–9.
22. Curtis E, Fernandez R, Lee A. The effect of topical medications on radial artery spasm in patients undergoing transradial coronary procedures: a systematic review. JBI Database System Rev Implement Rep. 2018;16(3):738–51.
23. Johnson S. Sedation and analgesia in the performance of interventional procedures. Semin Intervent Radiol. 2010;27(04):368–73. © Thieme Medical Publishers.

Chapter 4
Procedure Suite Setup

Kristina Prachanronarong and Vivian Bishay

Abbreviations

RA	Radial artery
TFA	Transfemoral arterial approach
TRA	Transradial arterial approach

Introduction: Prior to Entering the Angiography Suite and Angiography Suite Setup

Prior to entering the angiography suite, a physical exam of the wrist should be performed, and the Barbeau test should be used to assess ulnopalmar arch patency, as described in Chap. 2 [1–3]. Briefly, a pulse oximeter is positioned on the patient's ipsilateral thumb or forefinger, and the waveform is analyzed [2, 4]. Waveform types A-C signify ulnopalmar arch patency, meaning that transradial access can be safely performed [4]. Waveform type D indicates that the ulnopalmar arch is not patent, which can be a contraindication to a transradial arterial approach (TRA). Relative contraindications to a TRA include radial artery (RA) occlusion, subclavian artery occlusion or stenosis, RA having a diameter smaller than the outer diameter of the sheath, and current or future hemodialysis [2, 5]. The RA can also be prepared for radial access using a topical vasodilator [6]. For example, in the PRE-DILATE protocol, 30 mg nitroglycerin ointment and 40 mg of lidocaine cream are applied to the RA access site 30 minutes before catheterization and secured with a small Tegaderm™ or bandage, which can increase RA cross sectional area by a mean of 16.5% [2, 6–8]. EMLA™ cream (lidocaine 2.5% and prilocaine 2.5%) can also be used [2].

K. Prachanronarong · V. Bishay (✉)
Department of Diagnostic, Molecular and Interventional Radiology,
Icahn School of Medicine at Mount Sinai, New York, NY, USA
e-mail: vivian.bishay@mountsinai.org

A. M. Fischman et al. (eds.), *Transradial Access in Interventional Radiology*,
https://doi.org/10.1007/978-3-030-81678-0_4

Table 4.1 Equipment/medication list for TRA

Pulse oximeter	Access kit (e.g., Cook® 21G Micropuncture® Kit)
Ultrasound	Access sheath (e.g., Cook® 5Fr Shuttle® Sheath)
30 g nitroglycerin ointment	Heparinized saline infusion for sheath side flush
40 g lidocaine cream	Medication cocktail: 3000 IU heparin 200 μg nitroglycerin 2.5 mg of verapamil
Small Tegaderm™	
Arm board with padding and straps	
Folded sheet or towel roll	

All monitors, medication, and equipment should be available in the angiography suite prior to bringing the patient into the suite. Supplies that are recommended for a TRA setup are listed in Table 4.1. Once the patient is in the suite, the patient can be positioned, and RA patency and caliber can be re-confirmed. A pulse oximeter should be placed on the thumb or index finger and remain in place for the entire procedure [7]. Determination of a left versus right radial approach can then be considered, and for most interventional procedures below the diaphragm, left RA access is preferred [1, 2, 4, 7, 8]. The distance to target vessels from the left wrist is shorter [2]. Catheters and sheaths do not cross the origins of the great vessels during a left-sided approach, theoretically limiting the risk of thrombus formation or cerebral emboli from the great vessels, although catheters lie across the left vertebral artery. Additional angiography suite considerations include standard suite setup and modifications specifically for TRA procedures. Reducing scatter radiation in TRA procedures is important to ensure adequate radiation protection [4, 9]. Early evidence shows that once an operator overcomes the learning curve for using a TRA, differences between radiation exposure between a transfemoral arterial approach (TFA) vs a TRA are minimal [5, 10–13].

Equipment List

Technical Considerations: Patient Positioning and Obtaining Radial Access

The patient can be positioned in various ways to optimize access and patient comfort [2]. Often, the patient is supine, but the patient can also be in the prone position, such as for patients with chronic back pain [1, 2, 7, 8]. The patient's arm can be positioned 0–15° from the patient's side in a similar position to that of the patient's groin (Fig. 4.1) [2]. In this configuration, catheters and drapes can be arranged similarly to when they are used for TFA procedures (Fig. 4.2) [2]. The patient's arm can also be positioned 75–90° from the patient's side [2]. This type of positioning permits easier access, but

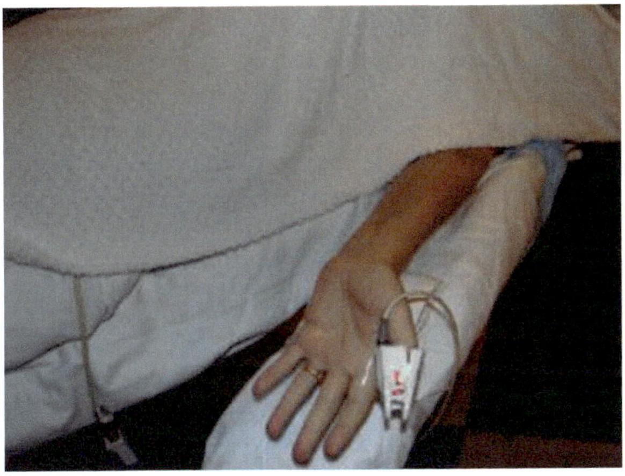

Fig. 4.1 The arm is at an acute angle for easier access. The towel roll provides support for the wrist [2]

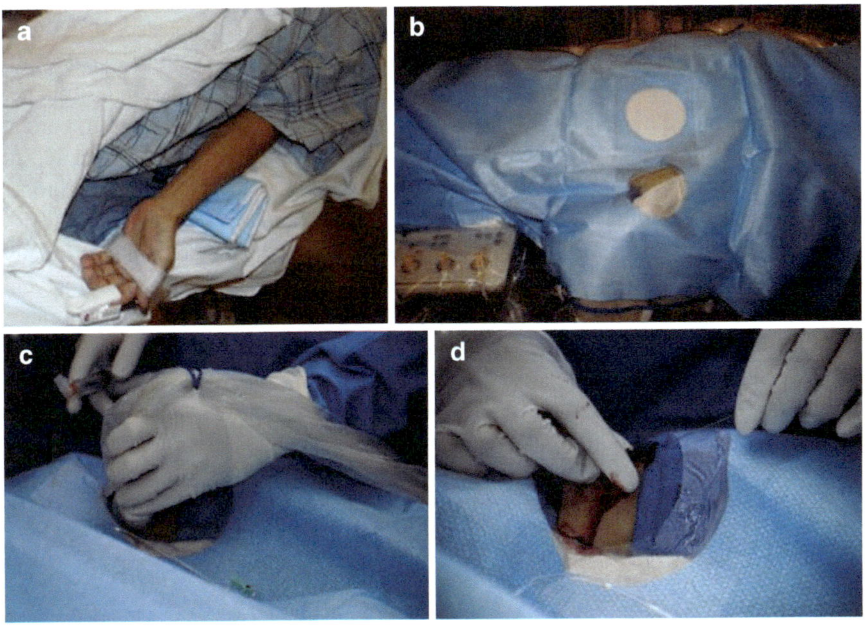

Fig. 4.2 (**a**) Arm positioning parallel to the Table. (**b**) The arm position allows for more ergonomic wire and catheter exchange and use of standard TFA access drapes. (**c**) Example of ultrasound-guided access to the radial artery with a 21-G micropuncture needle. (**d**) The radial artery is accessed with a 0.021-in wire and with finger pressure over the access site as the sheath is advanced [2]

catheter exchanges may be unwieldy [2]. A long moveable arm board, with padding and/or memory foam, is recommended to increase comfort for the patient and is helpful when the patient's arms need to be raised during a procedure, such as for cone beam computed tomography, and specific arm boards are designed to reduce radiation scatter [4]. Once the patient's arm is in correct position, the wrist can be supinated and hyperextended with a folded sheet or towel roll inserted under the distal forearm for support and with the hand secured to the arm board (Fig. 4.2a) [1, 2, 7, 8].

The steps for obtaining radial access are similar to the approach taken for obtaining other types of ultrasound-guided access. First, the patient is prepped and draped in usual sterile surgical fashion [8]. Guidewires, sheaths, and catheters are prepared. Monitors should be placed on the patient, including a pulse oximeter that should be placed on the thumb or forefinger of the wrist being accessed. If the patient's arm is positioned parallel to the patient's body, standard femoral access drapes can be used, with one of the openings positioned over the RA (Fig. 4.2b) [8]. The RA can be identified and examined using ultrasound (a high frequency linear transducer) to assess for anatomy, patency, and caliber [7, 8]. The access area can then be anesthetized with lidocaine and a 21-gauge needle [8], and access can be obtained with ultrasound guidance and using Seldinger technique [2]. A wire (e.g., a 0.021-in wire) can then be advanced into the RA, and if there is any resistance, the wire is pulled back and readjusted. If the wire cannot be advanced, fluoroscopy and direct visualization with contrast can be performed. Use of a single-wall puncture technique and placement of the smallest-diameter hydrophilic sheath available to successfully complete the procedure are important considerations for limiting trauma to the RA [7]. Once access is obtained, specialized radial access sheaths with hydrophilic coating can then be used to facilitate the procedure [2]. Catheter, sheath, and wire selection are discussed in subsequent chapters [4, 7].

After sheath placement, a medication "cocktail" is administered intra-arterially directly through the access sheath to dilate the RA, prevent arterial spasm, prevent thrombus formation, and reduce vascular tone [2, 14]. This cocktail can include nitrates, calcium channel blockers, and heparin. There is no consensus on the ideal combination of medications, but one example includes 3000 IU heparin, 200 μg of nitroglycerin, and 2.5 mg of verapamil [5, 11, 14]. Before injection of the cocktail, blood is withdrawn into the syringe to "hemodilute" the medication cocktail, and a slow rate of injection of 1 mL/second can be used to minimize the burning sensation felt with these medications [2, 7, 8, 14]. A continuous side flush of heparinized saline infusion can also be started to prevent clot formation between the sheath and catheter [7, 8].

References

1. Posham R, Biederman DM, Patel RS, Kim E, Tabori NE, Nowakowski FS, et al. Transradial approach for noncoronary interventions: a single-center review of safety and feasibility in the first 1,500 cases. J Vasc Interv Radiol. 2016;27(2):159–66.
2. Fischman AM, Swinburne NC, Patel RS. A technical guide describing the use of transradial access technique for endovascular interventions. Tech Vasc Interv Radiol. 2015;18(2):58–65.

3. Titano JJ, Biederman DM, Zech J, Korff R, Ranade M, Patel R, et al. Safety and outcomes of transradial access in patients with international normalized ratio 1.5 or above. J Vasc Interv Radiol. 2018;29(3):383–8.
4. Thakor AS, Alshammari MT, Liu DM, Chung J, Ho SGF, Legiehn GM, et al. Transradial access for interventional radiology: single-centre procedural and clinical outcome analysis. Can Assoc Radiol J. 2017;68(3):318–27.
5. Isaacson AJ, Fischman AM, Burke CT. Technical feasibility of prostatic artery embolization from a transradial approach. AJR Am J Roentgenol. 2016;206(2):442–4.
6. Beyer AT, Ng R, Singh A, Zimmet J, Shunk K, Yeghiazarians Y, et al. Topical nitroglycerin and lidocaine to dilate the radial artery prior to transradial cardiac catheterization: a randomized, placebo-controlled, double-blind clinical trial: the PRE-DILATE study. Int J Cardiol. 2013;168(3):2575–8.
7. Bishay VL, Biederman DM, Ward TJ, van der Bom IM, Patel RS, Kim E, et al. Transradial approach for hepatic radioembolization: initial results and technique. AJR Am J Roentgenol. 2016;207(5):1112–21.
8. Patel A, Naides AI, Patel R, Fischman A. Transradial intervention: basics. J Vasc Interv Radiol. 2015;26(5):722.
9. Iqtidar AF, Jeon C, Rothman R, Snead R, Pyne CT. Reduction in operator radiation exposure during transradial catheterization and intervention using a simple lead drape. Am Heart J. 2013;165(3):293–8.
10. Loewenstern J, Welch C, Lekperic S, Bishay V, Ranade M, Patel RS, et al. Patient radiation exposure in transradial versus transfemoral yttrium-90 radioembolization: a retrospective propensity score-matched analysis. J Vasc Interv Radiol. 2018;29(7):936–42.
11. Liu LB, Cedillo MA, Bishay V, Ranade M, Patel RS, Kim E, et al. Patient experience and preference in transradial versus transfemoral access during transarterial radioembolization: a randomized single-center trial. J Vasc Interv Radiol. 2019;30(3):414–20.
12. Becher T, Behnes M, Unsal M, Baumann S, El-Battrawy I, Fastner C, et al. Radiation exposure and contrast agent use related to radial versus femoral arterial access during percutaneous coronary intervention (PCI)-Results of the FERARI study. Cardiovasc Revasc Med. 2016;17(8):505–9.
13. Jolly SS, Cairns J, Niemela K, Steg PG, Natarajan MK, Cheema AN, et al. Effect of radial versus femoral access on radiation dose and the importance of procedural volume: a substudy of the multicenter randomized RIVAL trial. JACC Cardiovasc Interv. 2013;6(3):258–66.
14. Resnick NJ, Kim E, Patel RS, Lookstein RA, Nowakowski FS, Fischman AM. Uterine artery embolization using a transradial approach: initial experience and technique. J Vasc Interv Radiol. 2014;25(3):443–7.

Chapter 5
Recovery Room and Post-procedure Care

Kristina Prachanronarong and Vivian Bishay

Abbreviations

RA	Radial artery
TFA	Transfemoral arterial approach
TRA	Transradial arterial approach

Introduction: Hemostasis

One of the most important considerations in the recovery room and during post-procedure care is the achievement of RA hemostasis. At the end of the procedure before transitioning to the post-procedure recovery room, the radial pulse should be identified, and the last catheter used during the procedure should be removed slowly over a soft wire to reduce potential trauma to the artery [1]. Once the catheter and wire are removed, the sheath can be withdrawn a few centimeters, and a hemostasis band can be placed over the access site [2–4]. Non-occlusive "patent" hemostasis is critical for reducing the risk of post-procedural RA thrombosis [4]. The PROPHET study demonstrated that "patent" hemostasis is better than occlusive pressure in promoting hemostasis while preserving RA patency [4, 5]. Non-occlusive hemostasis is most often achieved with a wrist band device, with several examples listed in Table 5.1 [4].

To achieve hemostasis, the wrist band is placed over the arteriotomy site while continuing to monitor the pulse oximeter waveform, and then the wrist band is inflated (Fig. 5.1). Following device inflation, the ulnar artery is compressed, and then air is gradually released from the band device in a controlled manner until an oximeter waveform returns, which signifies RA patency [1]. The band can be maximally inflated with an accompanying syringe, and air can be removed in 1 mL increments until bleeding is seen at the access site. Then, 1 mL of air can be added to the

K. Prachanronarong · V. Bishay (✉)
Department of Diagnostic, Molecular and Interventional Radiology,
Icahn School of Medicine at Mount Sinai, New York, NY, USA
e-mail: vivian.bishay@mountsinai.org

A. M. Fischman et al. (eds.), *Transradial Access in Interventional Radiology*,
https://doi.org/10.1007/978-3-030-81678-0_5

Table 5.1 Radial compression devices approved in the United States in 2020 [4, 6]

Device name	Company
RadAR™	Advanced Vascular Dynamics (Milwaukie, OR)
VasoStat™	Forge Medical (Bethlehem, PA)
Rayband™	Lepu Medical Technology (Beijing, CN)
SyvekRadial™	Marine Polymer Technologies (Danvers, MA)
TRAcelet™	Medtronic Vascular (Danvers, MA)
RADstat®, Finale®, PreludeSync™, PreludeSync Distal™, PreludeSync Evo™, SafeGuard Radial™	Merit Medical Systems, Inc (South Jordan, UT)
VASOBand	VASOInnovations, Inc (South Pasadena, CA)
TR Band®	Terumo Interventional Systems (Elkton, MD)
ARC Adjustable Radial Cuff	TZ Medical, Inc (Portland, OR)
D-Stat® Rad-Band	Vascular Solutions, LLC (Maple Grove, MN)

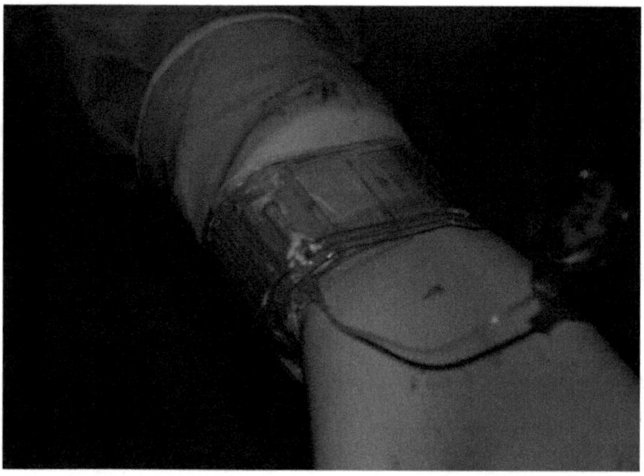

Fig. 5.1 The TR Band® (Terumo Interventional Systems) on a patient demonstrating the "patent" hemostasis technique [4]

cuff to prevent bleeding while maintaining an oximeter waveform [3]. A physical exam can also be performed periodically to assess for circulation within the hand [2, 3]. Throughout the hemostasis period, which can last from 30 to 120 minutes, depending on procedure complexity, a distal RA pulse should be present [4]. The band can then be incrementally deflated and released [7]. The failure rate of inflatable wrist bands, such as the TR Band®, is lower than transfemoral vascular closure devices, and these bands offer benefits such as rapid exchange, re-deployment, or parallel usage in cases of failure [8, 9]. In addition, the use of prophylactic ipsilateral ulnar artery compression in the PROPHET-II trial to increase flow in the radial artery post-procedurally has shown improved patent hemostasis and decreased risk of post-procedural complications such as RA occlusion [10].

Equipment List

Technical Considerations: Post-procedure Care and Post-procedural Complications

After achieving hemostasis, the inflatable wrist band can be removed, and a sterile dressing can be applied. The patient should be observed for 30 minutes before discharge [2, 4, 8, 11]. Patients are able to sit up in bed and ambulate immediately after a procedure using a TRA [1, 4, 7, 12, 13]. Repeat evaluation of the radial pulse and access site should be completed before discharge and during a follow-up outpatient visit [11]. Physical exams, including a neurologic motor and sensory exam and evaluation of radial pulse and capillary refill, should also be performed frequently to ensure the patient is neurovascularly intact. On discharge, patients should be instructed to avoid unnecessary wrist flexion or extension, avoid heavy lifting for 24 hours, avoid blood pressure measurements and blood draws from the procedural arm for 24 hours, keep the dressing in place for 24 hours, and avoid soaking the wound for 24–72 hours [1, 11]. Patients should be instructed on what steps to take if bleeding or swelling occurs, such as holding manual pressure and reporting to a hospital for further evaluation. If there is pain at the access site, acetaminophen and/or NSAIDs, elevation, compression, and ice packs can be recommended [4].

Studies show that access-site related complications are reduced using a TRA versus a transfemoral arterial approach (TFA) [8, 11, 14–18]. One of the most common complications from using a TRA, although rare, is localized access site hematoma and bruising, which is often asymptomatic, occurs with a frequency of <1%, is more common in females, and is much less common compared to procedures that use a TFA [4, 13, 19]. Bertrand et al. proposed a grading system for the severity of post TRA hematomas and associated treatment guidelines [20]. If a hematoma begins to form, a second wrist band/cuff can be applied in parallel to the first device [2, 3]. A blood pressure cuff can also be used more proximally to aid in hemostasis [20]. Additional considerations for managing a hematoma are to control blood pressure, which is associated with adequate pain management, and consider withdrawing anti-coagulation/anti-platelet treatment if necessary [20]. During management, a pulse oximeter should be used continuously to monitor RA patency and oxygenation to prevent ischemia.

Another possible complication of a TRA is RA occlusion, which is almost always asymptomatic due to a patent ulnopalmar arch but may have an occurrence of up to 6–10% [5, 11]. The PROPHET study demonstrated that factors associated with decreased incidence of RA occlusion include smaller sheath size, use of a hydrophilic sheath, and increased heparin dose [5]. Some rare complications after using a TRA include RA pseudoaneurysm, radial arteritis, perforation, spasm, and RA dissection [4, 7]. Pseudoaneurysms are rare with an incidence rate of <1% and can be treated with thrombin. It is also rare for complications from procedures using a TRA to require management by open surgical intervention [11]. Permanent or temporary neurologic or ischemic complications in the hand are rare [1, 4, 11, 13, 14, 21, 22]. Another potential rare complication is stroke, with an unknown incidence rate (≪1%) [23, 24]. Procedures using a TRA from the left upper extremity avoid manipulation of the aortic arch [11]. However, by using a left-sided TRA during sub-diaphragmatic interventions, catheters rest across the origin of the left vertebral artery from the left subclavian artery, which theoretically could cause an ischemic event [4]. A retrospective analysis of a database of PCIs from the British Cardiovascular Intervention Society, which included 124,616 radial and 223,476 femoral procedures, discovered that there was no statistically significant association between the occurrence of neurologic complications and the use of TRA, with a frequency of 0.11% in each cohort [3, 21].

References

1. Thakor AS, Alshammari MT, Liu DM, Chung J, Ho SGF, Legiehn GM, et al. Transradial access for interventional radiology: single-centre procedural and clinical outcome analysis. Can Assoc Radiol J. 2017;68(3):318–27.
2. Patel A, Naides AI, Patel R, Fischman A. Transradial intervention: basics. J Vasc Interv Radiol. 2015;26(5):722.
3. Bishay VL, Biederman DM, Ward TJ, van der Bom IM, Patel RS, Kim E, et al. Transradial approach for hepatic radioembolization: initial results and technique. AJR Am J Roentgenol. 2016;207(5):1112–21.
4. Fischman AM, Swinburne NC, Patel RS. A technical guide describing the use of transradial access technique for endovascular interventions. Tech Vasc Interv Radiol. 2015;18(2):58–65.
5. Pancholy S, Coppola J, Patel T, Roke-Thomas M. Prevention of radial artery occlusion-patent hemostasis evaluation trial (PROPHET study): a randomized comparison of traditional versus patency documented hemostasis after transradial catheterization. Catheter Cardiovasc Interv. 2008;72(3):335–40.
6. Prepared by Division of Small Manufacturers Assistance OoT, Assistance. Premarket notification, 510(k) : regulatory requirements for medical devices: Rockville, MD: U.S. Dept. of Health and Human Services, Public Health Service, Food and Drug Administration, Center for Devices and Radiological Health. Washington, DC: For sale by the Supt. of Docs., U.S. G.P.O.; 1990.
7. Isaacson AJ, Fischman AM, Burke CT. Technical feasibility of prostatic artery embolization from a transradial approach. AJR Am J Roentgenol. 2016;206(2):442–4.
8. Biederman DM, Marinelli B, O'Connor PJ, Titano JJ, Patel RS, Kim E, et al. Transradial access for visceral endovascular interventions in morbidly obese patients: safety and feasibility. J Vasc Access. 2016;17(3):256–60.

9. Nathan S, Rao SV. Radial versus femoral access for percutaneous coronary intervention: implications for vascular complications and bleeding. Curr Cardiol Rep. 2012;14(4):502–9.
10. Pancholy SB, Bernat I, Bertrand OF, Patel TM. Prevention of radial artery occlusion after transradial catheterization: the PROPHET-II randomized trial. JACC Cardiovasc Interv. 2016;9(19):1992–9.
11. Posham R, Biederman DM, Patel RS, Kim E, Tabori NE, Nowakowski FS, et al. Transradial approach for noncoronary interventions: a single-center review of safety and feasibility in the first 1,500 cases. J Vasc Interv Radiol. 2016;27(2):159–66.
12. Resnick NJ, Kim E, Patel RS, Lookstein RA, Nowakowski FS, Fischman AM. Uterine artery embolization using a transradial approach: initial experience and technique. J Vasc Interv Radiol. 2014;25(3):443–7.
13. Liu LB, Cedillo MA, Bishay V, Ranade M, Patel RS, Kim E, et al. Patient experience and preference in transradial versus transfemoral access during transarterial radioembolization: a randomized single-center trial. J Vasc Interv Radiol. 2019;30(3):414–20.
14. Jolly SS, Yusuf S, Cairns J, Niemela K, Xavier D, Widimsky P, et al. Radial versus femoral access for coronary angiography and intervention in patients with acute coronary syndromes (RIVAL): a randomised, parallel group, multicentre trial. Lancet. 2011;377(9775):1409–20.
15. Valgimigli M, Gagnor A, Calabro P, Frigoli E, Leonardi S, Zaro T, et al. Radial versus femoral access in patients with acute coronary syndromes undergoing invasive management: a randomised multicentre trial. Lancet. 2015;385(9986):2465–76.
16. Posham R, Young LB, Lookstein RA, Pena C, Patel RS, Fischman AM. Radial access for lower extremity peripheral arterial interventions: do we have the tools? Semin Intervent Radiol. 2018;35(5):427–34.
17. Titano JJ, Biederman DM, Zech J, Korff R, Ranade M, Patel R, et al. Safety and outcomes of transradial access in patients with international normalized ratio 1.5 or above. J Vasc Interv Radiol. 2018;29(3):383–8.
18. Feldman DN, Swaminathan RV, Kaltenbach LA, Baklanov DV, Kim LK, Wong SC, et al. Adoption of radial access and comparison of outcomes to femoral access in percutaneous coronary intervention: an updated report from the national cardiovascular data registry (2007-2012). Circulation. 2013;127(23):2295–306.
19. Romagnoli E, Biondi-Zoccai G, Sciahbasi A, Politi L, Rigattieri S, Pendenza G, et al. Radial versus femoral randomized investigation in ST-segment elevation acute coronary syndrome: the RIFLE-STEACS (Radial Versus Femoral Randomized Investigation in ST-Elevation Acute Coronary Syndrome) study. J Am Coll Cardiol. 2012;60(24):2481–9.
20. Bertrand OF. Acute forearm muscle swelling post transradial catheterization and compartment syndrome: prevention is better than treatment. Catheter Cardiovasc Interv. 2010;75(3):366–8.
21. Ratib K, Mamas MA, Routledge HC, Ludman PF, Fraser D, Nolan J. Influence of access site choice on incidence of neurologic complications after percutaneous coronary intervention. Am Heart J. 2013;165(3):317–24.
22. Pandie S, Mehta SR, Cantor WJ, Cheema AN, Gao P, Madan M, et al. Radial versus femoral access for coronary angiography/intervention in women with acute coronary syndromes: insights from the RIVAL trial (Radial Vs femor AL access for coronary intervention). JACC Cardiovasc Interv. 2015;8(4):505–12.
23. Raposo L, Madeira S, Teles RC, Santos M, Gabriel HM, Goncalves P, et al. Neurologic complications after transradial or transfemoral approach for diagnostic and interventional cardiac catheterization: a propensity score analysis of 16,710 cases from a single centre prospective registry. Catheter Cardiovasc Interv. 2015;86(1):61–70.
24. Al-Hakim R, Gandhi RT, Benenati JF. Incident of stroke after transradial arterial access for subdiaphragmatic intervention. J Vasc Interv Radiol. 2017;28(9):1287–8.

Chapter 6
Access Complications and Management

Naveen Galla and Rajesh I. Patel

Introduction

As cardiologists have adopted the transradial approach (TRA) as their preferred access for diagnostic and interventional coronary angiography, the TRA has become an increasingly popular option for visceral and peripheral endovascular procedures. Several large prospective multicenter trials, predominantly studying the TRA for percutaneous coronary interventions, have demonstrated high patient satisfaction scores and decreased complication rates [1–4]. In a large-scale retrospective analysis of 1500 patients who underwent the TRA for noncoronary interventions, the TRA was described as a well-tolerated approach with a major complication rate of 0.1% and minor complication rate of 2.4% [5].

As the TRA has become more widely adopted for noncoronary interventions, many interventional practices have transitioned to a predominantly TRA model. There is a significant learning curve associated with the TRA, with literature reporting that approximately 30–50 TRA procedures are needed before procedural metrics and complication rates plateau for new TRA operators [6]. Despite its safety profile, it is important to remember that the TRA is not without risk and has its own unique complications. In this chapter, we detail potential complications and roadblocks operators may face when using the TRA during IR procedures (Table 6.1), preventive measures, and the appropriate procedural and post-procedural management of these complications.

N. Galla (✉) · R. I. Patel
Department of Diagnostic, Molecular and Interventional Radiology,
Icahn School of Medicine at Mount Sinai, New York, NY, USA
e-mail: naveen.galla@mountsinai.org

A. M. Fischman et al. (eds.), *Transradial Access in Interventional Radiology*,
https://doi.org/10.1007/978-3-030-81678-0_6

Table 6.1 Incidence of complications from transradial catheterization

Complication	Incidence
Radial artery spasm	5–10% [7–9]
Radial artery occlusion	2–18% [10–13]
Access-site hematoma	1–6% [14–19]
Radial artery perforation	0.1–1.0% [15, 20–22]
Radial artery dissection	0.1–1.3% [8]
Pseudoaneurysm	0.1–0.2% [8, 15]
AV fistula	Extremely rare
Compartment syndrome/hand ischemia	Extremely rare
Neurologic deficits	Extremely rare
Catheter/sheath entrapment	Extremely rare
Catheter granuloma	Extremely rare

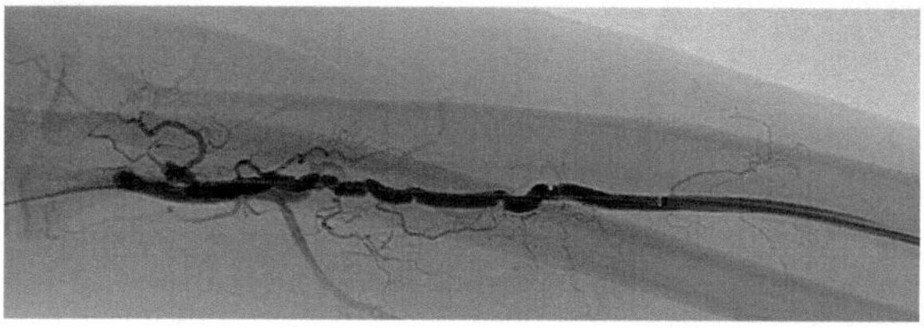

Fig. 6.1 Radial artery angiography revealing multifocal radial artery spasm

Radial Artery Spasm

Radial artery spasm (RAS) is the most common complication of the TRA, occurring in approximately 5–10% of cases (Fig. 6.1) [10–13]. RAS can manifest as forearm or upper arm pain or resistance while inserting sheaths or advancing wires and catheters. The small arterial diameter, thick arterial media, and high density of alpha-adrenergic receptors to the smooth muscle cells in the radial artery contribute to its high vasospastic potential. RAS is associated with female sex, diabetes, low BMI, smaller radial artery diameters, increased number of catheter exchanges, and the use of large catheter sizes [23]. RAS most commonly occurs at the onset of a transradial procedure with initial puncture and sheath placement, but can also occur later during the procedure from local release of catecholamines, endothelin-I, and angiotensin-II from shear stress.

Tactics to Minimize RAS

An effective prophylactic method to minimize RAS when obtaining access involves application of topical lidocaine-prilocaine cream (EMLA) and nitroglycerin ointment covered with an adhesive 30 minutes prior to the start of the procedure.

Because the majority of procedures do not require general anesthesia, it is important to administer adequate sedation prior to arterial puncture to dampen catecholamine release from pain and anxiety. After the vascular sheath is in place, administration of an intra-arterial cocktail consisting of verapamil, nitroglycerin, and heparin prior to guidewire and catheter insertion reduces the rate of RAS. In addition, the use of specially designed hydrophilic coated sheaths is crucial to minimize RAS during the insertion and removal of sheaths. While many visceral and peripheral interventions require 5–7 French sheaths, the operator should attempt to use the smallest sheath feasible.

Procedural Management of RAS

The overwhelming majority of TRA procedures will have smooth and seamless advancement of the guidewire and catheter from the puncture site to the descending aorta. If RAS presents when obtaining radial artery access, ensure that adequate time has elapsed since administration of sedation. Subcutaneous injection of nitroglycerine in the peri-arterial region can assist with radial artery cannulation. When RAS manifests as catheter resistance, it is important to restrain from further catheter manipulation to prevent additional release of local inflammatory mediators. In many cases, RAS spontaneously resolves within a few minutes, and the procedure can continue without issue. Administration of verapamil or nitroglycerin as well as increasing sedation and pain control in awake patients can mitigate RAS and allow operators to proceed in the vast majority of cases.

It is important to ensure that resistance associated with transradial catheter advancement is not prematurely labeled as RAS instead of variant anatomy such as remnant radial arteries, curvatures, or loops. When RAS is suspected and not relieved with medication, operators should maintain a low threshold to perform a radial angiography via the catheter or side port of the introducer sheath to define the anatomy. If RAS is confirmed, the operator can attempt to cross the region of RAS with a hydrophilic guidewire to minimize shear stress. After successfully traversing the area of spasm, a catheter can be negotiated over the wire using gentle cork-screw forward movements instead of a pushing movement, and the procedure can proceed in the usual manner.

Take-Home Points

While its incidence can be dependent on operator experience, RAS is an inevitable occurrence even for the most experienced operators. Although permanent effects from RAS are rare, it can cause significant patient discomfort and prolonged procedure times and potentially result in conversion to alternative access sites in cases of spasm refractory to medication. With appropriate management, RAS will subside, and operators can proceed with the procedure in the regular manner.

Radial Artery Occlusion

Radial artery occlusion (RAO) has been reported to occur in 2–18% of TRA procedures, with the majority of the literature reporting RAO rates of 5–10% [10–13]. RAO arises from a combination of factors, including local vascular inflammatory mediators from endothelial shear stress, disruption of normal antegrade flow, and inappropriate post-procedure compression. Although RAO generally has a benign and clinically silent course due to the protective effects of retrograde flow from the ulnar artery, proper patient selection and appropriate hemostasis are of the utmost importance in minimizing this complication.

Risk Factors for RAO

Introducer sheath size has been reported to be a predictor for RAO. The radial artery has a mean intraluminal diameter of 2.7 ± 0.4 mm in males and 2.4 ± 0.4 mm in females [24], in comparison to 5 French radial introducer sheaths with outer diameters measuring approximately 2.4 mm. For patients with smaller radial arteries, it is important to minimize the sheath size when possible. Saito et al. demonstrated that the RAO rate when the ratio of the radial artery inner diameter to sheath outer diameter is <1.0 is 4% compared to 13% when the ratio is >1.0 [19]. Diabetes, female gender, and low BMI are associated with increased rates of RAO [25].

Techniques to Reduce RAO

Administration of adequate systemic anticoagulation (50 IU/kg or 5000 U UFH) is the simplest method to minimize the risk of RAO. Studies have demonstrated that patients undergoing TRA procedures with suboptimal doses of unfractionated heparin develop RAO in up to 30% of cases [26]. Some operators inject subcutaneous nitroglycerin at the puncture site to reduce rates of RAO [27].

The PROPHET study demonstrated that patent hemostasis decreases the risk of RAO compared to the traditional occlusive hemostasis technique [11]. The vast majority of IR practices have adopted the principles of patent hemostasis with commercially available transradial (TR) bands, allowing antegrade blood flow through the radial artery and decreasing the likelihood of local thrombus formation. In addition, shorter duration of hemostatic compression is associated with decreased rates of RAO [28]. Nursing staff in the post-procedure recovery area should frequently assess and relieve pressure from the TR band to minimize the duration of compression. Some studies have demonstrated that prophylactic ipsilateral ulnar artery compression reduces RAO, presumably from increasing blood flow in the radial artery [29].

Treatment of RAO

Duplex ultrasound examinations have demonstrated spontaneous recanalization of occluded radial arteries after 3 months in the majority of cases [30]. Because of the clinically silent nature of RAO, the predominance of providers do not treat RAO with anticoagulation. Focal ulnar compression is a tactic used by some providers after detecting RAO, by placing a TR band over the ulnar artery for 1–2 hours, thereby preferentially increasing flow through the occluded radial artery [31].

Consequences of RAO

Histopathological studies have demonstrated that patients undergoing TRA procedures can have non-occlusive radial artery injuries in the segments corresponding to the sheath location. Radial artery intimal hyperplasia, intima-media thickening, and smaller mean radial artery diameter were demonstrated in short-term follow-up in one study, while another study demonstrated resolution after 1 year [32, 33]. Despite non-occlusive injuries and RAO, studies of repeated transradial catheterization report technical success rates ranging from 95% to 98% [34–37]. However, another study reported that failed repeat TRA and conversion to TFA were primarily attributed to radial artery luminal narrowing and RAO [38]. Although clinical symptoms and conversion rate to TFA on repeat procedures are low, strategies to minimize RAO should be taken for patients to benefit from subsequent TRA procedures.

TRA procedures resulting in symptomatic ischemia are very rare due to the dual blood supply to the hand. Proper patient selection using pre-procedure Barbeau testing should routinely be done to ensure adequate ulnar collateral flow. Even with abnormal pre-procedure testing (Barbeau C and D), hand ischemia is still unlikely because of the recruitment of collaterals from the interosseous arterial system [39]. There are rare case reports detailing distal ischemia after TRA in patients undergoing cardiac catheterization [40]. In this particular case report, the operator did not perform a pre-procedure Barbeau test, and it was later determined that the ulnar artery was not present, leading to ischemia after RAO.

Hematomas

Access-Site Hematoma

Due to the radial artery's small caliber and superficial location, access-site complications are infrequently encountered using the TRA. When a hematoma is detected near the puncture site with a TR band already placed, it is important to assess for appropriate location of the TR band. If the TR band has migrated, placing an additional TR band or BP cuff proximal to the arteriotomy site can temporarily occlude blood flow while readjusting the TR band to the appropriate position. If the TR band is well positioned with swelling proximal to the device, an additional proximal TR band can be applied.

Radial Artery Perforation

Radial artery perforation is a rare incident, most commonly the result of forceful pushing of a wire into variant anatomy, such as radial artery side branches. When extravasation is observed (Fig. 6.2), it is important to attempt to cross the lesion and advance a catheter to occlude the extravasation site. In the majority of these situations, the catheter will seal the perforation and the extravasation will subside. In fact, many operators have achieved resolution of radial artery perforation even when proceeding with full anticoagulation throughout the case [21]. Additional tactics include inserting a long sheath across the extravasation site for tamponade or placement of a covered stent for refractory bleeding [41]. Even if extravasation is not present on subsequent angiograms prior to sheath removal, strict post-procedure observation is required to screen for hematomas and forearm compartment syndrome.

Failure to recognize perforations without treatment can lead to gradual intramuscular bleeding. A hematoma classification system was designed by investigators in the EASY trial to guide operators and nursing staff [42]. In this system, hematoma <5 cm (grade 1) and <10 cm (grade II) are related to the access site, while hematomas distal to the elbow (grade III) (Fig. 6.3) and proximal to the elbow (grade IV) are thought to result from vessel perforation from wire damage. For grade III and IV hematomas, arm elevation, external compression of the brachial artery with a blood pressure cuff, and application of an ace compression bandage should be used to prevent hematoma growth. Grade V is reserved for compartment syndrome.

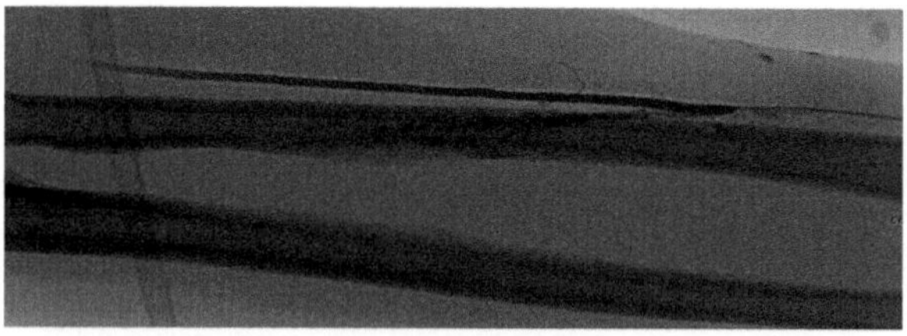

Fig. 6.2 Radial artery angiogram demonstrating radial artery perforation with contrast extravasation

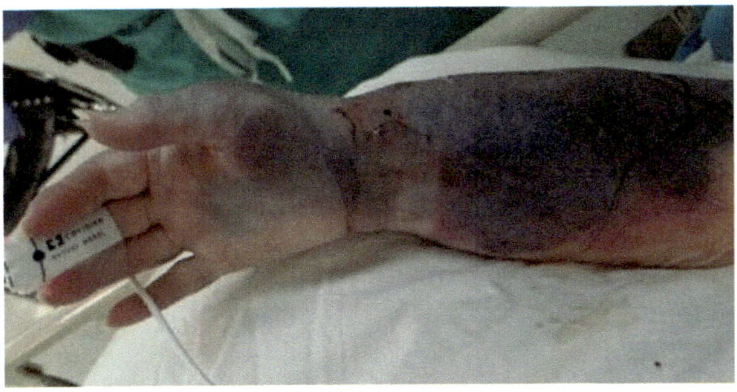

Fig. 6.3 Photograph of a grade III hematoma with extensive ecchymosis extending from the access site to the hand and forearm

Compartment Syndrome

Forearm compartment syndrome is an extremely rare occurrence, occurring in fewer than 0.01% of cases [43]. When a forearm hematoma is present, there should be very frequent monitoring for signs of perfusion, such as skin color, pulse, pain, paresthesia, and capillary refill. Signs of compartment syndrome such as expanding hematoma, extreme pain with passive movement of the forearm and hemodynamic changes should be promptly recognized with immediate action and surgical consultation. Surgical fasciotomy is the definitive treatment for compartment syndrome.

Hand compartment syndrome without involvement of the forearm is an exceptionally rare phenomenon with unclear etiology that has been described in a single case report [44].

Miscellaneous Vascular Complications

Dissection

Radial artery dissection is an uncommon complication, with the majority of cases occurring with hydrophilic guidewires negotiating through difficult anatomy such as curvatures and loops. It is important to understand that TRA-related dissections are retrograde and the dissection flap is unlikely to propagate. The operator should attempt to cross the dissection plane with a soft 0.014 inch wire to limit further dissection. Once the lesion is traversed, advancement of a catheter over the dissection plane will likely seal the dissection, and the case should proceed without expectation of any clinical manifestation of the dissection.

Pseudoaneurysm

TRA-related pseudoaneurysms are very rare occurrences due to the small vessel calibers (Fig. 6.4). Pseudoaneurysms commonly present days to weeks following the procedure and can present as a painful pulsating localized swelling. The majority of pseudoaneurysms resolve spontaneously. Ultrasound-guided compression, thrombin injections, or surgical ligation can be performed depending on the size and severity of symptoms.

AV Fistula

AV fistulas resulting from TRA are exceptionally rare occurrences, with most AV fistulas being clinically asymptomatic and managed conservatively. Placement of a covered stent has been described for large and symptomatic AV fistulas [45].

Radial Arteritis

After TRA procedures, soreness and mild pain at the access site and forearm is common. When a patient has post-procedure forearm pain that is out of proportion of what is expected with normal post-procedure pulses and an unremarkable ultrasonographic evaluation, a diagnosis of radial arteritis is made. The vast majority of

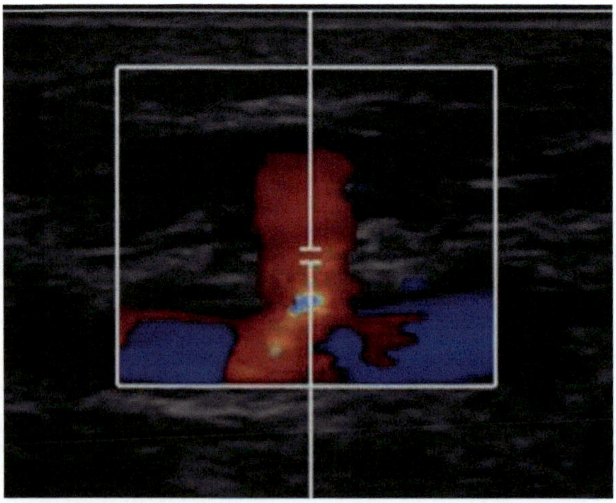

Fig. 6.4 Duplex ultrasound demonstrating a radial pseudoaneurysm after transradial catheterization in the longitudinal view

cases resolve with the use of NSAIDs, with few requiring treatment with oral steroids.

Neurologic Complications

Risk of Stroke

As the TRA involves catheters and wires traversing across the origins of the great vessels, there is a theoretical risk of periprocedural stroke. When performing subdiaphragmatic TRA procedures, the left radial approach is the strongly preferred side as it minimizes aortic arch manipulation and passage adjacent to the great vessels. As the TRA is routinely used for patients with atherosclerosis, it is important to understand this potential risk.

Although cardiology literature has explored the risk of stroke from the right radial approach, which involves aortic arch manipulation across the great vessels, multivariate analysis of observational data and large-scale meta-analyses have not demonstrated an increased risk of stroke with the TRA [46]. The incidence of cerebral embolization when using the left TRA for subdiaphragmatic procedures is exceptionally rare and is limited to case reports [47].

With the left TRA approach, caution should be used when passing the origin of the left vertebral and left subclavian arteries. With the increased scope and complexity of procedures that can be performed via the TRA, a variety of catheters and microcatheters have been designed to be used at specific stages of a procedure. As the number of catheter exchanges increases, it becomes increasingly important to flush every catheter to prevent air emboli. Operators should take special precaution when removing a catheter that may have residual embolic material or debris. In order to prevent the catheter from inadvertently cannulating the left vertebral artery and releasing embolic material, the operator should remove the catheter over a wire.

By using the left TRA with appropriate catheter technique and meticulous attention to detail when traversing the left vertebral and left subclavian arteries, the risk of clinically significant cerebral infarctions is overwhelmingly rare.

Neuromuscular Complications

It is not uncommon for patients to have minor numbness and tingling in the hands or wrists following TRA procedures, with symptoms generally resolving within a few hours. Rare case reports of complex regional pain syndromes after TRA procedures have been described, with treatment options including oral pain medication, steroid injections, antidepressants, nerve blocks, and occupational therapy depending on severity [48, 49].

There is limited data exploring the relationship between radial access-site complications and hand and limb dysfunction. The majority of reported cases of limb dysfunction are transient and resolve over time. In one study, there was diminished hand sensitivity in certain dermatomes using monofilament testing, which did not correlate with patient-reported hand symptoms [50]. In a large-scale meta-analysis, indicators of hand dysfunction including grip strength change and power loss were observed in 0.26% of cases, with the majority of symptoms resolving within 30 days [51]. This transient and rare phenomenon should be considered for individuals requiring fine-motor hand movement in the short-term after the procedure.

Device-Related Complications

Sheath Entrapment

Radial artery spasm can result in device entrapment in very extreme circumstances and has been greatly minimized with the use of hydrophilic sheaths. When faced with device entrapment, the operator should hydrate the patient, apply warm towels to the forearm, and administer antispasmodics, sedation, and pain medication. While attempting to remove the catheter, the operator should slowly retract the catheter in a cork-screw fashion. When forceful rapid retraction of catheters or sheaths is applied without success, worsening of the RAS is likely and may lead to radial artery intussusception or radial artery rupture. In these exceptional situations, radial endarterectomy with general anesthesia and regional nerve blocks will be required for removal of the entrapped device (Fig. 6.5).

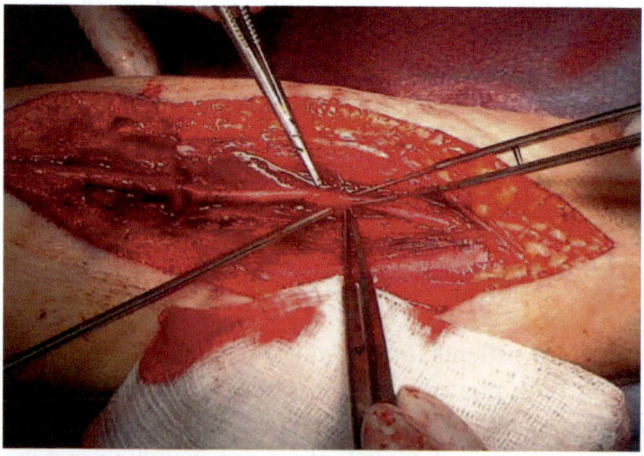

Fig. 6.5 Photograph of a radial endarterectomy procedure to remove an entrapped sheath

Catheter Granuloma

Certain sheaths have been reported to cause granulomatous skin reactions. The skin reaction follows a benign course and is usually self-limited without intervention [52].

Conclusion

The TRA has a demonstrated history of safety and patient satisfaction across heterogeneous populations in a broad range of peripheral and visceral endovascular interventions. Although clinically significant complications with the TRA are rare, it is important to recognize common pitfalls and complications unique to the TRA as it becomes more widely adopted throughout the practice of interventional radiology.

References

1. Romagnoli E, Biondi-Zoccai G, Sciahbasi A, et al. Radial versus femoral randomized investigation in ST-segment elevation acute coronary syndrome: the RIFLE-STEACS (radial versus femoral randomized investigation in ST-elevation acute coronary syndrome) study. J Am Coll Cardiol. 2012;60:2481–9.
2. Mehta S, Jolly S, Cairns J, et al. Effects of radial versus femoral artery access in patients with acute coronary syndromes with or without ST-segment elevation. J Am Coll Cardiol. 2012;60:2490–9.
3. Valgimigli M, Gagnor A, Calabro P, et al. Radial versus femoral access in patients with acute coronary syndromes undergoing invasive management: a randomized multicenter trial. Lancet. 2015;385:2465–76.
4. Kok M, Weernick M, Von Birgelen C, et al. Patient preference for radial versus femoral vascular access for elective coronary procedures: the PREVAS study. Catheter Cardiovasc Interv. 2018;91:17–24.
5. Posham R, Biederman D, Patel R, et al. Transradial approach for noncoronary interventions: a single-center review of safety and feasibility in the first 1,500 cases. J Vasc Interv Radiol. 2016;27:159–66.
6. Hess C, Peterson E, Neely M, et al. The learning curve for transradial percutaneous coronary intervention among operators in the United States: a study from the National Cardiovascular Data Registry. Circulation. 2014;129:2277–86.
7. Kiemeneij F. Prevention and management of radial artery spasm. J Invasive Cardiol. 2006;18:159–60.
8. Jolly S, Yusef S, Cairns J, et al. Radial versus femoral access for coronary angiography and intervention in patients with acute coronary syndromes (RIVAL): a randomized, parallel group, multicentre trial. Lancet. 2011;377:1409–20.
9. Rathore S, Stables R, Pauriah M, et al. Impact of length and hydrophilic coating of the introducer sheath on radial artery spasm during transradial coronary intervention: a randomized study. JACC Cardiovasc Interv. 2010;3:475–83.

10. Sanmartin M, Gomez M, Ramon J, et al. Interruption of blood flow during compression and radial artery occlusion after transradial catheterization. Catheter Cardiovasc Interv. 2007;70:185–9.
11. Pancholy S, Coppola J, Patel T, et al. Prevention of radial artery occlusion- patent hemostasis evaluation trial (PROPHET study): a randomized comparison of traditional versus patency documented hemostasis after transradial catheterization. Catheter Cardiovasc Interv. 2008;72:335–40.
12. Pancholy S. Impact of two different hemostatic devices on radial artery outcomes after transradial catheterization. J Invasive Cardiol. 2009;21:101–14.
13. Cubero J, Lombardo J, Pedrosa C, et al. Radial compression guided by mean artery pressure versus standard compression with a pneumatic device (RACOMAP). Catheter Cardiovasc Interv. 2009;73:467–72.
14. Hildick-Smith D, Lowe M, Jm W, et al. Coronary angiography from the radial artery-- experience, complications and limitations. Int J Cardiol. 1998;64:231–9.
15. Sanmartin M, Cuevas D, Goicolea J, et al. Vascular complication associated with radial artery access for cardiac catheterization. Rev Esp Cardiol. 2004;57:581–4.
16. Kumar V, Balaji R, Anupam B, et al. Mid-forearm hematomas in transradial procedures. Indian Heart J. 2005;57:181.
17. Cao Z, Zhou Y, Zhao Y, et al. Transradial approach for coronary angioplasty in Chinese elderly patients. Chin Med J (Engl). 2008;121:1121–9.
18. Lim Y, Chan C, Kwok V, et al. Transradial access for coronary angiography and angioplasty: a novel approach. Singap Med J. 2003;44:563–9.
19. Saito S, Ikei H, Hosokawa G, et al. Influence of the ratio between radial artery inner diameter and sheath outer diameter on radial artery flow after transradial coronary intervention. Catheter Cardiovasc Interv. 1999;44:173–8.
20. Bazemore E, Man J. Problems and complications of the transradial for coronary interventinos: a review. J Invasive Cardiol. 2005;57:581–4.
21. Calvino-Santos R, Vasquez R, Salgado-Fernandez J, et al. Management of iatrogenic radial artery perforation. Catheter Cardiovasc Interv. 2004;61:74–8.
22. Kanei Y, Kwan T, Nakra N, et al. Transradial cardiac catheterization: a review of access site complications. Catheter Cardiovasc Interv. 2011;78:840–6.
23. Jia D, Zhou Y, Shi D, et al. Incidence and predictors of radial artery spasm during transradial coronary angiography and intervention. Chin Med J (Engl). 2010;123:843–7.
24. Loh Y, Nakao M, Tan W, et al. Factors influencing radial artery size. Asian Cardiovasc Thorac Ann. 2007;15:324–6.
25. Zhou Y, Zhao Y, Cao Z, et al. Incidence and risk factors of acute radial artery occlusion following transradial percutaneous coronary intervention. Zhonghua Yi Xue Za Zhi. 2007;87:1531–4.
26. Stella P, Kiemeneij F, Laarman G, et al. Incidence and outcome of radial artery occlusion following transradial artery coronary angioplasty. Catheter Cardiovasc Diagn. 1997;40:156–8.
27. Chen Y, Ke Z, Xiao J, et al. Subcutaneous injection of nitroglycerine at the radial artery puncture site reduces the risk of early radial artery occlusion after transradial coronary catheterization: a randomized, placebo-controlled clinical trial. Circ Cardiovasc Interv. 2018;11:e006571.
28. Pancholy S, Patel T. Effect of duration of hemostatic compression on radial artery occlusion after transradial access. Catheter Cardiovasc Interv. 2012;79:78–81.
29. Pancholy S, Bernat I, Bertrand O, et al. Prevention of radial artery occlusion after transradial catheterization: the PROPHET-II randomized trial. JACC Cardiovasc Interv. 2016;9:1992–9.
30. Nagai S, Abe S, Sato T, et al. Ultrasonic assessment of vascular complications in coronary angiography and angioplasty after transradial approach. Am J Cardiol. 1999;83:180–6.
31. Tian J, Chu Y, Sun J, et al. Ulnar artery compression: a feasible and effective approach to prevent the radial artery occlusion after coronary intervention. Chin Med J (Engl). 2015;128:795–8.
32. Madssen E, Haere P, Wiseth R. Radial artery diameter and vasodilatory properties after transradial coronary angiography. Ann Thorac Surg. 2006;82:1698–703.

33. Burstein J, Giderewicz D, Hutchinson S, et al. Impact of radial artery cannulation for coronary angiography and angioplasty on radial artery function. Am J Cardiol. 2007;99:457–9.
34. Charalambous M, Constantinides S, Talias M, et al. Repeated transradial catherization: feasibility, efficacy, and safety. Tex Heart Inst J. 2014;41:575–8.
35. Caputo R, Simons A, Giambartolomei A, et al. Safety and efficacy of repeat transradial access for cardiac catheterization procedures. Catheter Cardiovasc Interv. 2001;54:188–90.
36. Yoo B, Lee S, Ko J, et al. Procedural outcomes of repeated transradial coronary procedure. Catheter Cardiovasc Interv. 2003;58:301–4.
37. Valsecchi O, Vassileva A. Radial artery: how many times? Indian Heart J. 2010;62:226–9.
38. Chen S, Brunet M, Sur S, et al. Feasibility of repeat transradial access for neuroendovascular procedures. J Neurointerv Surg. 2019. https://doi.org/10.1136/neurointsurg-2019-015438.
39. Ghuran A, Dixon G, Holmberg S, et al. Transradial coronary intervention without prescreening for a dual palmar blood supply. Int J Cardiol. 2007;121:320–2.
40. De Bucourt M, Teichgraber U. Digital ischemia and consecutive amputation after emergency transradial cardiac catheter examination. Cardiovasc Intervent Radiol. 2012;35:1242–4.
41. Chatterjee A, White J, Leesar M. Management of radial artery perforation during transradial catheterization using a polytetrafluoroethylene-covered coronary stent. Cardiovasc Revasc Med. 2017;18:133–5.
42. Agostoni P, Biondi-Zoccai G, de Benedictis M, et al. Radial versus femoral approach for percutaneous coronary diagnostic and interventional procedures; systematic overview and meta-analysis of randomized trials. J Am Coll Cardiol. 2004;44:349–56.
43. Tizon-Marcos H, Barbeau G. Incidence of compartment syndrome of the arm in a large series of transradial approach for coronary procedures. J Interv Cardiol. 2008;21:380–4.
44. Jue J, Karam J, Mejia A, et al. Compartment syndrome of the hand: a rare sequela of transradial cardiac catheterization. Tex Heart Inst J. 2017;44:73–6.
45. Summaria F, Romagnoli E, Preziosi P. Percutaneous antegrade transarterial treatment of iatrogenic radial arteriovenous fistula. J Cardiovasc Med. 2012;13:50–2.
46. Patel V, Brayton K, Kumbhani D, et al. Meta-analysis of stroke after transradial versus transfemoral artery catheterization. Int J Cardiol. 2013;168:5234–8.
47. Al-Hakim R, Gandhi R, Benenati J. Incident of stroke after transradial arterial access for subdiaphragmatic intervention. J Vasc Interv Radiol. 2017;28:1287–8.
48. Padadimos T, Hofmann J. Radial artery thrombosis, palmar arch systolic blood velocities, and chronic regional pain syndrome following transradial cardiac catheterization. Catheter Cardiovasc Interv. 2002;57:537–40.
49. Sasano N, Tsuda T, Sasano H, et al. A case of complex regional pain syndrome type II after transradial coronary intervention. J Anesth. 2004;18:310–2.
50. Van der Heijden D, Leeuwen M, Ritt M, et al. Hand sensibility after transradial arterial access: an observational study in patients with and without radial artery occlusion. J Vasc Interv Radiol. 2019;30:1832–9.
51. Haq M, Rashid M, Kwok C, et al. Hand dysfunction after transradial artery catheterization for coronary procedures. World J Cardiol. 2017;9:609–19.
52. Zellner C, Ports T, Yeghiazarians Y, et al. Sterile radial artery granuloma after transradial procedures:a unique and avoidable complication. Catheter Cardiovasc Interv. 2010;76:673–6.

Chapter 7
Transradial Access for Renal and Mesenteric Artery Disease

Nicholas Voutsinas and Robert A. Lookstein

Introduction

While renal and mesenteric interventions have been traditionally performed from a femoral approach, advances in technology allow interventionalists the ability to safely treat a multitude of disease processes affecting these regions with a transradial approach [1].

The acute angle of origin of the superior mesenteric artery off of the aorta allows for easier access by a transradial approach compared to a transfemoral approach [2]. Transradial access for mesenteric procedures include angioplasty, stent placement, and a variety of embolization procedures (aneurysms, tumors, gastrointestinal bleeds) [3, 4]. Performing these procedures with a transradial approach is possible due to recent advances in technology allowing for longer microcatheters, longer coil delivery systems, and longer shafts to deliver stents. The mesenteric arterial system can be accessed with an appropriately sized catheter that allows for delivery of appropriate treatment options, usually 5 or 6 French lumen size, for example, a 5 French Sarah Radial Catheter (Terumo). Additionally, guide catheters, such as the JR4 guide catheter (Cordis), can be used to have extra ability to perform angiograms while positioning potential stents or coils. Multiple medical companies manufacture a variety of coils, stents, microvascular plugs, pressure wires, and embolic agents that can be deployed after a transradial approach within the mesenteric arterial system.

As with mesenteric artery interventions, technology allowing for interventions to be performed despite traveling a longer distance has led to the ability to perform renal artery interventions after transradial access. Accessing the renal arteries from a superior approach within the aorta can allow for a more atraumatic approach when compared to transfemoral access, especially for renal arteries that have a down

N. Voutsinas (✉) · R. A. Lookstein
Department of Diagnostic, Molecular and Interventional Radiology, Icahn School of Medicine at Mount Sinai, New York, NY, USA
e-mail: nicholas.voutsinas@mountsinai.org

A. M. Fischman et al. (eds.), *Transradial Access in Interventional Radiology*, https://doi.org/10.1007/978-3-030-81678-0_7

sloping origin [5]. Employing a "no touch" technique with a guide catheter or multipurpose catheter can potentially reduce traumatic entry into the renal artery, especially in cases of severe ostial stenosis, preventing distal calcific embolization or spasm [6]. This co-axial guide catheter approach can allow for easier positioning of stents with the ability to perform angiograms as the stent is being deployed. This transradial guide catheter approach is comparable to using larger and longer sheaths from a transfemoral approach with a lower profile of intervention at the access site. Stabilizer wires can be used for securing access to the distal arteries while interventions are performed more proximally. Guide catheters should be connected to a side flush, similar to any arterial sheath, in order to prevent clot formation and distal embolization to the target organs.

The following case examples are just a few of the many procedures that are in the arsenal of interventionalists from a transradial approach.

Case 1

A 73-year-old male with hypertension, recently started on ACE inhibitor, presented due to acute renal injury. Subsequent renal Doppler ultrasound demonstrated left renal artery stenosis, leading to patient presenting for angiogram and stent placement. The left radial artery was accessed, Barbeau waveform A, and a 5/6 French hydrophilic slender sheath was placed. The left renal artery was cannulated using a 6 French JR4 guide catheter (Cordis) over a 0.014 stabilizer wire. Left renal angiogram (Fig. 7.1a) demonstrated severe ostial stenosis. A 7 × 15 mm Herculink (Abbott Medical) balloon expandable bare metal stent was deployed and after being successfully pre-dilated with a 3 × 20 mm Maverick balloon (Boston Scientific) (Fig. 7.1b). Post-stenting angiogram (Fig. 7.1c) showed improved flow through the origin of the left renal artery.

Case 2

A 70-year-old male presented for angiography due to incidentally detected 2.8 cm aneurysm at the origin of the inferior mesenteric artery (IMA). Following placement of a 5/6 French slender sheath, Barbeau waveform B, a 0.014 stabilizer wire and JR4 guide catheter were advanced into the IMA, and angiography (Fig. 7.2a) showed the known IMA aneurysm. Coil embolization was performed with numerous 0.035 coils, including 19 packing coils, 5 non-fibered coils, and 9 fibered coils. Post-coiling angiography (Fig. 7.2a) demonstrated complete occlusion of the IMA. Superior mesenteric artery angiography revealed collateral filling of the distal IMA branches via a prominent Arc of Riolan indicating adequate collateral supply to the bowel supplied by the IMA.

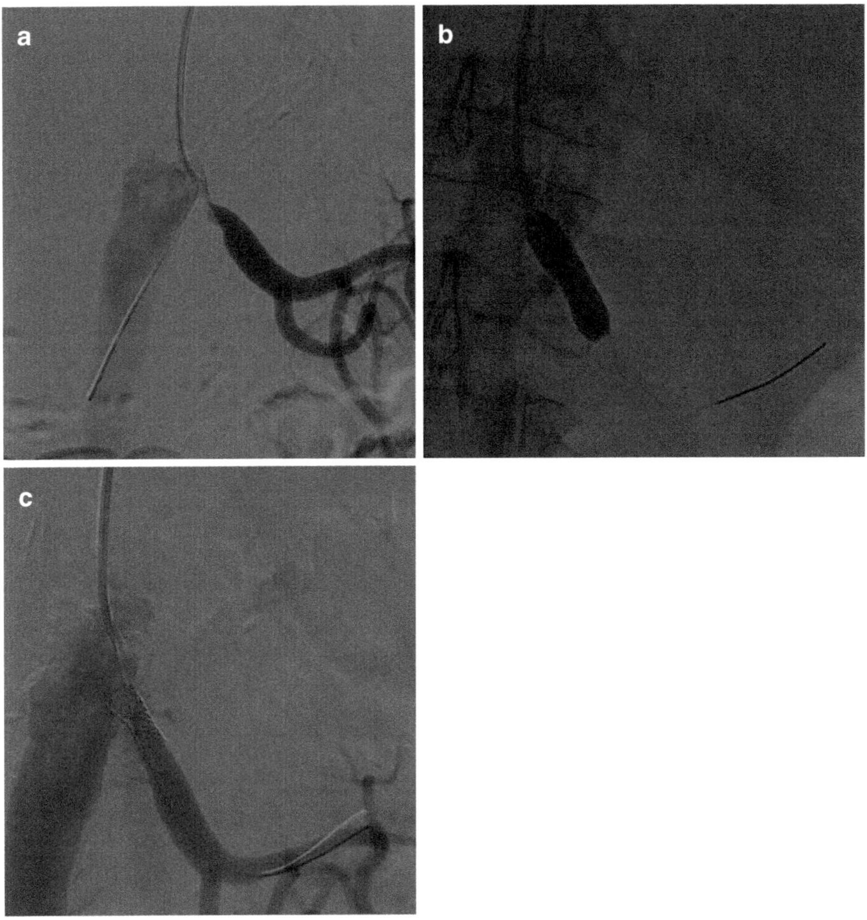

Fig. 7.1 (**a**) angiographic image of the left renal artery demonstrating severe ostial stenosis after left radial artery access. (**b**) demonstrates placement of a balloon expandable stent in the ostium, with (**c**) demonstrating post-stenting angiogram with improved flow through the renal artery

Case 3

A 64-year-old female presented for embolization of a left renal mass, found to be a 5.7 cm angiomyolipoma arising from the lower pole of the kidney. After a 5/6 French hydrophilic sheath was placed into the radial artery, Barbeau waveform B, a 5 French 110 cm Sarah Radial catheter (Terumo) was used to catheterize the left renal artery, with the angiogram (Fig. 7.3a) showing a vascular mass arising off a lower pole branch of the renal artery. A Progreat 2.4F 150cm microcatheter (Terumo) was advanced into the lower pole artery (Fig. 7.3b), and 1 mL of Onyx-18 co-polymer (Medtronic) was injected slowly through the catheter. Post-embolization angiogram

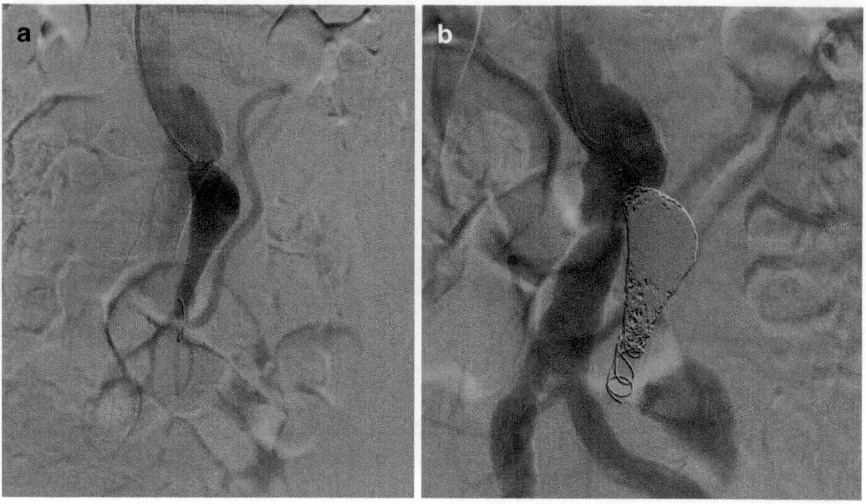

Fig. 7.2 (**a**) angiographic image demonstrating a large inferior mesenteric artery aneurysm after left radial artery access. Multiple packing coils, non-fibered coils, and fibered coils were placed into the aneurysm sac showing occlusion of the artery in (**b**)

(Fig. 7.3c) demonstrates the Onyx cast in the lower pole branch and lack of flow into the angiomyolipoma.

Conclusion and Future Direction

Angioplasty, stenting, and embolization procedures of the renal and mesenteric arteries can be safely performed from the left radial artery and in some case more easily than from transfemoral access. Unfortunately, limitations of size of the radial artery prevent deployment of covered stents, as all currently available covered stents are too large to fit through a 6 French system, and further research is needed to develop new technologies. Additional future needs include pre-shaped guide sheaths. As transradial access becomes more widely adopted, innovation will develop more available technologies to assist in performing these procedures.

Author Equipment List

- JR4 Guide Catheter (Cordis) or Sarah Radial Catheter (Terumo)
- Appropriately sized microcatheters, including Progreat Microcatheter (Terumo) or Truselect Microcatheter (Boston Scientific)
- 0.014 stabilizer wire

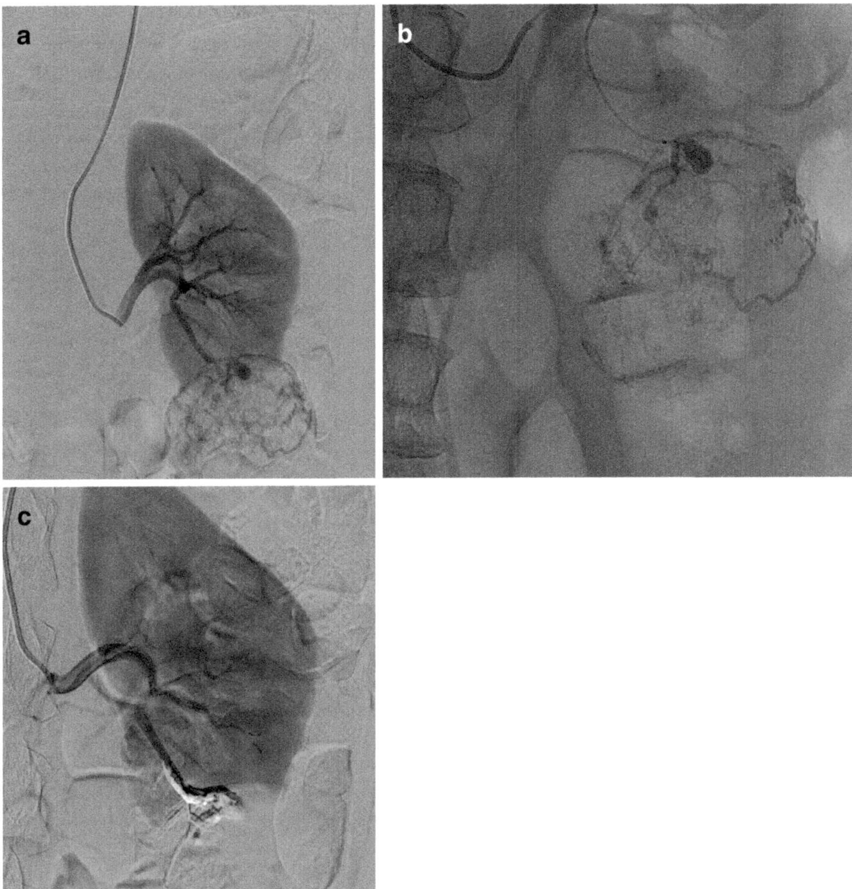

Fig. 7.3 (**a**) demonstrates a left renal angiogram with a large angiomyolipoma arising from the lower pole after left radial artery access. A microcatheter was advanced into the vascularity of the mass to inject an embolic agent, as seen in (**b**), with post-embolization angiogram in (**c**) demonstrating occlusion of the vessels supplying the angiomyolipoma

Procedure Menu

- Angioplasty and stenting of renal/mesenteric artery stenosis
- Embolization of renal/mesenteric aneurysm
- Embolization of renal/mesenteric masses or hemorrhage

Tips

1. Over 95% of renal and mesenteric procedures can be performed with a 6 French guide catheter.

2. Pre-shaped guide catheters can navigate through any renal/mesenteric anatomy to position the operator in the immediate proximity to the target lesion.
3. Use low profile (0.014/0.018) equipment to ensure technical success and allow equipment delivery through 6 French guide catheter.
4. Always obtain completion angiography, including venous phase, to evaluate for potential complications.
5. For complex procedures, test guide wire and microcatheter systems on the bench to ensure compatibility with 6 French guide catheter.

References

1. Posham R, Biederman DM, Patel RS, et al. Transradial approach for noncoronary interventions: a single-center review of safety and feasibility in the first 1,500 cases. J Vasc Interv Radiol. 2016;27(2):159–66.
2. Oderich GS, de Souza LR. Techniques of endovascular mesenteric revascularization. In: Oderich GS, editor. Mesenteric vascular disease: current therapy. New York: Springer; 2015. p. 165–86.
3. Voutsinas N, Patel RS, Bishay VL, Ranade M, Nowakowski FS, Kim E, Fischman AM, Divino CM, Marin ML, Lookstein RA. Pre-operative endovascular occlusion for unresectable metastatic carcinoid tumor: technique and initial results. Abdom Radiol (NY). 2020;45(8):2554–60. https://doi.org/10.1007/s00261-020-02534-2.
4. van Dijk LJD, van Noord D, van Mierlo M, Bijdevaate DC, Bruno MJ, Moelker A. Single-center retrospective comparative analysis of transradial, transbrachial, and transfemoral approach for mesenteric arterial procedures. J Vasc Interv Radiol. 2020;31(1):130–8.
5. Ruzsa Z, Tóth K, Jambrik Z, et al. Transradial access for renal artery intervention. Interv Med Appl Sci. 2014;6(3):97–103.
6. Sanghvi K, Coppola J, Patel T. Cranio-caudal (transradial) approach for renal artery intervention. J Interv Cardiol. 2013;26(5):530–5.

Chapter 8
Transradial Access for Interventional Oncology: Chemoembolization and Radioembolization Applications

Samuel Z. Maron, Nickolas Dreher, Joseph J. Titano, and Edward Kim

Abbreviations

HCC	Hepatocellular carcinoma
IO	Interventional oncology
IR	Interventional radiology
MAA	Macroaggregated albumin scanning
TACE	Transarterial chemoembolization
TARE	Transarterial radioembolization
TFA	Transfemoral access
TRA	Transradial access

Introduction

Many interventional oncology (IO) procedures have traditionally employed transfemoral artery access (TFA). A growing body of evidence, however, has shown transradial access (TRA) to be effective, safe, and potentially associated with higher patient satisfaction in several IO interventions. This chapter will briefly review common IO applications, discuss the TRA technique for these procedures, and contrast TRA and TFA on the basis of technical success rates, adverse events, costs, radiation exposure, and patient preferences.

S. Z. Maron (✉) · N. Dreher · J. J. Titano · E. Kim
Department of Diagnostic, Molecular and Interventional Radiology, Icahn School of Medicine at Mount Sinai, New York, NY, USA
e-mail: samuel.maron@icahn.mssm.edu

A. M. Fischman et al. (eds.), *Transradial Access in Interventional Radiology*, https://doi.org/10.1007/978-3-030-81678-0_8

Indications and Associated Epidemiology

Hepatocellular Carcinoma and Liver Metastasis

TRA is an increasingly common technique in interventional procedures in general and IO specifically. The mainstay of IO is the treatment of liver malignancies, especially HCC and metastases. In 2018, HCC was the sixth most common neoplasm and the third leading cause of cancer death [1].

Regardless of the etiology, intra-arterial IO treatments for liver tumors are chemoembolization (TACE), radioembolization (TARE), and bland embolization [2, 3]. The use of TRA in abdominal and pelvic interventions has increased in recent years, and several studies have shown its safety and efficacy in TACE and TARE specifically [4–7]. Both of these techniques utilize the preferential recruitment of arteries of hypervascular malignancies for delivery of flow directed therapies. Tumors receive blood supply primarily from the hepatic artery, while the liver parenchyma is relatively spared due to its reliance on portal blood supply. In TACE, an emulsification of Lipiodol/ethiodized oil and drug or a drug eluting platform is administered directly into a branch of the hepatic artery in conjunction with embolic substances. In TARE, Yttrium-90 microspheres deliver radiation to the tumor. These glass or resin microspheres emit beta particles that stimulate apoptosis and subsequent shrinkage of the tumor. Prior to TARE, macroaggregated albumin (MAA) mapping is used to assess tumor blood supply, identify vessels that may allow for nontarget embolization and assess lung shunt fraction.

Procedural Methodology

Access

Prior to the procedure, MRI or CT should be reviewed to assess thoracic and abdominal aorta anatomy as well as the arterial supply to the liver, evaluating for any anatomical variants. Preoperatively, the evaluation in TRA for IO is completed in line with that of other IR procedures. The Barbeau waveform and the size of the radial artery are assessed in order to ensure sufficient collateral flow to the hand and safe access. In some institutions, TACE and TARE are completed as ambulatory same-day procedures [6, 7]. A complete technical guide to transradial access can be found by Fischman et al. [7].

The left radial artery is preferably used in order to reduce the required catheter lengths and to minimize the manipulation of the aortic arch vessels. Once TRA is achieved, and appropriate intra-arterial vasodilators and anticoagulation have been administered, a wire and catheter – typically 110 cm in length – are advanced to navigate the aortic arch and select the target mesenteric vessel. A 5Fr Sarah Radial Optitorque (Terumo Medical, Somerset, NJ) catheter with a 0.035-inch Bentson wire is typically the combination utilized at our institution to advance beyond the transverse arch toward the descending thoracic aorta and ultimately the mesenteric arteries. In cases with variant or tortuous vascular anatomy, a reverse curve catheter such as a Glidecath Simmons-2 (Terumo Medical, Somerset, NJ) in combination with an exchange-length 0.035-inch wire can be used to select the descending aorta. With the exchange-length wire in the abdominal aorta, the reverse curve catheter can be exchanged for the intended base-catheter, and the mesenteric vessels are selected. After performing angiography in the superior mesenteric artery and the celiac axis, a 150–155 cm microcatheter is utilized to subselect the vessels supplying the liver and the tumor. Angiograms and cone-beam CTs are then performed in order to assess liver and tumor perfusion, and the appropriate intra-arterial therapy is subsequently delivered.

After the intervention is completed, all wires and catheters are removed. A compression device, such as a TR band (Terumo Medical, Somerset, NJ), is placed for 90 minutes in order to achieve hemostasis. During this time, a pulse-oximeter is used, and the arterial waveform is monitored to ensure adequate blood flow to the wrist and hand.

Benefits of Transradial Access (TRA) in Interventional Oncology

Numerous studies have found no significant difference in success rate between TRA and TFA in IO indications. A meta-analysis of 1096 patients undergoing hepatic procedures by Chen et al. showed that TRA had a 99.2% success rate that was not significantly different from the TFA success rate [4]. Further, a number of studies have found that TRA has non-inferior rates of morbidity than TFA in a variety of interventions, including IO procedures. Chen et al. found that the overall complication rate for hepatic interventions in the TRA cohort did not differ significantly from the TFA cohort (7.6% vs 10.4%, $P = 0.32$) [4]. In chemoembolization specifically, Wu et al. found TRA to be associated with fewer complications when compared to TFA. They reported fewer incidents of abdominal distention (42.85% vs. 87.97%, $P > 0.001$), lumbago (1.59% vs. 97.46%, $P < 0.001$), vomiting (53.17% vs. 77.22%, $P < 0.001$), and dysuria (0% vs. 62.03%, $P < 0.001$) [8, 9]. In radioembolization however, there is no reported difference between major or minor complications in TRA compared to TFA [10]. Overall, TRA is safe and well tolerated in all IO applications that have been studied to date with several studies confirming its utility in liver malignancy [2, 3, 11].

Furthermore, in IO procedures, TRA is associated with lower cost and shortened length of stay [8, 10]. Kis et al. reported that, at their institution, they saved an average of about $100 in procedural supplies (catheters, vasodilator cocktail, etc.) per procedure when utilizing TRA vs. TFA ($669.10 vs. $767.40) in a cohort of 50 patients [10]. The authors of the study argue that the savings are likely underestimated given that the post-operative care was half the time in TRA procedures as compared to those using TFA (2 hours vs. 1 hour). In their preliminary study, Wu et al. reported similar findings that TRA was associated with lower costs [8].

In general, patients also prefer TRA to TFA due to significantly lower pain scores during the procedure and shorter recovery times afterward [9, 12]. In TARE procedures, overall pain during the procedure, pain at the access site during the procedure, and overall pain after the procedure were all lower following TRA compared to TFA ($P = 0.0046$, $P = 0.0004$, and $P = 0.0357$, respectively) [12]. Patients undergoing a TRA approach also had shorter recovery times (108 min for TRA, 153 min for TFA, $P = 0.0193$), allowing them to ambulate and perform basic activities sooner after the procedure [12]. Similar findings in TRA have also been reported for TACE with less discomfort at the access site after the procedure and greater post-procedure independence ($P < 0.001$) [9]. These findings align with results found by Liu et al. that 73.3% of patients had a preference for TRA [12]. Similarly, Chen et al.'s meta-analysis confirmed that 86.5% ($P < 0.00001$) of patients prefer TRA to TFA when given the choice [4].

However, in addition to the benefits of TRA, there are several potential tradeoffs that exist when TRA is applied in IO. While there is some conflicting evidence, there is concern that TRA can lengthen procedure time and also increase radiation exposure. Some studies have found that TRA is associated with increased fluoroscopy time and radiation dose in IO procedures [9, 10, 13, 14]. In addition, the learning curve associated with providers' transitioning to TRA can also contribute to increased procedure time and radiation dose in cases performed early in an operator's experience [9].

References

1. Forner A, Reig M, Bruix J. Hepatocellular carcinoma. Lancet. 2018;391(10127):1301–14.
2. van Dam L, Geeraedts T, Bijdevaate D, van Doormaal PJ, The A, Moelker A. Distal radial artery access for noncoronary endovascular treatment is a safe and feasible technique. J Vasc Interv Radiol. 2019;30(8):1281–5.
3. Posham R, Biederman DM, Patel RS, Kim E, Tabori NE, Nowakowski FS, et al. Transradial approach for noncoronary interventions: a single-center review of safety and feasibility in the first 1,500 cases. J Vasc Interv Radiol. 2016;27(2):159–66.
4. Chen Y-Y, Liu P, Wu Y-S, Lin H, Chen X. Transradial vs transfemoral access in patients with hepatic malignancy and undergoing hepatic interventions: a systematic review and meta-analysis. Medicine (Baltimore). 2018;97(52):e13926.
5. Shiozawa S, Tsuchiya A, Endo S, Kumazawa K, Ogawa K. Transradial approach for transcatheter arterial chemoembolization in patients with hepatocellular carcinoma. Nihon Shokakibyo Gakkai Zasshi. 2002;99(12):1450–4.
6. Bishay VL, Biederman DM, Ward TJ, van der Bom IMJ, Patel RS, Kim E, et al. Transradial approach for hepatic radioembolization: initial results and technique. AJR Am J Roentgenol. 2016;207(5):1112–21.
7. Fischman AM, Swinburne NC, Patel RS. A technical guide describing the use of transradial access technique for endovascular interventions. Tech Vasc Interv Radiol. 2015;18(2):58–65.
8. Wu T, Sun R, Huang Y, Wang Z, Yin X, Zhu Z, et al. Transradial arterial chemoembolization reduces complications and costs in patients with hepatocellular carcinoma. Indian J Cancer. 2015;52(Suppl 2):e107–11.

9. Iezzi R, Pompili M, Posa A, Annicchiarico E, Garcovich M, Merlino B, et al. Transradial versus transfemoral access for hepatic chemoembolization: intrapatient prospective single-center study. J Vasc Interv Radiol. 2017;28(9):1234–9.
10. Kis B, Mills M, Hoffe SE. Hepatic radioembolization from transradial access: initial experience and comparison to transfemoral access. Diagn Interv Radiol. 2016;22(5):444–9.
11. Pan P, Lee EW, Eghbalieh N, Trieu H. Ipsilateral transradial access in transarterial embolization of upper extremity bony metastases. J Vasc Access. 2019;20(2):202–8.
12. Liu LB, Cedillo MA, Bishay V, Ranade M, Patel RS, Kim E, et al. Patient experience and preference in transradial versus transfemoral access during transarterial radioembolization: a randomized single-center trial. J Vasc Interv Radiol. 2019;30(3):414–20.
13. Loewenstern J, Welch C, Lekperic S, Bishay V, Ranade M, Patel RS, et al. Patient radiation exposure in transradial versus transfemoral yttrium-90 radioembolization: a retrospective propensity score-matched analysis. J Vasc Interv Radiol. 2018;29(7):936–42.
14. Lekperic S, Livshits I, Tabori N, Patel R, Lookstein R, Kim E, et al. Patient radiation exposure in hepatic chemoembolization utilizing cone-beam CT: comparison of transradial and transfemoral approaches. J Vasc Interv Radiol. 2017;28(5):775.

Chapter 9
Transradial Access for Peripheral Arterial Disease: Aortoiliac Applications

Alex Sher, Raghuram Posham, Samuel Z. Maron, and Rami O. Tadros

Abbreviations

CFA	Common femoral artery
CLI	Chronic limb ischemia
DCB	Drug-coated balloon
OTW	Over-the-wire
PAD	Peripheral arterial disease
SFA	Superior femoral artery
TASC	Inter-Society Consensus for the Management of Peripheral Arterial Disease
TFA	Transfemoral arterial approach
TRA	Transradial arterial approach
USA	United States
USPSTF	United States Preventive Services Task Force

Introduction

Peripheral arterial disease (PAD) is a common medical condition affecting tens of millions of individuals in the United States (US) and Europe, with three million new cases in the USA each year alone [1]. Its worldwide prevalence is estimated to be between 3% and 12% [2]. Even with these numbers, since screening is not recommended by the United States Preventive Services Task Force (USPSTF), it is likely

A. Sher · R. Posham · S. Z. Maron
Department of Diagnostic, Molecular and Interventional Radiology,
Icahn School of Medicine at Mount Sinai, New York, NY, USA

R. O. Tadros (✉)
Department of Surgery, Division of Vascular Surgery, Icahn School of Medicine
at Mount Sinai, New York, NY, USA
e-mail: rami.tadros@mountsinai.org

A. M. Fischman et al. (eds.), *Transradial Access in Interventional Radiology*,
https://doi.org/10.1007/978-3-030-81678-0_9

underdiagnosed and undertreated [3, 4]. In PAD, there is progressive narrowing of the vasculature often caused by atherosclerosis. Some individuals have no significant symptoms, while others present with claudication that can progress to chronic limb ischemia (CLI) as a result of severe atherosclerosis. The presence of PAD in symptomatic and asymptomatic individuals is a general marker for increased cardiovascular risk. Risk factors for PAD mirror other cardiovascular diseases and include both dietary and behavioral factors, such as tobacco and high cholesterol, and comorbidities including hypertension and diabetes [1]. PAD patients can benefit from behavioral changes such as the cessation of smoking and exercise. Pharmaceutical interventions available for these patients include risk factor modification through blood pressure control, statin therapy to lower cholesterol, antiplatelet therapy, and vasodilatory medications such as cilostizol [3].

A significant proportion of patients will experience progression of their symptoms despite medical and behavior management and require endovascular or surgical intervention (atherectomy, stenting, endarterectomy, or bypass) in order to revascularize limbs and restore blood flow [4–6]. Given that PAD patients are often high-risk candidates for surgery, there has been an increasing focus on endovascular interventions as the first choice for treating PAD patients. Classically, endovascular interventions for peripheral arterial disease and lower extremity interventions have been completed using a transfemoral arterial approach (TFA). However, there are many benefits to employing TRA for PAD interventions. In cases of unfavorable TFA such as prior aortoiliac intervention such as aorto-bifemoral graft, severe iliac vessel tortuosity, femoral artery stenting, endarterectomy, adjacent bypass, or diseased artery, TRA may be preferred. In addition, any patient with a recent groin infection or prior surgery, abundance of soft tissue, or high bifurcation of the femoral vessels. Other benefits include higher patient satisfaction, ability to sit up and ambulate immediately following the procedure, less bleeding risk, and lower overall costs as compared to TFA [7–10]. A list of some relative indications and contraindications can be seen in Table 9.1.

In order to understand the available tools required to perform lower extremity interventions from the radial artery, we must first discuss two important factors: (1)

Table 9.1 Relative indications and contraindications to TRA

Relative indications	Relative contraindications
Steep or tortuous iliac arteries	Barbeau D waveform
Previous stent, endarterectomy, or bypass involving or adjacent to the femoral artery	Radial loop
Recent groin surgery or access	Radial artery <2 mm
Obesity	ESRD and potential for future HD access or functional upper extremity HD access
CFA above inguinal ligament	Aortic arch atherosclerosis/thrombosis/calcification
Groin infection	
Unable to discontinue anticoagulation	

CFA common femoral artery, *ESRD* end-stage renal disease, *HD* hemodialysis distance from the radial artery and (2) vessel diameter, with increased importance given to the latter for aortoiliac applications. The size of the radial artery and the target vessel is important in device selection and for determining feasibility. It is estimated that the radial artery diameter in the US population is approximately 3.2 ± 0.6 mm in men and 2.7 ± 0.5 mm in women [11]. Thus, a standard 6Fr sheath (approximate outer diameter 2.6–2.81) [12] could be used to cannulate the radial artery in approximately 90% of men and 75% of women. Lower profile sheaths, such as the 6Fr Terumo Destination Slender sheaths, which have an outer diameter of 2.46 mm would allow for an increased population of patients eligible for TRA. This is particularly important for PAD interventions as a 6Fr sheath is often required for interventions, and the majority of tools required for aortoiliac interventions require larger sheath sizes. Careful consideration should be made to measuring the radial artery under ultrasound before procedures to limit complications, including arterial spasm and radial artery occlusion.

Aortoiliac Disease

The femoral artery remains the preferred access site choice for aortoiliac arterial disease interventions, especially for complex endovascular procedures. The most notable advantages include relative proximity to the target lesions and the ability to introduce a wide range of tools through large bore sheaths such as stent grafts and covered stents. From a 6Fr sheath in the wrist, covered balloon expandable stent options are only available up to 7 mm in diameter (Lifestream, Bard) which precludes its use in the majority of patients with aortoiliac pathology. Additionally, aortoiliac stent grafts are unavailable in 6 Fr platforms, which limits the ability to perform complex aortic procedures via the radial artery. For most patients, the role of TRA as the sole access site for treating aortoiliac disease is limited to the iliac arteries to perform atherectomy, angioplasty, and deployment of bare metal stents. TRA can also be used as a secondary access site for internal iliac artery embolization for iliac limb extension for AAA or iliac artery aneurysms. TRA can also be used to achieve through-and-through access when unable to cross from a femoral approach.

Operators have had the tools to treat iliac artery disease with balloon angioplasty and bare metal stents for many years. In the largest two studies published on TRA to treat aortoiliac disease by Ruzsa et al. (n = 156) [13] and by Cortese et al. (n = 147) [14], the authors reach and image the target lesions using a standard guidewire and pigtail diagnostic angiographic catheter through a 5Fr or 6Fr short introducer sheath (Terumo, Japan). The pigtail and short sheath are removed and swapped for a dedicated long sheath (8.5Fr 100 cm or 6.5Fr 120 cm Sheathless Eaucath, Asahi, Japan or 7Fr 90 cm Destination Introducer, Terumo, Japan). The lesions were then traversed using a stiff guidewire followed by balloon expandable (Omnilink Elite, Abbot, USA) and self-expandable stents (Absolute, Abbot, USA) with shaft working lengths of 130–135 cm.

At present, the largest diameter stent which can be deployed via TRA is a 12 mm diameter self-expanding stent, which is available on a 6Fr × 120 cm platform, allowing stenting of the majority of external iliac arteries and also common iliac arteries in select patients. Overall, there are no drug-coated balloons indicated for treatment of the iliac arteries, and numerous plain angioplasty balloons are available on 6Fr platforms reaching up to 10 mm in diameter.

There is variability in the marketing of various catheter and sheath systems which can be confusing for operators. At present, the 6.5Fr and 7.5Fr 100 cm Sheathless Eaucath systems (Asahi, Japan) and very recently the 6Fr Destination Slender Sheath 119 cm and 149 cm systems (Terumo, Japan) have been approved for use in the USA. It is worth noting that the Asahi "sheathless" systems are marketed as catheters, and thus the sizing refers to the outer diameter, despite being used in practice as sheaths. Thus, in order to accommodate a 6Fr compatible stent or balloon, an 8.5Fr Sheathless Eaucath (not available in the USA) or 6Fr Destination Slender sheath would be required.

Transradial Access for Aortoiliac Peripheral Arterial Disease: Technical Considerations and Case Examples

This section describes techniques and tools specific to TRA for treating aortoiliac disease. Procedural steps common to both aortoiliac and infrainguinal cases are described below and are followed with several example cases. Important points specific to the cases presented are highlighted in the blue boxes at the end of every case. While the complications for TRA have been previously discussed (Chap. 6), there are several differences that come with PAD interventions. Compared to other interventions via TRA, PAD interventions typically require a larger and longer introducer sheath. This comes with a potential increased risk of radial artery occlusion, spasm, thromboembolism, arterial injury, and bleeding risk. As such careful manipulation of the aortic arch and monitoring of the introducer sheath while crossing lesions is important. Additionally, use of vasodilatory and anticoagulants can help reduce complications.

Radial Artery Access and Navigating to the Descending Aorta

The left radial artery is favored as it comes with a shorter distance, roughly 10–12 cm than the right radial artery, to the descending aorta, and fewer great vessels are crossed [15]. This is important as device length can be a limitation of TRA. The specific radial access technique is described in detail in Chap. 4.

TRA considerations for PAD is unique in that we recommend a 6Fr sheath to ensure adequate catheter and stent platform compatibility. Thus, preprocedural patient selection is key to ensure that the procedure can be performed successfully via the radial artery.

Slightly different than the radial cocktail described in Chap. 4, a solution consisting of 200 mcg of nitroglycerin and 2.5 mg of verapamil is diluted and administered slowly through the radial artery sheath to limit spasm. Various dosages for radial cocktails have been used. Use of intra-arterial vasodilatory agents is important as upper extremity arterial spasm will reduce the lumen around the catheter and may increase the risk of complications. Patients undergoing PAD interventions also receive anticoagulation with 80–100 mg/kg of unfractionated heparin. An Active Clotting Time (ACT) is assessed every 30–60 minutes, and the heparin is re-dosed to reduce the risk of thromboembolic events. When heparin is contraindicated (e.g., heparin-induced thrombocytopenia), it is recommended that Argatroban or Bivalirudin is used.

Operators have several available introducer systems involving sheaths and guiding catheters to treat aortoiliac and infrainguinal lesions (Table 9.2). The cases described below will highlight their use.

Aortoiliac Interventions

Case 1

Right Common Iliac and External Iliac Stenosis Causing Claudication

Procedure

1. Obtain radial access as described in Chap. 4. Unfractionated heparin is given at 80–100 mg/kg. Throughout the procedure an Active Clotting Time (ACT) is checked every 30–60 minutes, and heparin can be re-dosed at 1000 units to reduce risk of thromboembolic events.
2. Navigate to the infrarenal abdominal aorta using a 150 cm guidewire (Bentson Guidewire) and a guiding catheter (5Fr × 110 Optitorque Sarah Radial).
3. Perform aortography and right lower extremity angiography. Findings:
   (a) Patent Left Aortoiliac bypass
   (b) Right Lower Extremity – high grade stenosis at the proximal right common iliac artery due to eccentric calcified plaque. Moderate stenosis at the mid external iliac artery (Fig. 9.1a).
4. Exchange Bentson for a stiff support wire (0.035-inch × 260 cm Terumo Angled Glidewire) and exchange the 5Fr guiding catheter for a 6Fr × 90 cm MP Mach 1 guiding catheter within the aorta.
5. Advance a crossing support catheter over the support guidewire (3.2Fr × 150 cm Spectranetics Quick-Cross Select catheter) and cross the R CIA and mid R EIA lesions. After crossing the lesions, the Glidewire may be exchanged for a super stiff 0.035-inch × 260 cm Amplatz wire in preparation for stent deployment at the proximal R CIA.

Table 9.2 Devices Available for Transradial Lower Extremity Arterial Interventions

Device type	Manufacturer	Product	Dimensions	Comments
Sheaths and guiding catheter	Cook	Shuttle sheath	5 Fr; 110 cm	
	Boston Scientific	Guiding catheter	6 Fr; 110/125 cm	
	Cordis	Guiding catheter	5/6 Fr; 125 cm	
	Terumo	Glidecath	4 Fr; 150 cm	
	Terumo	R2P Destination Slender Sheath	5 Fr; 119/149 cm	
	R2P Slenguide catheter	Terumo	7 Fr (6 Fr ID); 120/150 cm	
	Asahi	Sheathless Eaucath	6.5–7.5 Fr (4–5 Fr ID); 100 cm	
	Asahi	Sheathless Eaucath	8.5 Fr (6 Fr ID); 120 cm	NA
Guidewires	Medtronic	Nitrix	0.035″	
	Cardiovascular Systems	Viper	0.014″; 335–475 cm	
	Terumo	Glidewire	0.035″; 350–450 cm	
	Boston Scientific	Novagold	0.018″; 480 cm	Off-label
Support catheter	Various		4–6 Fr; 135 cm, 150 cm	
Percutaneous transluminal angioplasty (PTA) balloons	Cook	Advance 14LP	4 Fr; 170 cm	
	Medtronic	Pacific Plus	4 Fr; 180 cm; 7 mm max OD	
	Bard	Ultraverse Rx	0.014″ 5 mm max OD; 4–5 Fr; 200 cm; REx	
	Terumo	Metacross	8 mm max OD;5 Fr; 200 cm; REx	
Drug-coated balloons	Various		For 6Fr system with shaft length >120 cm most DCBs have max 6 mm diameter	
	Bard	Lutonix	7 mm,130 cm shaft length	
Drug-eluting stents	Boston Scientific Cook	Eluvia Zilver	6–7 mm, 130 cm, 6Fr 5–8 mm, 125 cm, 6Fr	
Reentry devices	NA			
Self-expanding stents	Medtronic	Everflex Entrust	7 mm max OD; 5 Fr; 150 cm	Longest shaft
	OptiMed	Sinus SuperFlex 518	10 mm max OD; 5 Fr; 180 cm	NA
	Terumo	Metacross	8 mm max OD; 6 Fr; 200 cm; REx	FDA approved but NA

Table 9.2 (continued)

Device type	Manufacturer	Product	Dimensions	Comments
Atherectomy	Cardiovascular Systems	Diamondback	5 Fr; 200 cm	

Source: Table updated and adapted from previous sources [16, 17]
Abbreviations: *Fr* French, *ID* inner diameter, *NA* not available in the USA as of (August 2019), *OD* outer diameter, *Rex* rapid exchange

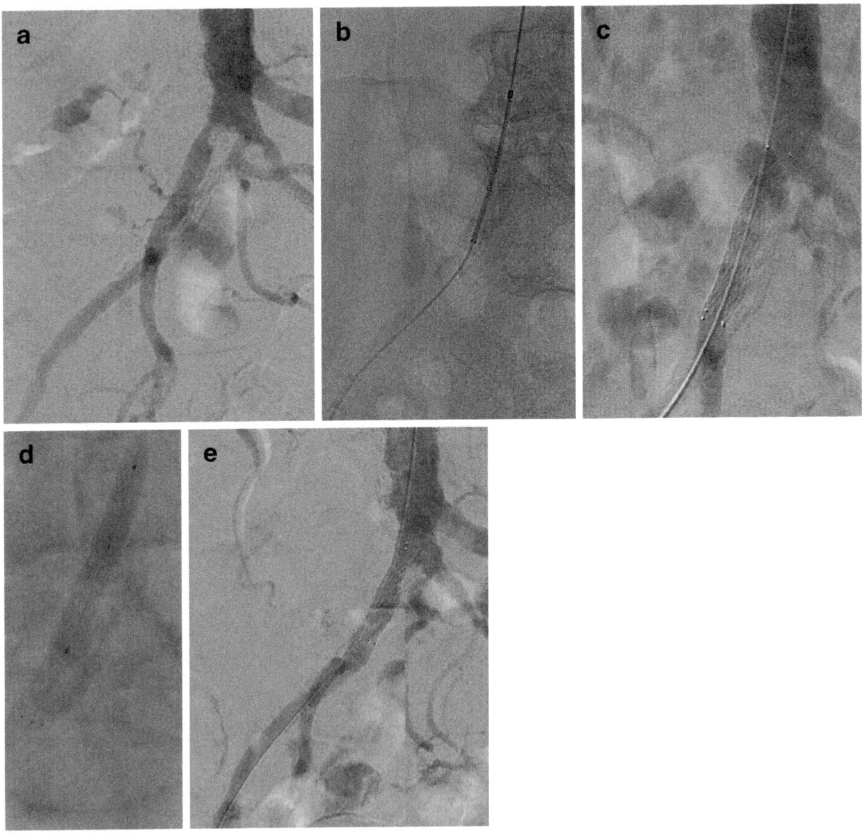

Fig. 9.1 Angiography images demonstrating stenosis at the proximal right common iliac artery the right mid-external iliac artery (**a**), stent placement and deployment (**b** and **c**), positioning of balloon (**d**), and final post intervention image (**e**)

6. Remove the Quick-Cross catheter and pre-dilate the stenosis with a balloon 1–2 mm smaller (e.g., 5- or 6-mm balloon) before stenting. Note from authors: it is recommended that the stenosis is dilated before stenting is performed.
7. Advance and deploy an appropriately sized stent across the proximal R CIA lesion (7 mm × 40 mm Everflex Entrust 150 cm shaft bare metal stent) (Fig. 9.1b).

(a) Post deployment images show a residual stenosis at the proximal aspect of the stent (Fig. 9.1c).

8. Advance an angioplasty balloon (6 mm diameter × 40 mm length Pacific Plus PTA 180 cm shaft length balloon) over the guidewire to the proximal aspect of the stent and angioplasty the stenosis in the native mid R EIA (not shown), and at the proximal aspect of the newly deployed stent at the R CIA under fluoroscopic guidance (Fig. 9.1d).
9. Repeat angiogram shows acceptable residual stenosis at the stent and good luminal gain at the mid R EIA stenosis (Fig. 9.1e). Distal angiogram shows preserved runoff to the right foot.
10. Remove the catheters, guidewire, and sheath from the arm and apply a radial hemostasis band for 60 minutes.

Case 2

Right External Iliac Artery Bypass Stenosis Causing Rutherford Grade III Claudication

Clinic Visit

71F with history of hypertension, hyperlipidemia, and peripheral arterial disease (history of right external iliac to SFA PTFE bypass) presenting with right lower extremity claudication (Rutherford Grade III), with preprocedural arterial duplex confirming a severe decrease in flow at the bypass anastomosis. Patient height: 5 feet 1 inches. Barbeau B.

Procedure

1. Obtain radial access as described in Chap. 4. Unfractionated heparin is given at 80–100 mg/kg. Throughout the procedure an ACT is checked every 30–60 minutes, and heparin can be re-dosed at 1000 units to reduce risk of thromboembolic events.
2. Navigate to the infrarenal abdominal aorta using a 150 cm guidewire (Bentson Guidewire) and a 5Fr × 110 cm Sarah Radial diagnostic catheter (Terumo)
3. Perform aortography and lower extremity angiography. Findings:

   (a) Patent distal aorta and bilateral common iliac arteries.
   (b) High grade flow limiting stenosis at proximal aspect of the right external iliac artery bypass graft (Fig. 9.2a).

4. Advance the Bentson wire and diagnostic catheter system to the right external iliac artery. Exchange the Bentson for a stiff support wire (0.035-inch × 260 cm Terumo Angled Glidewire).
5. Over the Glidewire, exchange the diagnostic catheter for a longer guiding sheath, 5Fr 110 cm shuttle sheath (Cook).

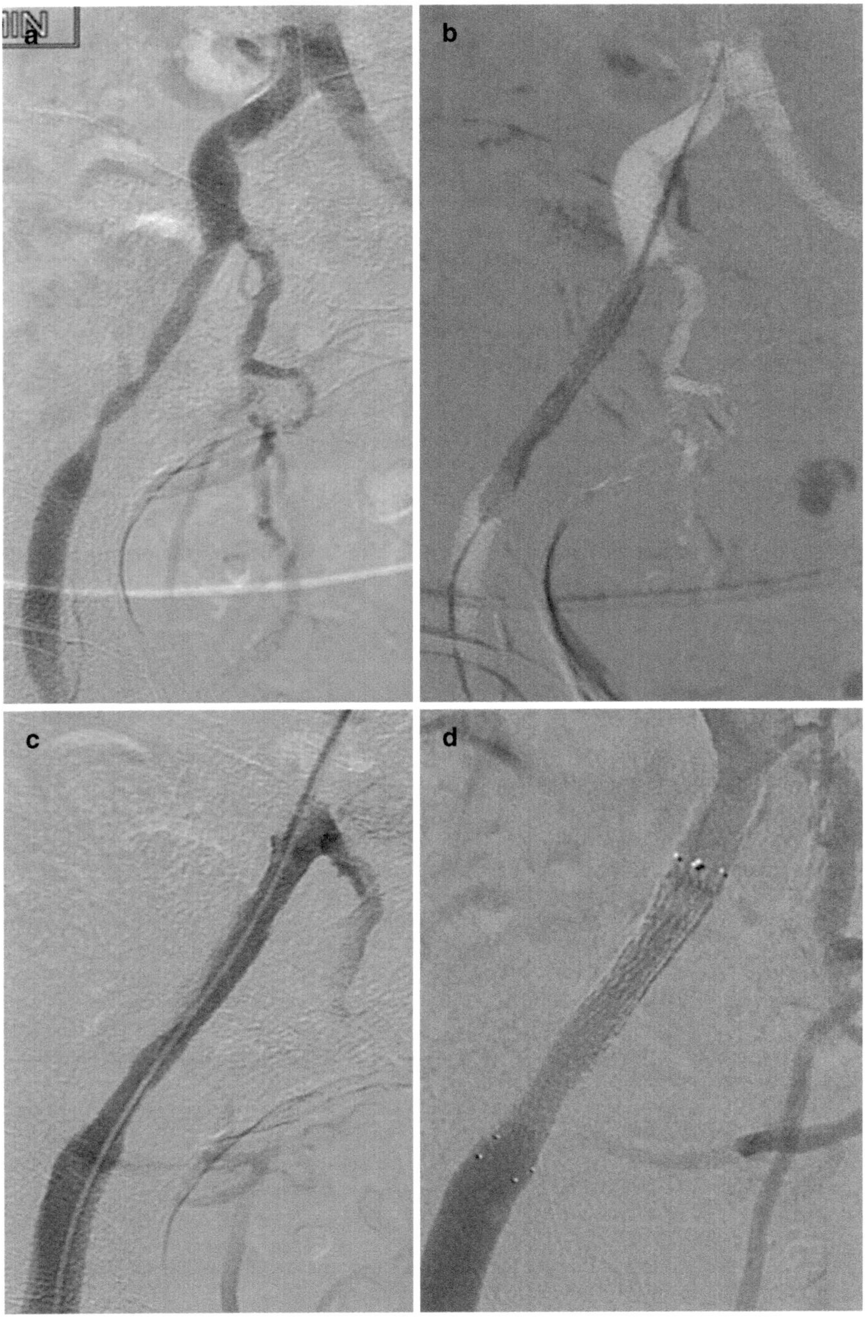

Fig. 9.2 Angiography images demonstrating stenosis at the external iliac artery (**a**), angioplasty of lesions (**b**), post angioplasty angiogram (**c**), post stent deployment angiogram (**d**)

6. Angioplasty the lesion. PTA balloons with working lengths capable of treating iliac artery lesions are compatible with both 0.035-inch and 0.018-inch wire systems.
   (a) Advance an angioplasty balloon over the guidewire (6 mm × 60 mm Boston Scientific Charger, 135 cm shaft). Angioplasty the lesion (Fig. 9.2b).
7. Deflate the balloon and perform a repeat angiogram, which shows significant residual stenosis at the right external iliac artery (Fig. 9.2c). A stent will be required to address this lesion.
8. Remove the balloon in preparation for a stent.
9. Advance and deploy an appropriately sized stent across the site of the lesion (7 mm × 40 mm Everflex Entrust 150 cm shaft self-expanding stent).
   (a) Remove the stent delivery system and balloon angioplasty the stent to ensure wall adherence, using the previously used angioplasty balloon.
10. Post-stent deployment angiogram demonstrates significantly improved flow to the right leg (Fig. 9.2d).
11. Remove the catheters, guidewire, and sheath from the arm and apply a radial hemostasis band for 60 minutes.

References

1. Sampson UKA, et al. Global and regional burden of death and disability from peripheral artery disease: 21 world regions, 1990 to 2010. Glob Heart. 2014;9:145–58.e21.
2. Fowkes FGR, et al. Comparison of global estimates of prevalence and risk factors for peripheral artery disease in 2000 and 2010: a systematic review and analysis. Lancet. 2013;382:1329–40.
3. Conte SM, Vale PR. Peripheral arterial disease. Heart Lung Circ. 2018;27:427–32.
4. US Preventive Services Task Force, et al. Screening for peripheral artery disease and cardiovascular disease risk assessment with the ankle-brachial index: US preventive services task force recommendation statement. JAMA. 2018;320:177–83.
5. Gerhard-Herman MD, et al. 2016 AHA/ACC guideline on the management of patients with lower extremity peripheral artery disease: executive summary: a report of the American College of Cardiology/American Heart Association task force on clinical practice guidelines. Circulation. 2017;135:e686–725.
6. Posham R, et al. Radial access for lower extremity peripheral arterial interventions: do we have the tools? Semin Intervent Radiol. 2018;35:427–34.
7. Le Corvoisier P, et al. Ambulatory transradial percutaneous coronary intervention: a safe, effective, and cost-saving strategy. Catheter Cardiovasc Interv. 2013;81:15–23.
8. Amin AP, et al. Costs of transradial percutaneous coronary intervention. JACC Cardiovasc Interv. 2013;6:827–34.
9. Kok MM, et al. Patient preference for radial versus femoral vascular access for elective coronary procedures: the PREVAS study. Catheter Cardiovasc Interv. 2018;91:17–24.
10. Cooper CJ, et al. Effect of transradial access on quality of life and cost of cardiac catheterization: a randomized comparison. Am Heart J. 1999;138:430–6.

11. Roberts J, et al. Radial artery to sheath size ratio in an American population – implications as to why real time ultrasound-guided radial access may decrease failure/crossover rates. J Am Coll Cardio. Abstract nos: 2018;72 (13_Supplement) B322–B323, 809–13.
12. Aminian A, et al. Comparison of a new slender 6 Fr sheath with a standard 5 Fr sheath for transradial coronary angiography and intervention: RAP and BEAT (Radial Artery Patency and Bleeding, Efficacy, Adverse evenT), a randomised multicentre trial. EuroIntervention. 2017;13:e549–56.
13. Ruzsa Z, et al. Transradial and transulnar access for iliac artery interventions using sheathless guiding systems: a feasibility study. Catheter Cardiovasc Interv. 2016;88:923–31.
14. Cortese B, et al. Transradial percutaneous iliac intervention, a feasible alternative to the transfemoral route. Cardiovasc Revasc Med. 2012;13:331–4.
15. Staniloae CS, Korabathina R, Coppola JT. Transradial access for peripheral vascular interventions. Catheter Cardiovasc Interv. 2013;81:1194–203.
16. Posham R, et al. Transradial approach for noncoronary interventions: a single-center review of safety and feasibility in the first 1,500 cases. J Vasc Interv Radiol. 2016;27:159–66.
17. Endovascular Today - Device Guide. Available at: https://evtoday.com/device-guide/. Accessed 15 Oct 2019.

Chapter 10
Transradial Access for Peripheral Arterial Disease: Infrainguinal Applications

Raghuram Posham, Alex Sher, Samuel Z. Maron, and Rami O. Tadros

Abbreviations

CFA	Common femoral artery
CLI	Chronic limb ischemia
DCB	Drug-coated balloon
OTW	Over-the-wire
PAD	Peripheral arterial disease
SFA	Superior femoral artery
TASC	Inter-Society Consensus for the Management of Peripheral Arterial Disease
TFA	Transfemoral arterial approach
TRA	Transradial arterial approach
US	United States
USPSTF	United States Preventive Services Task Force

Introduction

A brief introduction to peripheral arterial disease, relevant demographic information, and indications and contraindications to transradial access for PAD are presented in the prior chapter. Unique to transradial access for treating infrainguinal PAD is the potential to treat both lower extremities from the same access site. This chapter builds upon the prior chapter by discussing applications of treating infrainguinal PAD via transradial access (TRA).

R. Posham · A. Sher · S. Z. Maron
Department of Diagnostic, Molecular and Interventional Radiology, Icahn School of Medicine at Mount Sinai, New York, NY, USA

R. O. Tadros (✉)
Department of Surgery, Division of Vascular Surgery, Icahn School of Medicine at Mount Sinai, New York, NY, USA
e-mail: rami.tadros@mountsinai.org

A. M. Fischman et al. (eds.), *Transradial Access in Interventional Radiology*,
https://doi.org/10.1007/978-3-030-81678-0_10

In order to understand the available tools required to perform infrainguinal lower extremity interventions from the radial artery, we must again discuss two important factors: (1) distance from the radial artery and (2) vessel diameter, with increased importance given to the former. In discussing these variables, it is important to understand that differences exist based on patient gender, height, and limb length. It has been estimated from anthropometric measurements that the distance from the left radial artery to the common iliac arteries is approximately 105–115 cm and 200 cm to the foot [1]. A map of distances from the left wrist to lower extremity vasculature as well as approximate vessel diameters can be seen in Fig. 10.1. The size of the radial artery and the target vessel is also important in device selection and for determining feasibility, as described in the prior chapter. Careful consideration should be made to measuring the radial artery under ultrasound before procedures to limit complications, including arterial spasm and radial artery occlusion.

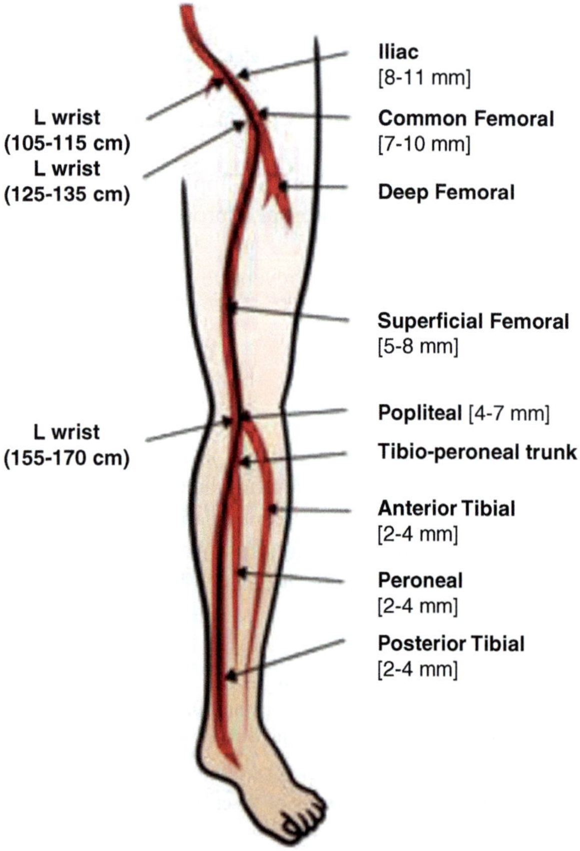

Fig. 10.1 Lower extremity arterial anatomy with distances from the left wrist and estimated vessel diameters. L left

Infrainguinal Disease

Similar to aortoiliac disease, the femoral artery remains the gold standard access site given its proximity to infrainguinal lesions. Unlike aortoiliac interventions via the wrist which is limited by vessel diameter and sheath size required for larger balloons and stents, the major limiting factor for infrainguinal disease remains the working length of the tools available. Relative to aortoiliac interventions, infrainguinal interventions are more challenging and have a steeper learning curve. In order to cross heavily calcified lesions seen in PAD, adequate pushability and support is needed. Reinforced stiff support sheaths up to 110 cm and reinforced support catheters up to 150 cm have facilitated the crossing of more simple (TASC A-C) lower extremity lesions down to the popliteal artery [2–4]. Introducer sheaths used in one of the studies included a 8.5 Fr 120 cm Sheathless Eucath (Asahi, Japan) or a 6 Fr 125 cm guiding catheter (Cordis, USA), and lesions were angioplastied using a Pacific Plus balloon (Medtronic, USA) and stented using a 5 Fr self-expandable Sinus-SuperFlex-518 (OptiMed, Germany, not available in the USA) both 180 cm in shaft length. Patients with more complex lesions such as TASC D SFA lesions were excluded from most studies as the guiding catheters available typically do not have the support and pushability to cross longer total occlusions. However, with recently introduced tools such as the 6 Fr 119 and 149 cm Destination Slender sheath (Terumo, Japan), operators now have improved support that may help cross more difficult lesions as far as the foot.

Despite these improvements, we still do not have all the tools to provide interventions comparable to transfemoral access. For most patients, the lengths and sizes of drug-coated balloons (DCB) and drug eluting stent (DES) options are inadequate to treat infrainguinal lesions. This is because most available DCBs compatible with 5 or 6 Fr introducer sheaths have a maximum balloon diameter of 6 mm with one balloon available up to 7 mm (130 cm length Lutonix, Bard). With the median diameter of the proximal SFA of 8 mm at mean length of approximately 135 cm, devices may under dilate the proximal SFA and are of insufficient length to treat more distal lesions for most patients [5]. Other tools to help cross lesions such as re-entry devices are not yet available. This is important as subintimal paths to crossing lesions may be encountered from a TRA and operators may have difficulty re-entering the true lumen from the wrist. Theoretically in a very select patient population, one might be able to use a covered stent (catheter lengths up to 135 cm) in the proximal SFA; however, this would require an extremely short patient with a large enough radial artery to accommodate a 6 Fr sheath. As such, above the knee infrainguinal disease is typically amenable to treatment with atherectomy, plain balloon angioplasty, as well as bare metal stenting using TRA, while for below the knee lesions, we are limited to atherectomy and angioplasty. At the present time, the longest available stent shaft in the USA is the 150 cm Everflex (Medtronic), and thus stenting is limited to above the knee for most patients. Atherectomy can be performed with the 200 cm length Diamondback orbital atherectomy device (CSI) which is compatible with a 470 cm Viperwire. It is important to note that long over-the-write (OTW) devices up to 200 cm shaft length require at least 360 cm wires which is technically cumbersome and difficult (Table 9.2, prior chapter). Future industry support for tools on rapid exchange platforms with adequate shaft length to reach the infrainguinal region may help alleviate this challenge. Whether stents with longer shaft lengths are needed is still unclear as stenting below the knee is still considered off label. Upcoming trials are attempting to elucidate the role of stenting in this area. Along with limited options for bare metal stenting below the knee, there are no covered stent options for possible complications below the knee. At the present time, management of vessel perforation from the wrist is limited to prolonged balloon tamponade, and dissection can only be managed with stenting as distal as the popliteal artery for most patients. Preparation of the groin for additional femoral artery access should be done for this scenario.

The use of TRA for infrainguinal disease in combination with a second access site such as pedal access can help treat lesions not amenable to TRA alone. Several studies have demonstrated that using both radial and pedal access can help treat more complex lesions in this area [6, 7]. However, this approach comes with its own risks as unlike the upper extremity vasculature the lower extremity may lack significant collateral circulation to the foot and these vessels may be diseased themselves.

Transradial Access for Infrainguinal Peripheral Arterial Disease: Technical Considerations and Case Examples

This section describes techniques and tools specific to TRA for treating infrainguinal disease. Procedural steps common to both aortoiliac and infrainguinal cases are described below and are followed with several example cases. Important points specific to the cases presented are highlighted in the blue boxes at the end of every case. While the complications for TRA have been previously discussed (Chap. 6), there are several differences that come with PAD interventions. Compared to other interventions via TRA, PAD interventions typically require a larger and longer introducer sheath. This comes with a potential increased risk of radial artery occlusion, spasm, thromboembolism, arterial injury, and bleeding risk. As such careful manipulation of the aortic arch and monitoring of the introducer sheath while crossing lesions is important. Additionally, use of vasodilatory and anticoagulants can help reduce complications.

Radial Artery Access and Navigating to the Descending Aorta

The left radial artery is favored as it comes with a shorter distance, roughly 10–12 cm, to the descending aorta and fewer great vessels are crossed [1]. This is important as device length can be a limitation of TRA. The specific radial access technique is described in detail in Chap. 4.

TRA considerations for PAD is unique in that we recommend a 6 Fr sheath to ensure adequate catheter and stent platform compatibility. Thus, preprocedural patient selection is key to ensure that the procedure can be performed successfully via the radial artery.

Slightly different than the radial cocktail described in Chap. 4, a solution consisting of 200mcg of nitroglycerin and 2.5 mg of verapamil is diluted and administered slowly through the radial artery sheath to limit spasm. Various dosages for radial cocktails have been used. Use of intra-arterial vasodilatory agents is important as upper extremity arterial spasm will reduce the lumen around the catheter and may increase the risk of complications. Patients undergoing PAD interventions also receive anticoagulation with 80–100 mg/kg of unfractionated heparin. An Active Clotting Time (ACT) is assessed every 30–60 minutes, and the heparin is re-dosed to reduce the risk of thromboembolic events. When heparin is contraindicated (e.g., heparin-induced thrombocytopenia), it is recommended that Argatroban or Bivalirudin is used.

Operators have several available introducer systems involving sheaths and guiding catheters to treat aortoiliac and infrainguinal lesions (Table 9.2). The cases described below will highlight their use. Of note, when a valveless introducer system is used, a hemostatic valve should be placed to prevent retrograde bleeding from the catheter; however this comes at the expense of some external length, particularly of importance in infrainguinal disease treatment via TRA.

Case 1

Superficial Femoral Artery In-Stent Neointimal Hyperplasia Causing Hemodynamically Significant Stenosis

Clinic Visit

59 M with history of hypertension, hyperlipidemia, current smoker (129+ pack years), PAD (s/p previous right EIA stent, left SFA angioplasty, and stenting ~1 year prior) presenting with evidence of intimal hyperplasia formation in left SFA stent causing hemodynamically significant stenosis above the knee. Patient height: 5 feet 4 inches. Barbeau C.

Procedure

1. Obtain radial access as described in Chap. 4. Unfractionated heparin is given at 80–100 mg/kg. Throughout the procedure an ACT is checked every 30–60 minutes, and heparin can be re-dosed at 1000 units to reduce risk of thromboembolic events.
2. Navigate to the infrarenal abdominal aorta using a 150 cm guidewire (Bentson Guidewire) and a guiding catheter (6 Fr × 110 cm RunWay Guide MP1).
3. Perform aortography and left lower extremity angiography. Findings:
   (a) Tortuous iliac arteries. Patent right EIA stent and left EIA.
   (b) Left lower extremity – patent left SFA stent, with focal in-stent intimal flap at the proximal SFA (Fig. 10.2a). Patent distal native SFA, popliteal artery, and three vessel runoff.

4. Exchange Bentson for a stiff support wire (0.035-inch × 260 cm Terumo Angled Glidewire), and navigate to the left proximal SFA for intervention.
   (a) Over the Glidewire, exchange the short introducer sheath and diagnostic catheter for stiff long introducer sheath (6 Fr × 45 cm Terumo Pinnacle Destination Guiding Sheath) and support guiding catheter (5 Fr × 100 cm Terumo Glidecath).
5. Advance a crossing support catheter to the proximal SFA (3.2 Fr × 150 cm Spectranetics Quick-Cross Select catheter), and cross the proximal SFA intimal flap with the glidewire, advancing the support catheter forward as the glidewire is advanced.
6. Angioplasty the lesion. All currently available over-the-wire PTA balloons with long working lengths compatible with radial access require no more than a 0.018-inch diameter guidewire.
   (a) Exchange the Glidewire for a 0.018″ stiff guidewire (0.018-inch × 300 cm Boston Scientific V-18 Control steerable guidewire), and advance the wire to the distal SFA/popliteal artery.
   (b) Remove the crossing catheter (Quick-Cross), and advance an angioplasty balloon over the guidewire (6 mm diameter × 80 mm length Pacific Plus PTA 180 cm shaft length balloon) to the site of the lesion and dilate the balloon under fluoroscopic guidance (Fig. 10.2b).
7. Repeat angiogram shows a persistent intimal flap. A stent will be required to address the intimal flap (Fig. 10.2c).
8. Remove the balloon in preparation for a stent.
9. Advance and deploy an appropriately sized stent across the intimal flap (6 mm × 80 mm Everflex Entrust 150 cm shaft stent) (Fig. 10.2d). Only self-expanding uncovered stents are available for working shaft lengths of 150 cm or greater).
   (a) Remove the stent delivery system and balloon angioplasty the stent to ensure wall adherence.
10. Repeat angiogram shows restoration of flow without focal luminal narrowing in the left lower extremity (Fig. 10.2e). Distal angiogram shows preserved runoff to the left foot.
11. Remove the catheters, guidewire, and sheath from the arm and apply a radial hemostasis band for 60 minutes.

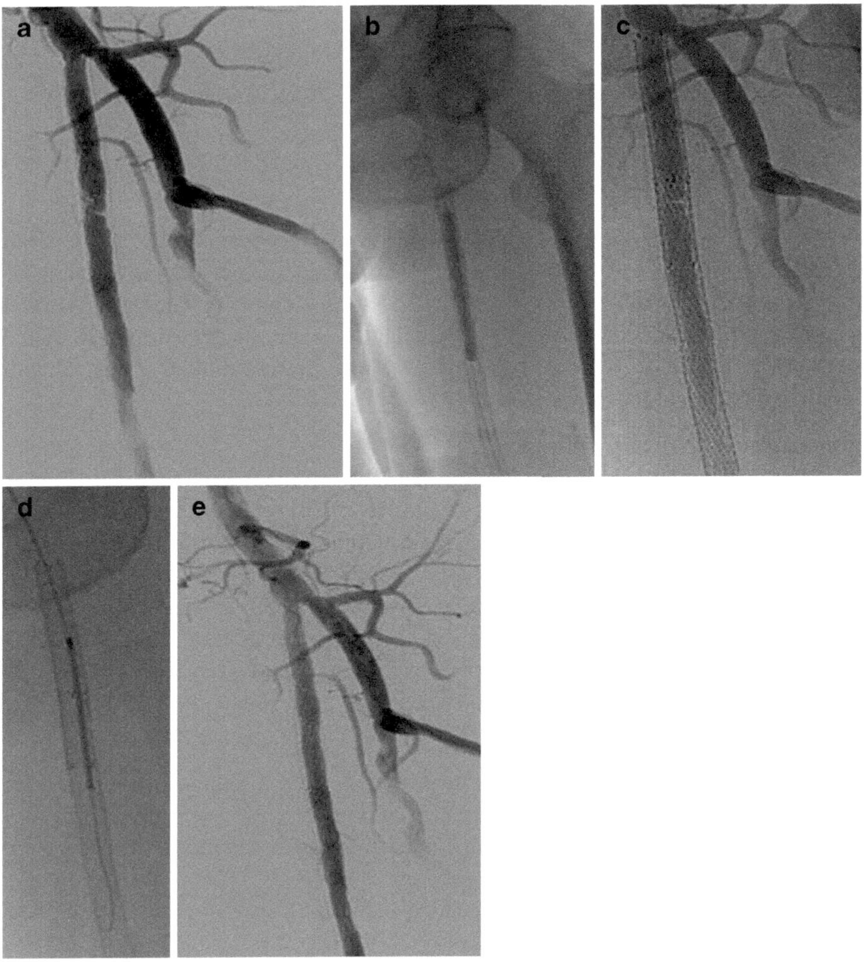

Fig. 10.2 Angiogram demonstrating focal in-stent intimal flap at the proximal left SFA (**a**), angioplasty of lesion (**b**) and persistence of intimal flap (**c**), positioning of stent (**d**), final angiogram demonstrating resolution of lesion (**e**)

Case 2

Occluded Popliteal Artery and Posterior Tibial Artery Causing Nonhealing Toe Ulcers

Clinic Visit

83 y.o. male with history of CKD stage III, coronary artery disease s/p CABG, COPD, former smoker (75 pack years), hyperlipidemia, hypertension, thrombocythemia, and PAD who presents with right second toe ulcer for 2 months. Arterial duplex studies show a multifocal severe atherosclerotic plaque formation of the distal SFA, occlusion of the popliteal artery and posterior tibial artery. Patient height: 5 Feet 9 inches. Barbeau B.

Procedure

1. Obtain radial access as described in Chap. 4. Unfractionated heparin is given at 80–100 mg/kg. Throughout the procedure an ACT is checked every 30–60 minutes, and heparin can be re-dosed at 1000 units to reduce risk of thromboembolic events.
2. Navigate to the infrarenal abdominal aorta using a 150 cm guidewire (Bentson Guidewire) and a guiding catheter (5 Fr × 110 cm Sarah Radial)
3. Perform aortography. Findings: tortuous iliac arteries, widely patent. Patent left profunda femoris artery and proximal SFA.
4. Exchange for a stiff support sheath and a working wire/catheter.

   (a) Exchange the Bentson guidewire for a stiff support wire (0.035-inch × 260 cm Terumo Angled Glidewire).
   (b) Remove both the catheter and short introducer sheath, holding pressure over the arteriotomy.
   (c) Advance the 6 Fr × 149 cm R2P Destination Slender Guiding Sheath. Note that at least 150 cm of the support wire must be outside of the patient to safely advance the long sheath.
   (d) Advance the 5 Fr × 150 cm Spectranetics Quick-Cross Select Catheter and navigate to the right proximal SFA.

5. Perform a right lower extremity angiography. Findings:

   (a) Tortuous iliac arteries, widely patent. Patent profunda femoris artery. Patent SFA, with multifocal calcifications throughout the mid and distal SFA, without significant luminal narrowing.
   (b) 2 cm chronic total occlusion of the mid popliteal artery which reconstitutes via collateral circulation by the geniculate arteries, and severe 2.5 cm stenosis of the distal popliteal artery (Fig. 10.3a).
   (c) Two vessel runoff to the foot predominantly via the anterior tibial artery.

6. Noting that the lesion is in the popliteal artery, a longer crossing catheter will be required. Through the long R2P sheath, exchange the system for a 5

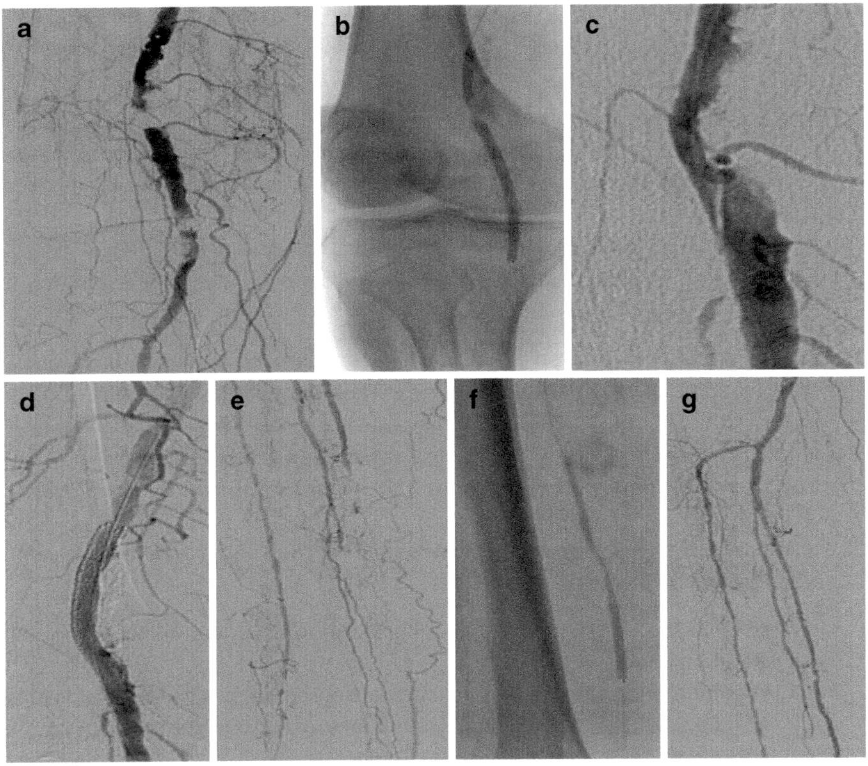

Fig. 10.3 Angiogram demonstrating chronic occlusion of mid popliteal artery and severe stenosis of distal popliteal artery (**a**), angioplasty of lesion (**b**), post angioplasty focal dissection (**c**), stenting of dissection area (**d**), repeat angiogram without dissection (**e**), angiogram with balloon in place for focal stenosis (**f**), final angiogram with three vessel runoff (**g**)

Fr × 200 cm Vipercath XC support catheter and a specialized crossing wire (0.14″ × 475 cm ViperWire Advance). Note that greater than 200 cm of the wire must be outside of the patient to safely advance the catheter.

7. Advance the crossing wire and catheter to the popliteal artery, just proximal to the occlusion.
8. Cross the occlusion using the Viperwire, advancing the support catheter forward for support as the wire is advanced. Once the identified popliteal artery lesions are crossed, advance the wire to the distal posterior tibial artery in preparation for atherectomy.
9. Leaving the Viperwire in position, remove the support catheter and advance the atherectomy device over the wire (200 cm shaft length 1.5 mm crown, CSI Diamondback Atherectomy).
10. After ensuring adequate distal positioning of the Viperwire, atherectomy can be performed under direct fluoroscopic guidance.

11. Following adequate atherectomy of the target lesions, angioplasty may be performed. Note that the stiff 0.014″ Viperwire can be used as the support wire for angioplasty.
    (a) Advance an angioplasty balloon over the guidewire (5 mm diameter × 120 mm length Pacific Plus PTA 180 cm shaft length balloon) to the site of the lesion, and dilate the balloon under fluoroscopic guidance (Fig. 10.3b).
    (b) Repeat angiogram shows a patent popliteal artery; however, a focal dissection (Fig. 10.3c) is noted at the treated lesion in the mid popliteal artery. A stent is required.
12. Leaving the Viperwire in position, an appropriately sized stent with an adequate shaft working length to reach the lesion is required (6.0 mm × 60 mm, 150 cm shaft Everflex Entrust Self-Expanding stent). The previously used balloon is utilized following stent delivery to ensure wall adherence (Fig. 10.3d).
13. Repeat angiogram shows no dissection or filling defect of the treated lesions (Fig. 10.3e).
14. Infrapopliteal angiogram shows focal stenosis of the mid posterior tibial artery, which can be treated with angioplasty.
    (a) Advance the Viperwire to the distal posterior tibial artery to the level of the lateral malleolus.
    (b) Angioplasty the stenotic lesion using an appropriately sized balloon with a shaft length that can reach the lesion (3 mm × 100 mm, 200 cm shaft length Ultraverse Rx PTA catheter) (Fig. 10.3f).
15. Repeat angiogram shows restoration of three vessel runoff to the left foot with predominant supply via the posterior tibial artery (Fig. 10.3g).
16. Remove the catheters, guidewire, and sheath from the arm and apply a radial hemostasis band for 60 minutes.

Case 3

Nonhealing Foot Wound

Procedure

1. Obtain radial access as described in Chap. 4. Unfractionated heparin is given at 80–100 mg/kg. Throughout the procedure an ACT is checked every 30–60 minutes, and heparin can be re-dosed at 1000 units to reduce risk of thromboembolic events.
2. Navigate to the infrarenal abdominal aorta using a 150 cm guidewire (Bentson Guidewire) and a guiding catheter (4 Fr Glidecath).
3. Perform aortography and right lower extremity angiography. Findings:

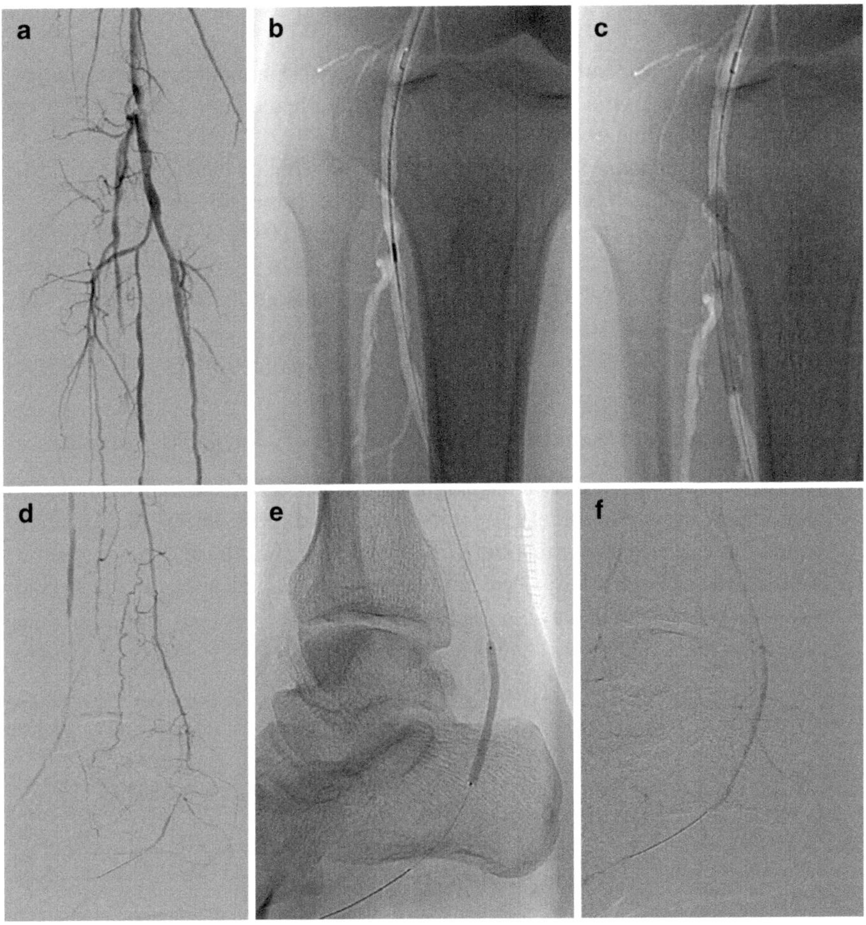

Fig. 10.4 Angiogram demonstrating severe stenosis of distal popliteal and tibio-peroneal trunk (**a**), atherectomy device in place at site of lesion (**b**), angioplasty of lesion (**c**), distal angiogram showing stenosis of lateral plantar artery (**d**), angioplasty of the lateral plantar artery (**e**), post angioplasty angiogram with improved flow (**f**)

(a) Patent right common femoral, profunda femoris, superficial femoral, and popliteal arteries.
(b) Stenotic P3 segment and tibioperoneal trunk. Occluded right anterior tibial artery and peroneal artery. Single vessel run-off to right foot via the posterior tibial artery (Fig. 10.4a). Severe stenosis of lateral plantar artery.

4. Exchange the Bentson wire for a stiff support wire (0.035-inch × 260 cm Terumo Angled Glidewire) and advance to the distal popliteal artery.
5. Exchange the short sheath for a 119 cm 6 Fr R2P Destination sheath (Terumo) down to the proximal SFA.

6. Exchange the guidewire for a 400 cm Viperwire (CSI) and carefully advance into the right posterior tibial artery.
7. Advance a 200 cm orbital atherectomy device (Diamondback Atherectomy, CSI Systems) over the Viperwire, and perform atherectomy at the level of the focal stenosis of the tibioperoneal trunk (Fig. 10.4b).
8. Post atherectomy angiogram demonstrates improved flow and reduced stenosis; however angioplasty is recommended to achieve further luminal gain.
9. Remove the atherectomy device, and advance a 0.014″ 5 Fr 200 cm length 4 mm Ultraverse rapid exchange balloon (Bard) to tibioperoneal trunk and angioplasty the lesion (Fig. 10.4c). Repeat angiogram shows significantly improved flow at the angioplasty site.
10. Advance the Viperwire to the level of the lateral plantar artery and perform a repeat angiogram.

    (a) A high-grade stenosis of the lateral plantar artery is noted (Fig. 10.4d).

11. Exchange for a 2.0 mm × 200 cm length Ultraverse rapid exchange balloon, and angioplasty the lateral plantar stenosis (Fig. 10.4e). Post lateral plantar artery angioplasty demonstrates markedly improved flow (Fig. 10.4f).
12. Remove the catheters, wires, and sheath from the arm and apply a radial hemostasis band for 60 minutes.

References

1. Staniloae CS, Korabathina R, Coppola JT. Transradial access for peripheral vascular interventions. Catheter Cardiovasc Interv. 2013;81:1194–203.
2. Hanna EB, Ababneh BA, Amin AN. Endovascular therapy of the superficial femoral artery via a stand-alone transradial access: a single-center experience. Vasc Endovasc Surg. 2018;52(2):107–14.
3. Coscas R, de Blic R, Capdevila C, Javerliat I, Goeau-Brissonniere O, Coggia M. Percutaneous radial access for peripheral transluminal angioplasty. J Vasc Surg. 2015;61(2):463–8.
4. Lorenzoni R, et al. Radial artery access for above the knee angioplasty: a feasibility study. EuroIntervention. 2011;7:924–9.
5. Lorbeer R, Grotz A, Dorr M, Volzke H, Lieb W, Kuhn JP, et al. Reference values of vessel diameters, stenosis prevalence, and arterial variations of the lower limb arteries in a male population sample using contrast-enhanced MR angiography. PLoS One. 2018;13(6):e0197559.
6. Hanna EB, Prout DL. Combined radial-pedal access strategy and radial-pedal rendezvous in the revascularization of complex total occlusions of the superficial femoral artery (the 'no femoral access' strategy). J Endovasc Ther. 2016;23:321–9.
7. Ruzsa Z, et al. Combined transradial and transpedal approach for femoral artery interventions. JACC Cardiovasc Interv. 2018;11:1062–71.

Chapter 11
Aortic Endoleak Following Endovascular Aortic Repair

Wayne Martin Bauknight and Rahul S. Patel

Introduction

Aortic aneurysm is defined as >50% increase in aortic diameter relative to normal aorta. Repair of abdominal aortic aneurysm (AAA) is indicated in patients who are symptomatic (tenderness and back pain), have a AAA ≥5.5 cm or has expanded by more than 0.5 cm within a 6-month interval, or is associated with infection or arterial disease. Endovascular aortic repair (EVAR) is generally preferred for repair of infrarenal AAA or descending thoracic aortic aneurysm (TAA) in patients with suitable anatomy due to decreased perioperative and 1-year morbidity and mortality versus open repair, though reintervention rates are twice as high in EVAR treated patients [1–6]. Juxtarenal AAA typically requires fenestrated stent-graft with suprarenal fixators. Suprarenal AAA, small caliber vessels, circumferential calcification, or extensive tortuosity are generally anatomic contraindications to EVAR necessitating open repair, though next gen devices are under development for suprarenal AAA [6].

Successful EVAR excludes the aneurysm sac from systemic arterial pressure, preventing continued expansion or rupture. Failure to completely exclude the aneurysm, leading to persistent arterial perfusion of the aneurysm sac, defines endoleak. Endoleak has a reported frequency of 20–25% in recent studies (up to 50% in earlier studies), and is associated with continued risk of expansion and rupture [1–10]. Typically, <20% of all EVAR patients require reintervention for endoleak [1–7, 11–14]. Risk for endoleak, particularly type II, necessitates ongoing post-repair surveillance, typically with 3-phase CT angiography ("gold standard"),

W. M. Bauknight (✉)
Northwestern Medicine, Chicago, IL, USA

R. S. Patel
Department of Diagnostic, Molecular and Interventional Radiology, Icahn School of Medicine at Mount Sinai, New York, NY, USA
e-mail: rahul.patel@mountsinai.org

A. M. Fischman et al. (eds.), *Transradial Access in Interventional Radiology*, https://doi.org/10.1007/978-3-030-81678-0_11

contrast-enhanced duplex ultrasound (CEUS) at 1-month post-EVAR, and annually thereafter [11, 15]. MR angiography (MRA) may be useful in cases where the endoleak source is difficult to identify.

In this chapter, we discuss (1) endoleak classification (I–V), (2) endoleak management and approach, and (3) considerations for transradial approach to endoleak management.

Endoleak Classification

Incomplete aneurysm sac exclusion leads to five types of Endoleak (I–V), classified by the source of arterial leak. Endoleak types are summarized in Figs. 11.1 and 11.2. Frequency of endoleak at 6-year follow-up reported in the OVER trial was 30% overall, with Type I (12%), Type II (76%), Type III (3%), Type IV (3%), and Indeterminate/Type 5 (6%) [9]. Of note, OVER reported that 1/2 of endoleaks resolved spontaneously and 1/3 required secondary intervention [9].

Type I

Type I endoleak results from incompetent vessel to stent-graft apposition and seal at the proximal (Ia) or distal (Ib) attachment sites, and can occur either immediately following stent-graft deployment or during the post-repair surveillance period (Late

Type of Endoleak	Definition
Type I	Inadequate endograft seal
Ia	Inadequate seal at proximal end of endograft
Ib	Inadequate seal at distal end of endograft
Ic	Inadequate seal at iliac occluder plug
Type II	Backflow of blood from aortic collaterals into aneurysm sac
Type III	Component or fabric defect with flow from visceral vessels
IIIa: component disconnection	Flow from module disconnection
IIIb: stent fabric disturbance	Flow from fabric disruption (minor <2mm; major >2mm)
Type IV	Flow from porous fabric (<30 days post EVAR)
Type V: endoleak of undefined origin	Flow seen in sac but source unidentifiable

Fig. 11.1 Endoleak classification

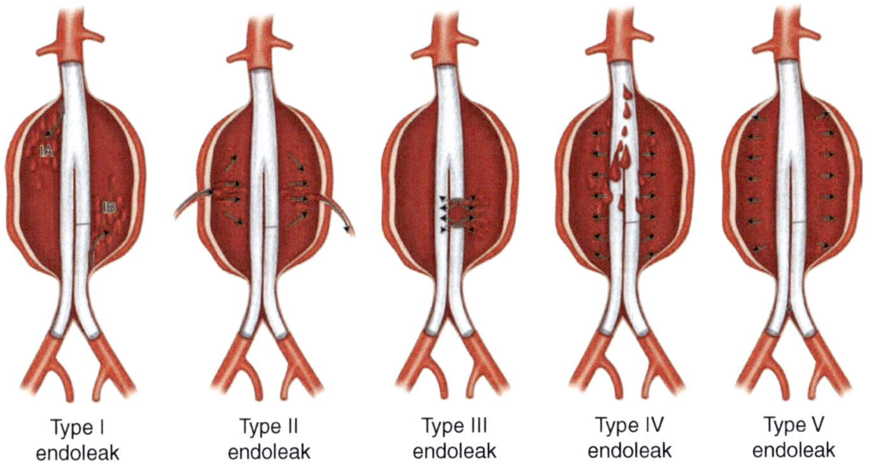

Fig. 11.2 Graphic depiction of endoleak classification types. (Source: Reprinted with permission Springer International Publishing AG; N.A. Keefe et al., IR Playbook, 2018)

Type I). Type I endoleak occurs most commonly with difficult anatomy, such as a short aortic neck, failing first-generation endografts, or small leaks detected on high quality imaging [8, 16]. EUROSTAR, the largest published registry of 3595 patients, reported an overall Type 1 incidence of 10%, most of which resolved [8, 17, 18]. In a more recent review of the Vascular Study Group of New England, among 2402 EVARs, only 3.3% had Type 1 endoleak (TIE) likely reflecting advances in stent-graft technology and operator experience. Factors associated with TIE included age, female sex, large endograft body, and unplanned graft extension. 90% of patients with TIE resolved without the need for reintervention at 1 year; however, persistent TIE was associated with increased mortality (OR 4.4) [19].

- *Type 1a* – Typical causes of Type Ia endoleak include aortic angulation, calcification or reverse taper, mural thrombus, or improper sizing of the stent-graft. Of note, risk of Type Ia endoleak does not significantly differ between endografts with or without suprarenal fixation [20]. See Fig. 11.3.
- *Type Ib* – Causes of Type Ib (distal) endoleak typically include incorrect sizing of the iliac limbs or excessive tortuosity of the more proximal external iliac vessels.
- *Late Ia/Ib* – Conformational change in the aneurysm sac, aneurysmal degeneration of the aortic neck or distal iliac arteries, progressive angulation at fixation sites, or graft migration are typical causes of late Ia/Ib endoleak [12–14]. Patients requiring large diameter devices to seal a dilated aortic neck (34–36 mm) or dilated iliac limb (>20 mm) have a higher risk of late Ia/Ib endoleak of 15% vs 3–4% for "normal" sized devices (<34 mm aortic neck, <20 mm iliac limb) [21, 22].

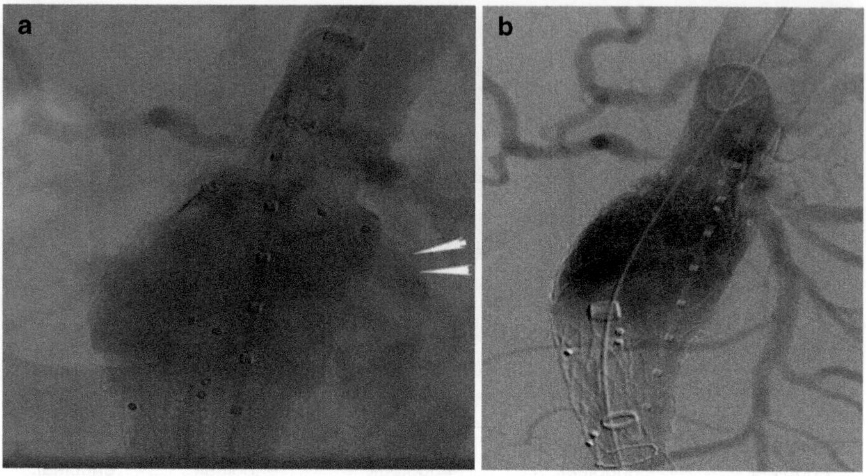

Fig. 11.3 Type Ia (proximal) endoleak before (**a**) and after Palmaz balloon deployment (**b**). (Source: Reprinted with permission Springer International Publishing AG; N.A. Keefe et al., IR Playbook, 2018)

Type II

Type II endoleak is commonly discovered during post-EVAR surveillance and occurs due to the presence of patent lumbar, IMA, aortic, sacral, accessory renal, or intercostal branches (in TAA) allowing retrograde flow into the sac. See Fig. 11.4. Risk of Type II endoleak has been positively correlated with number and size of patent branches present prior to exclusion, especially from the IMA, in multiple reviews [2, 8, 18, 19, 23–28]. In a review of 832 EVAR patients, 23% had persistent type 2 endoleak (>6 months), most positively correlated with patent IMA feeders (HR 4.0). These data support prophylactic pre- or intraoperative embolization as a reasonable method to reduce type II endoleak risk [28]. According to the Vascular Study Group of New England database, hypogastric embolization, distal graft extension, older age, and type of graft were also significant risk factors [29]. Lower risk of Type II endoleak was associated with small vessel disease, including smoking, peripheral vascular disease, and thrombus load [30, 31]. Clinical significance of persistent type II endoleak remains a source of debate, which we discuss in the management section below.

Type III

Type III endoleaks are high pressure junctional leaks due to disconnected endograft components (Type IIIa) or suture break, ring fracture, or endograft fabric holes (Type IIIb), and can occur at the time of EVAR or during the surveillance period

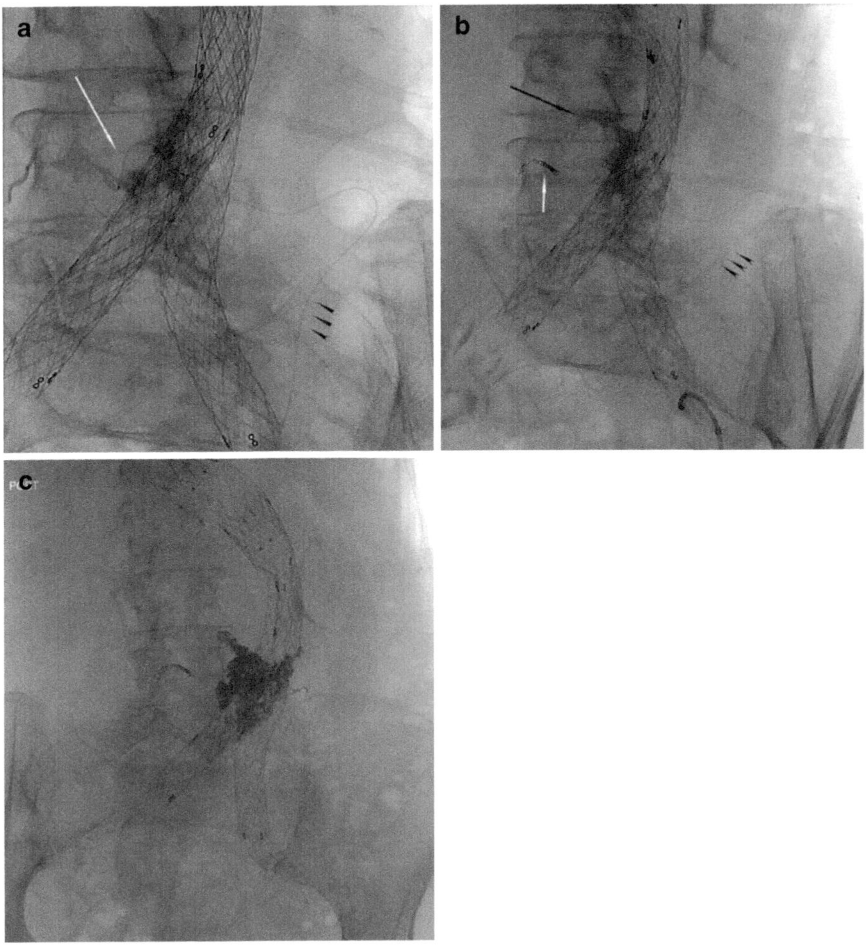

Fig. 11.4 Type II endoleak originating from a lumbar perforator (**a**) treated with coil embolization (**b**) and Onyx (**c**). (Source: Reprinted with permission Springer International Publishing AG; N.A. Keefe et al., IR Playbook, 2018)

[18, 19]. Type III endoleak warrants intervention [32, 33]. Late Type III endoleak is associated with change in conformation of the aneurysm sac, graft migration, dilation of the aortic or iliac sites of attachment, and increased endograft angulation [34–36]. Type III endoleak was more common with earlier generation endografts, but current estimates across multiple platforms suggest a rate of around 2–3% [36–38] as late generation endografts have very low material fatigue and longer overlap zones that decrease the likelihood of dissociation [34]. In the EUROSTAR registry, patients with Type III endoleak had a 9x increased risk of rupture vs all other EVAR pts. [39] See Fig. 11.5.

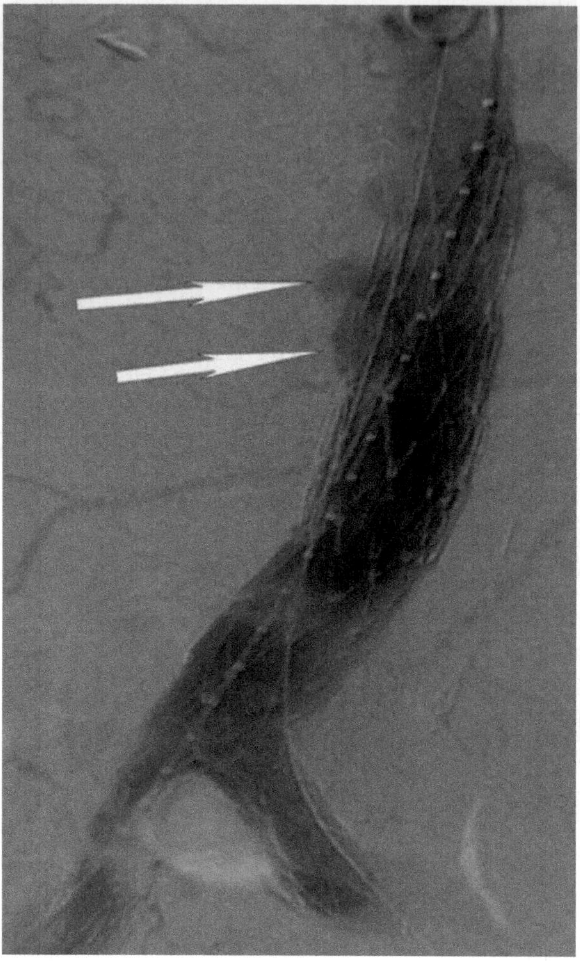

Fig. 11.5 Type III endoleak between graft components. (Source: Reprinted with permission Springer International Publishing AG; N.A. Keefe et al., IR Playbook, 2018)

Type IV

Type IV endoleak occurs due to endograft wall porosity leading to exudation of plasma across the graft wall. Type IV endoleak was commonly seen at completion angiography with early generation endografts with high permeability (i.e., polyester), but is much less common with current generation materials [33, 40, 41].

Type V

Type V endoleak, sometimes referred to as endotension, is a "catch-all" bucket for endoleak of undefined origin or aneurysm sac expansion without a demonstrable endoleak by imaging [14].

As we will discuss in the next sections, there is little controversy over the natural history and need for treatment for Types I and III endoleak; however, optimal timing and treatment of Type II endoleak is still debated.

Diagnosis/Post-EVAR Surveillance

Endoleak is frequently discovered during completion angiography (especially Type I and III as Type II requires delayed imaging) but may also be seen during post-EVAR imaging surveillance. Though blood in the sac is usually apparent, the source of leak can be difficult to determine. Additionally, though most endoleaks are asymptomatic (outside of overt rupture), new onset back or flank pain should raise suspicion and may warrant further interrogation [42, 43].

Timing and Modality

Routine surveillance is mandatory to ensure endograft integrity and monitor for endoleak, sac enlargement, stent migration, and component dissociation. Updated guidelines from the Society for Vascular Surgery recommend baseline CTA ("gold standard") and duplex ultrasound at 1 month followed by annual CTA or CEUS [44–50]. FDA-approved pivotal device trials required CTA or duplex ultrasound at 6 months; however, evidence has shown that eliminating 6-month follow-up is reasonable in patients without evidence of sac expansion or device abnormality at 1 month [47–50]. Even in the presence of a Type II endoleak, most do not recommend 6-month follow-up given the likelihood of conservative treatment and spontaneous resolution [44, 47–49, 51]. MRA may be considered as an alternative imaging modality due to increased sensitivity for detecting endoleak [52]. Some recommend initiating CEUS follow-up for all patients with stable or shrinking aneurysms instead of CTA to reduce radiation exposure [47]. Digital subtraction angiography is helpful to measure aneurysm sac pressure, while wireless pressure sensors have also been occasionally used [39, 49, 53–56].

Endoleak Management and Approach

The most common endoleak types (I/II/III) are typically managed with additional stent component placement or feeder embolization. However, while management recommendations for Types I and III endoleak are relatively established (necessitate reintervention), optimal follow-up and treatment for Type II endoleak remains controversial. See Fig. 11.6 for a representative algorithm of endoleak management.

Type I

Consensus recommendation is immediate repair of Type I endoleak upon discovery as Type I is a high-pressure endoleak associated with significant risk of rupture, open conversion, and death [57, 58]. For Type I endoleak discovered at the time of endograft placement, initial management consists of reballooning the endograft fixation site or potential reversal of intraoperative anticoagulation.

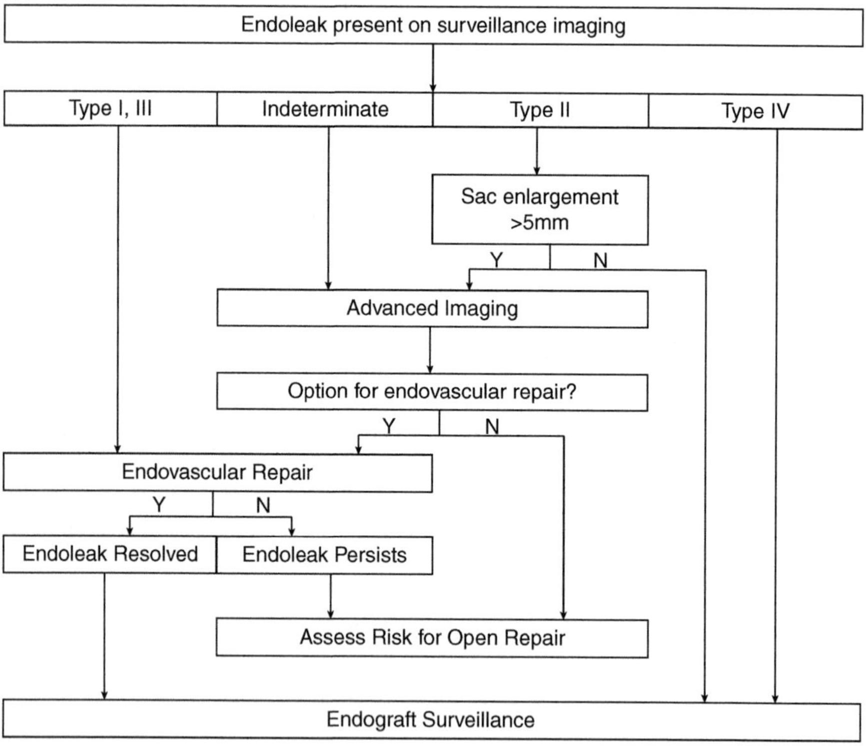

Fig. 11.6 Algorithm for endoleak management

- *Type Ia:* For persistent or late proximal (Ia) endoleaks, placement of additional aortic cuffs or balloon-expandable stents (e.g., Palmaz) through radial or femoral access maximize graft-aortic neck apposition by increasing radial force [59, 60]. Observation of small, persistent Type I endoleak with 1-month CT follow-up is reasonable in cases where the graft is seated flush with the lowest renal artery as most will resolve [59, 60].
- *Type Ib:* Persistent or late distal type I endoleak is typically managed through femoral access with iliac limb extensions. If the original iliac limb was undersized, a flared iliac extension can be deployed. If the distal common iliac cannot accommodate an extension, a branched device may be considered. If the extension will cover the ipsilateral hypogastric (internal iliac) artery, then hypogastric embolization should be performed prior to stent deployment to prevent Type II endoleak, but may be associated with pelvic ischemia in 25% or more of patients [61–63].
- *Refractory Type I:* Persistent Type I endoleak despite the above methods represents a challenge. Placement of stents in the renal artery or SMA in combination with endograft extension (Chimney Technique) has shown reasonable results with limited follow-up [64–66]. Fenestrated (F-EVAR) or additional branched extension cuffs may also be considered, and have better mortality than open surgery, but require advanced technique to manage the challenges of the previously placed endograft [67]. No significant difference has been shown between Chimney and fenestrated endograft treated patients in 30-day mortality, renal impairment, or endoleak [65]. Endostaples may also be used preemptively to improve endograft apposition and seal but have shown mixed results in treating existing Type 1 endoleak. In the ANCHOR trial using Heli-FX, 34% of patients continued to have Type 1a endoleak post treatment [68, 69]. If visceral branches preclude graft extension, glue, Onyx, or coils can be deployed between the graft and endograft wall, though these can create beam hardening artifacts on follow-up CT that may limit surveillance [53] . These advanced techniques may be attempted from transradial or femoral approaches. Open conversion is rarely required for delayed Type 1 endoleak and may be associated with increased morbidity and mortality [70].
  - If rescue approaches described above are unsuccessful, watchful waiting of low-flow Type I endoleak is reasonable as a high-resolution rate of >90% has been reported by multiple groups [16, 19, 71]. Resolution is potentially due to gradual aortic neck remodeling and improved aortic wall apposition over time. However, clinically significant, high flow Type I endoleaks are clearly associated with ongoing risk of rupture and should be evaluated for open repair [19, 57].

Type II

Type II represents a low-pressure endoleak that may present as simple inflow-outflow pattern or may appear as a complex nidus resembling an AVM [7, 30, 72]. Post-EVAR, incidence is highest at 1 and 6 months, but may occur up to 5 years following repair [7, 73–75]. Rate of Type II endoleak decreases to <10% after 2 years of follow-up [25, 76].

- *Criteria for Treatment:* Type II endoleak has a relatively benign natural history with only ~1% associated with rupture and 60% spontaneous resolution rate within 6-months post EVAR [77, 78]. Patients with underlying small vessel disease or hypercoagulable states are more likely to have spontaneous resolution, while those with internal iliac occlusion or anticoagulation are more likely to persist [24, 29, 78–80]. Thus, prevailing consensus is continued observation and surveillance in the case of persistent Type 2 endoleak without sac expansion, and consideration of intervention only in the case of sac expansion >5 mm during interval follow-up [1, 3]. This is further supported by the findings that patients with persistent Type II endoleak have no increase in aneurysm-related mortality, and some patients may see their aneurysm shrink [77, 78]. Patients with persistent Type II endoleak for more than 6 months, however, do have up to 55% chance of some aneurysm sac expansion [24, 78–82]. In the EUROSTAR registry, cumulative 2-year incidence of rupture was 1.8% in patients with Type II endoleak, which despite being numerically higher, was not statistically significantly different from the 0.9% in patients without endoleak [73]. Furthermore, a large meta-analysis of >1500 Type II endoleaks post-EVAR showed a rupture rate of only 0.9%, and 43% of these had no evidence of sac expansion [26]. These data call into question the utility of >5 mm sac expansion as an indication for reintervention in Type II endoleak given the large portion of patients with rupture and no sac expansion.
- *Treatment Technique:* Repair of Type II endoleaks through transarterial and translumbar embolization is common to eliminate side branch perfusion. Choice of approach primarily depends on operator preference.

  - Transarterial embolization is the most common technique utilizing a coaxial system with microcatheters through femoral or radial access to cannulate the IMA or lumbar arteries and embolize Type II endoleak feeders. Selection through the internal iliac (superior gluteal) or SMA (middle colic and marginal) arteries is common. Microcoils are common, but glue, thrombin, and Onyx are also used with no clear evidence to support one over the other [7].
  - Translumbar embolization with the patient in the prone position may also be considered as an alternative to transradial access when femoral access is not feasible, but is relatively uncommon [80, 83–85]. Following aneurysm sac access from a paraspinal approach, a "sacogram" is performed through a long needle (20 g) prior to 5F catheter insertion, angiography, and subsequent microcatheter interrogation of the sac and target arteries for embolization.
  - Transcaval and ventral approaches have also been described with limited data [80, 86]. Transcaval approach is typically used in patients with an aneurysm sac located to the right of midline limiting transarterial or translumbar approaches. After obtaining a venogram of the iliac vein and IVC, a TIPS needle is directed into the IVC and exchanged for a catheter to perform angiography and identify the afferent and efferent branches. Care must be taken not to deploy embolization material into the IVC.

– Success, defined as no recurrence of Type II endoleak during follow-up, was not significantly different between transarterial and translumbar approaches in a study of 386 pts. from 2006 to 2015 [87]. Recurrence and need for reintervention are not uncommon, however, and continued expansion despite technical endovascular success can necessitate laparoscopic or open ligation associated with increased morbidity and mortality [88–90].
– *Pre- or Intraoperative Embolization:* Given Type II endoleak is correlated with number and size of patent branches, prophylactic embolization of IMA or lumbar feeders prior to endograft deployment is reasonable, and has been shown to significantly lower the need for secondary intervention [91].

Type III

Consensus recommendation is to treat Type III endoleak immediately to prevent not only aortic rupture, but also obstruction of aortic blood flow due to graft uncoupling leading to ischemia [36, 58].

- *Treatment Technique:* Cannulation of the main body gate through femoral access can be challenging if offset, but once achieved, standard treatment typically consists of additional stent-graft component deployment to seal fabric defects or bridge disconnections between components. Alternatively, an entirely new bifurcated endograft may be deployed within the existing device, particularly appropriate when the endograft has migrated significantly from the proximal attachment site or in the case of multiple component dissociation [34].

Type IV

Type IV endoleak is self-limited by thrombosis of endograft material defects, typically within 24 hours post-EVAR [34, 35]. Type IV endoleak is not associated with long-term adverse effects and does not necessitate treatment or intervention but can obscure more concerning Type I or III endoleak if seen at completion angiography [34, 35].

Type V

Type V endoleak or "endotension" of undefined origin or sac expansion without identifiable endoleak source is not well described, but in a limited number of cases, has been linked to an incomplete seal at the landing zone with laminated thrombus that prevents demonstration of an endoleak [86]. Original grafts with semiporous material (i.e., Excluder) were commonly associated with endoleak of undefined origin, with treatment consisting of relining the existing graft with a new lower-porosity material.

Given the sensitivity of MRA over CTA, MRA may be reasonable to aid in endoleak source identification. Treatment of Type V endoleak typically involves extending the endograft limbs or relining the original endograft with a new endograft. If unsuccessful, explantation of the endograft and open surgical repair may be necessary.

A Word on Anti-thrombotic Therapy and Endoleak

Consideration for temporarily withholding antithrombotic therapy to resolve endoleak (mostly Type II) is highly controversial and may depend on multiple factors such as patient history, device type, and significance of the endoleak [34, 35, 79, 89–94]. There is some data that correlate antithrombotic therapy with lack of aneurysm sac shrinkage and endoleak persistence [79]. A systematic review showed antithrombotic therapy increased risk of any type of endoleak (OR 1.8) and increased risk of persistence of Type II endoleak (OR 1.6), but risk/benefit must be carefully weighed in the context of the patient [79].

TEVAR Endoleak Management

TEVAR endoleak management mirrors that of AAA EVAR, though there is less supporting data. The European Talent Thoracic Retrospective Registry identified Type I or III endoleak in 10%, with other series demonstrating similar incidence [95–99], relatively in-line with AAA EVAR. As with AAA EVAR, Types I and III TEVAR endoleak necessitate definitive repair. Type III endoleak can be simply treated with a bridging graft, but Type I endoleak can be more challenging if proximal or distal landing zones are short or aneurysmal [100–103]. If endovascular treatment of Type 1 endoleak is not feasible, debranching of the supraaortic vessels may be required to extend the seal zone for additional endografting [104]. As with AAA EVAR, current consensus recommends intervention in Type II endoleak associated with aneurysm sac expansion. If related to the origin of the left subclavian, Type II endoleak can be treated with ligation, plugging, or coiling of the subclavian artery with or without revascularization given the significant collateral supply around of the left upper extremity [104]. Other endoleak branch vessels can be embolized through translumbar or transthoracic approaches with coil or glue.

Complex Endograft Endoleak Management

Fenestrated (F-EVAR), branched, or chimney endografts enable customization of the proximal landing zone to optimize seal and are deployed in AAA involving visceral vessels with common or hypogastric artery aneurysms where preservation of flow is required. The Chimney or snorkel technique is often employed when suprarenal endograft placement to gain additional neck length is warranted [95]. While durable, their complexity lends to increased risk of component dissociation [105, 106]. Fenestrated or branched grafts incorporate side holes or stents for visceral or arch branches and were shown to have a low Type Ia endoleak incidence of 2.8% in a large series of 969 patients [106]; however the risk/benefit versus increased component instability is still debated. The Chimney technique deploys a covered stent into a vital aortic branch, extending the sealing zone of the stent-graft beyond the branch artery. However, Chimney grafts are at increased risk for Type 1 "gutter" endoleaks between the main aortic graft and side branch stent. A systematic review showed a 13% and 11% early Type I endoleak for visceral and arch chimneys, respectively, and 25% and 4% rate of Late Type I endoleak in visceral and arch chimneys reflecting risk for "gutter" endoleak [107]. Comparison between F-EVAR and Chimneys has not shown significant differences in rates of endoleak [65].

Endoleak Prevention

Endoleak prevention starts with careful patient and device selection. Patients with less than 10–15 mm of aortic neck length, aortic neck angle >60°, suitable iliac arterial landing zone with diameter >7 mm, and without significant calcification are at high risk for either technical failure or endoleak. Consideration of laparoscopic or open repair in these patients is reasonable.

- *Type I and III* endoleak can generally be avoided by:
  - Proper stent-graft size selection (oversizing by 15–20% is common to ensure adequate radial force to prevent migration and generate seal). Both under and oversizing the device can lead to endoleak, with oversizing potentially causing incomplete device expansion or kinking leading to thrombus [35, 108].
  - Ensuring adequate proximal and distal landing zones.
  - Sufficient graft overlap with modular stent-grafts.
  - Appropriate balloon expansion at the attachment sites.
  - Correction of radiographic parallax to ensure proper positioning.
- *Type II endoleak prevention technique remains debated, but commonly includes:*
  - Pre-op or intraoperative embolization to occlude patent aortic side branches (commonly from IMA or large lumbar branches) appears to be an effective method to reduce Type II endoleak incidence [109–117]. Patients who did not receive embolization have a statistically significant increase in incidence of Type II endoleak and secondary intervention to treat Type II endoleak [91]. Note that prior to branched devices, hypogastric embolization was more common; however, today, this technique should generally be reserved in patients in whom external iliac extension is deemed necessary given the risk of pelvic ischemia.

– However, the decision to perform pre- or intraoperative embolization comes with risk, especially in inexperienced hands, as this generally increases fluoroscopy time and carries the risk of coil dislocation and higher overall cost [72].

Considerations for Radial Access in Treatment of Endoleak

EVAR is performed with bilateral femoral access to place endografts using standard guidewire access and progressive dilation to place the endograft sheath. Given most Type I and III endoleak are identified at the time of completion angiography, treatment via ballooning and additional endograft components can be performed through the existing femoral sheaths. Persistent Type II and delayed Type Ia endoleak may be attempted through radial access. In general, radial access is associated with lower cost, improved patient comfort, fewer vascular complications, and earlier ambulation when compared to femoral access [118]. Risks of transradial approach include radial artery injury or spasm and rarely perforation or compartment syndrome reported in 1% and 0.004%, respectively [119–122]. Typical approach following ultrasound guided radial puncture and sheath insertion includes positioning of a 6F glide catheter at the ostium of the type Ia endoleak, cannulating with a microcatheter system to interrogate the seal (e.g., Cera), and deploying coils and Onyx or an aortic cuff [123].

An early 2013 case report in an 80-year-old patient undergoing successful transradial repair of a large, posterior Type I endoleak with embolization release controlled spirals and Onyx concluded that a transradial approach appears to be a safe and effective alternative to femoral access [121]. Further reports of late Type Ia endoleak treated by transradial approach have shown similarly successful outcomes [123–125].

Deployment of advanced Chimney (snorkel) technique has also been described successfully utilizing transradial approach. A 2017 case report detailed a 71-year-old requiring a left renal snorkel to augment the proximal seal zone delivered transradially (6 Fr sheath and 6 mm iCast stent) [124]. Additionally, "gutter" embolization (coil and Onyx) of an existing snorkel was described in a complex renal and liver transplant patient with bilateral occluded renal snorkels [125].

Summary and Recommendations

- Endoleak post-EVAR remains a common complication in 20–50% of patients despite advances in technique and endograft device.
- Endoleak surveillance recommendations include 1-month CTA and baseline CEUS, followed by annual CTA or CEUS for patients without evidence of sac

expansion or device defect. Patients with sac expansion or device defect should receive additional 6-month imaging follow-up.

- Type I endoleak (proximal Ia or distal Ib seal defect) should be repaired immediately, typically with reballooning attachment sites and/or placement of additional stent components. Persistent low-flow type I endoleak can be monitored conservatively given the high likelihood for spontaneous resolution. Late Type Ia may be approached transradially, while Type 1b is typically not possible from a radial approach.
- Type II endoleak (IMA or other aortic branch feeders) is both common and a source of debate in terms of management. Spontaneous resolution is common and risk of rupture is low. Current treatment recommendation is in patients with >5 mm sac expansion on interval follow-up; however some reports suggest lack of expansion in many (>40%) of patients who rupture. More aggressive centers may treat all persistent Type II endoleak with any level of continuous expansion, while more conservative centers align with the 5 mm interval rule. Type II endoleak is correlated with number and size of patent branches; thus the best "treatment" for type II endoleak may be proactive, prophylactic IMA/Lumbar feeder embolization at the time of EVAR. Management of Type II endoleak may be attempted through transradial or femoral access.
- Type III or junctional endoleak due to component disconnection or fabric defect is uncommon due to improved endograft technology with longer overlap zones and improved material fatigue. Type III endoleak should be treated immediately through femoral access and typically involves placement of stent-graft components to bridge and seal the defect.
- Type IV endoleak due to graft porosity is self-limiting, resolves in 24 hours, and is not associated with long-term adverse events.
- Type V endoleak or endotension of undetermined origin has been linked to laminated thrombus that prevents clear endoleak expression and with early generation polyester grafts. MRA may be more sensitive than CTA in identifying an endoleak source in these patients. Treatment may consist of relining the old endograft with new stent-graft placement.
- Fenestrated, branched, or chimney endografts are advanced techniques that help preserve vital vessel flow and aid in the management of persistent endoleak, but come with an increased risk of component separation or failure.
- Transradial delivery of stent graft components or feeder embolization to treat post-EVAR delayed Type Ia and persistent Type II endoleak appears reasonable given improved outcomes, including patient comfort, earlier ambulation, and lower complications. Advanced techniques such as deployment of Chimney and F-EVAR and branched device have also been successfully managed transradially. Certainly, however, more complex cases or failure of transradial repair may require additional femoral access and/or open repair.

Case Images (Figs. 11.7, 11.8, and 11.9)

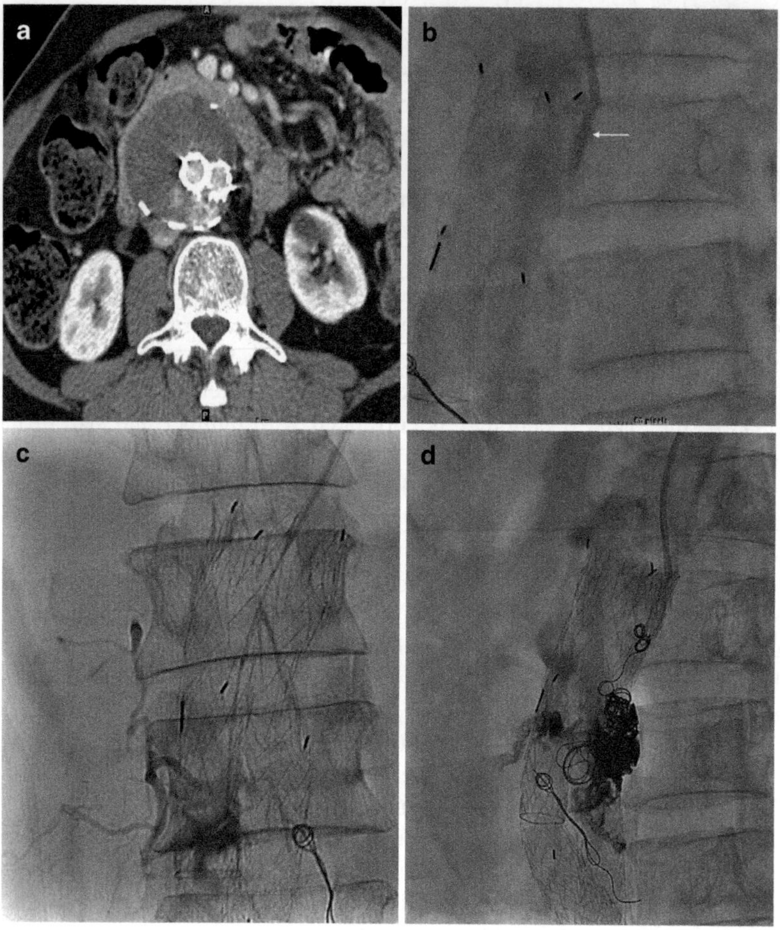

Fig. 11.7 Case 1: (**a**) Contrast enhanced CT angiogram demonstrating endoleak with enlarging aneurysmal sac. Findings on CT were consistent with a Type Ia leak. (**b**) Digital subtraction angiogram via 6fr MP guide catheter demonstrates a posterior Type Ia endoleak. (**c**) Digital subtraction angiogram via microcatheter demonstrates outflow lumbar arteries and filling of AAA sac. (**d**) Completion angiogram demonstrates EVOH and coils sealing Type Ia endoleak

Fig. 11.8 Case 2: (**a**) CT angiogram demonstrates contrast within the aneurysmal sac. This was consistent with a Type II endoleak. (**b**) Digital subtraction angiogram demonstrates Type II endoleak (arrow) arising from right iliolumbar artery. (**b**) Digital subtraction angiogram demonstrates Type II endoleak (arrow) arising from right iliolumbar artery. (**c**) Digital subtraction angiogram via microcatheter in a branch of the right iliolumbar artery demonstrating collateralized flow into right lumbar arteries and filling of aneurysm sac consistent with Type II endoleak. (**d**) Digital subtraction angiogram after microcatheter is advanced into aneurysm sac demonstrating endoleak and left lumbar artery outflow vessel. (**e**) Completion spot image demonstrating embolization of the Type II endoleak using a combination of EVOH and microcoils

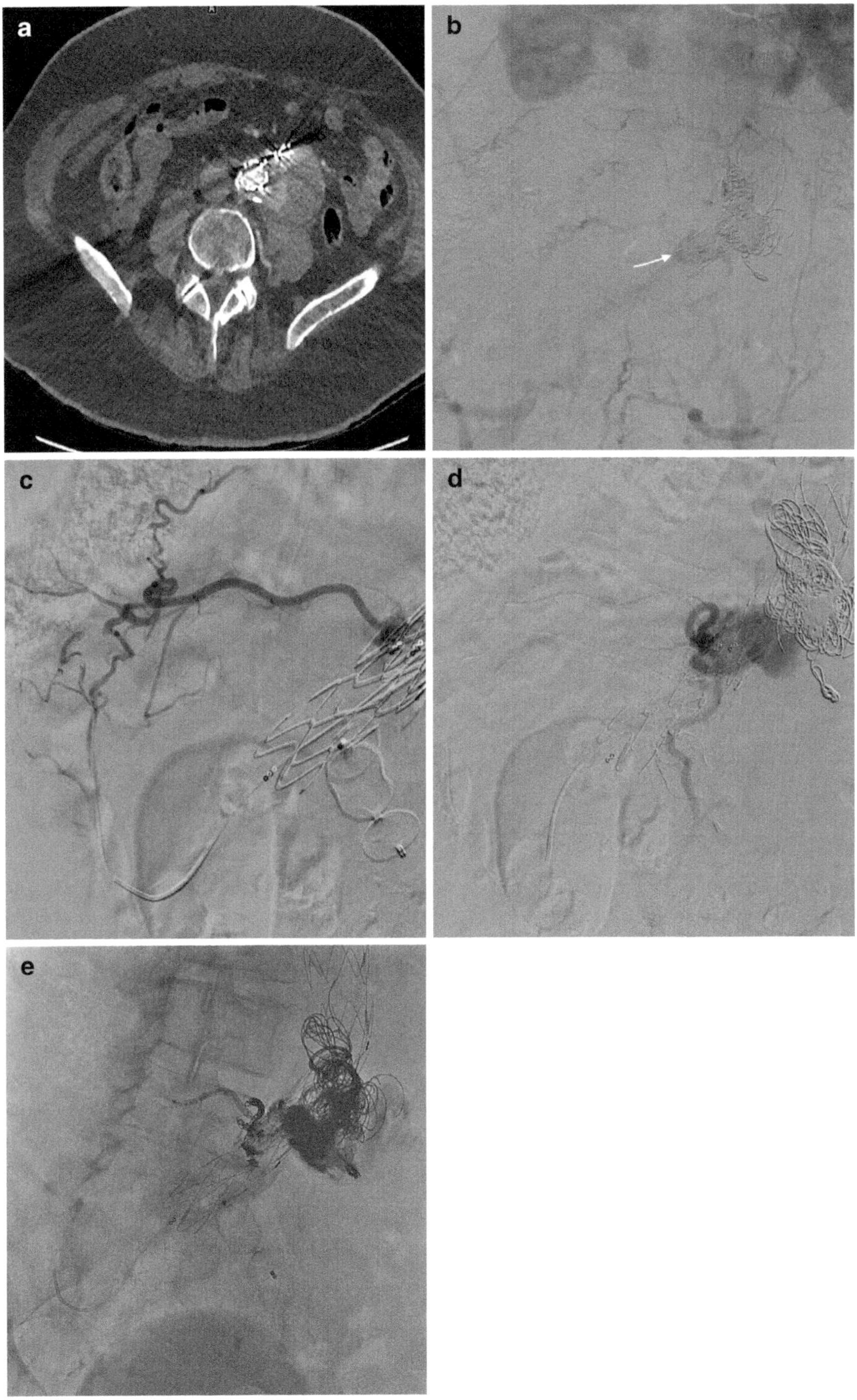
a
b
c
d
e

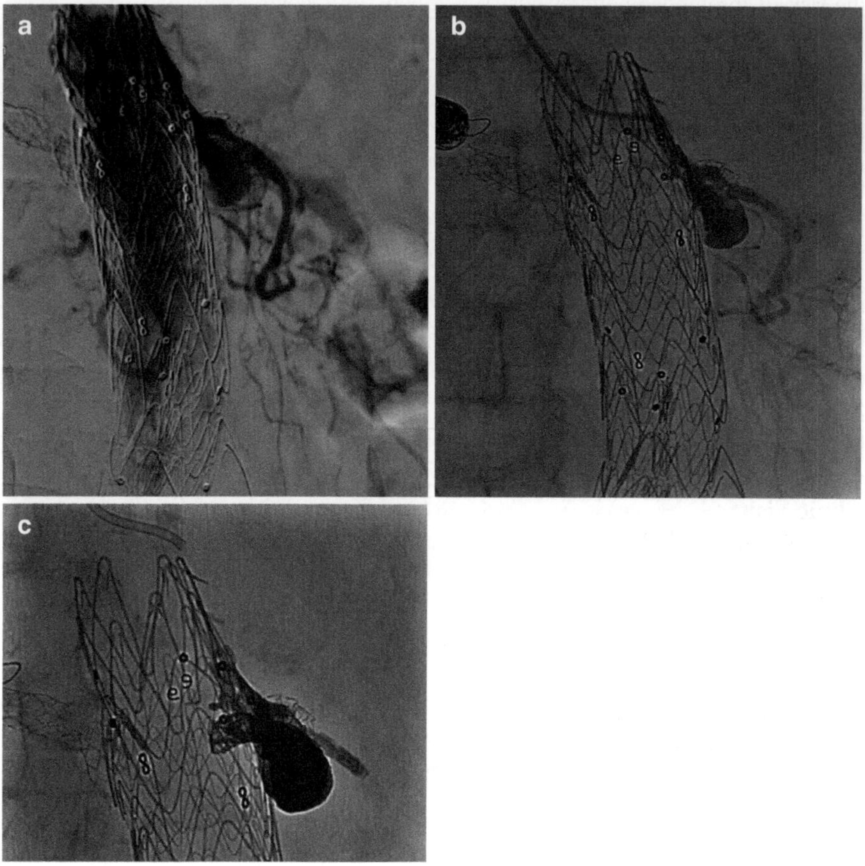

Fig. 11.9 Case 3: (**a**) Digital subtraction angiogram via 5Fr Sarah radial catheter demonstrates a gutter leak around the left renal snorkel. (**b**) Digital subtraction angiogram via microcatheter shows that the gutter leak also fills the left renal chimney possibly representing a fracture in the stent. (**c**) Completion spot image shows that the endoleak has been embolized using EVOH. Some of the EVOH went into the left renal stent, but this was not of concern as the kidney is non-functional

References

1. Chaikof EL, Brewster DC, Dalman RL, Makaroun MS, Illig KA, Sicard GA, et al. The care of patients with an abdominal aortic aneurysm: The Society for Vascular Surgery practice guidelines. Vasc Surg. 2009;50(4 Suppl):S2.
2. Dangas G, O'Connor D, Firwana B, Brar S, Ellozy S, Vouyouka A, et al. Open versus endovascular stent graft repair of abdominal aortic aneurysms: a meta-analysis of randomized trials. JACC Cardiovasc Interv. 2012;5(10):1071–80.
3. Moll FL, Powell JT, Fraedrich G, Verzini F, Haloun S, Waltham M, et al. Management of abdominal aortic aneurysms clinical practice guidelines of the European society for vascular surgery. Eur J Vasc Endovasc Surg. 2011;41(Suppl 1):S1–S58.

4. Stather PW, Sidloff D, Dattani N, Choke E, Bown MJ, Sayers RD, et al. Systematic review and meta-analysis of the early and late outcomes of open and endovascular repair of abdominal aortic aneurysm. Br J Surg. 2013;100(7):863–72.
5. Wyss TR, Brown LC, Powell JT, Greenhalgh RM. Rate and predictability of graft rupture after endovascular and open abdominal aortic aneurysm repair: data from the EVAR trials. Ann Surg. 2010;252(5):805–12.
6. Hiratzka LF, Bakris GL, Beckman JA, Bersin RM, Carr VF, Casey DE, et al. 2010 ACCF/AHA/AATS/ACR/ASA/SCA/SCAI/SIR/STS/SVM guidelines for the diagnosis and management of patients with thoracic aortic disease: a report of the American College of Cardiology Foundtion/American Heart Association task force on practice guidelines, American Association for Thoracic Surgery, American College of Radiology, American Stroke Association, Society of Cardiovascular Anesthesiologists, Society for Cardiovascular Angiography and Interventions, Society of Interventional Radiology, Society of Thoracic Surgeons, and Society for Vascular Medicine. Circulation. 2010;121(13):e266.
7. Avgerinos ED, Chaer RA, Makaroun MS. Type II endoleaks. J Vasc Surg. 2014;60(5):1386–91.
8. Buth J, Harris PL, van Marrewijk C, Fransen G. The significance and management of different types of endoleaks. Semin Vasc Surg. 2003;16(2):95–102.
9. Lal BK, Zhou W, Li Z, Kyriakides T, Matsumura J, Lederle FA, et al. Predictors and outcomes of endoleaks in the Veterans Affairs Open Versus Endovascular Repair (OVER) trial of abdominal aortic aneurysms. J Vasc Surg. 2015;62(6):1394–404.
10. White HA, Macdonald S. Estimating risk associated with radiation exposure during follow-up after endovascular aortic repair (EVAR). J Cardiovasc Surg. 2010;51(1):95.
11. Fransen GA, Vallabhaneni SR Sr, van Marrewijk CJ, Laheij RJ, Harris PL, Buth J. Rupture of infra-renal aortic aneurysm after endovascular repair: a series from EUROSTAR registry. Eur J Vasc Endovasc Surg. 2003;26(5):487.
12. Chaikof EL, Blankensteijn JD, Harris PL, White GH, Zarins CK, Vernhard VM, et al. Reporting standards for endovascular aortic aneurysm repair. J Vasc Surg. 2002;35(5):1048–60.
13. Mehta M, Sternbach Y, Taggert JB, Kreienberg PB, Roddy SP, Paty PS, et al. Long-term outcomes of secondary procedures after endovascular aneurysm repair. J Vasc Surg. 2010;52(6):1442.
14. Conrad MF, Adams AB, Guest JM, Paruchuri V, Brewster DC, LaMuraglia GM, et al. Secondary intervention after endovascular abdominal aortic aneurysm repair. Ann Surg. 2009;250(3):383–9.
15. Veith FJ, Baum RA, Ohki T, Amor M, Adiseshiah M, Blankensteijn JD, et al. Nature and significance of endoleaks and endotension: summary of opinions expressed at an international conference. J Vasc Surg. 2002;35(5):1029.
16. Görich J, Rilinger N, Sokiranski R, Kramer SC, Ermis C, Schutz A, et al. Treatment of leaks after endovascular repair of aortic aneurysms. Radiology. 2000;215(2):414.
17. Buth J, Laheij RJ. Early complications and endoleaks after endovascular abdominal aortic aneurysm repair: report of a multicenter study. J Vasc Surg. 2000;31(1 Pt 1):134–46.
18. Mohan IV, Laheij RJ, Harris PL, EUROSTAR COLLABORATORS. Risk factors for endoleak and the evidence for stent-graft oversizing in patients undergoing endovascular aneurysm repair. Eur J Vasc Endovasc Surg. 2001;21:344.
19. Arthurs ZM, Lyden SP, Rajani RR, Eagleton MJ, Clair DG. Long-term outcomes of Palmaz stent placement for intraoperative type Ia endoleak during endovascular aneurysm repair. Ann Vasc Surg. 2011;25(1):120–6.
20. Tan TW, Eslami M, Rybin D, Doros G, Zhang WW, Farber A, et al. Outcomes of patients with type I endoleak at completion of endovascular abdominal aneurysm repair. J Vasc Surg. 2016;63(6):1420–7.
21. Hager ES, Cho JS, Makaroun MS, Park SC, Chaer R, Marone L, et al. Endografts with suprarenal fixation do not perform better than those with infrarenal fixation in the treatment of patients with short straight proximal aortic necks. J Vasc Surg. 2012;55(5):1242–6.

22. McFarland G, Tran K, Virgin-Downey W, Sgroi MD, Chandra V, Mell MW, et al. Infrarenal endovascular aneurysm repair with large device (34- to 36-mm) diameters is associated with higher risk of proximal fixation failure. J Vasc Surg. 2019;69(2):385.
23. Gray D, Shahverdyan R, Reifferscheid V, Gawenda M, Brunkwall JS. EVAR with flared iliac limbs has a high risk of late type 1b endoleak. Eur J Vasc Endovasc Surg. 2017;54(2):170.
24. van Marrewijk CJ, Fransen G, Laheij RJ, Harris PL, Buth J, EUROSTAR Collaborators. Is a type II endoleak after EVAR a harbinger of risk? Causes and outcome of open conversion and aneurysm rupture during follow-up. Eur J Vasc Endovasc Surg. 2004;27(2):128–37.
25. Drury D, Michaels JA, Jones L, Ayiku L. Systematic review of recent evidence for the safety and efficacy of elective endovascular repair in the management of infrarenal abdominal aortic aneurysm. Br J Surg. 2005;92:937.
26. Sidloff DA, Stather PW, Choke E, Bown MJ, Sayers RD. Type II endoleak after endovascular aneurysm repair. Br J Surg. 2013;100(10):1262.
27. Ultee KHJ, Büttner S, Huurman R, Bastos Gonçalves F, Hoeks SE, Bramer WM, et al. Editor's choice - systematic review and meta-analysis of the outcome of treatment for type II endoleak following endovascular aneurysm repair. Eur J Vasc Endovasc Surg. 2018;56(6):794.
28. Makaroun M, Zajko A, Sugimoto H, Eskandari M, Webster M, et al. Fate of endoleaks after endoluminal repair of abdominal aortic aneurysms with the EVT device. Eur J Vasc Endovasc Surg. 1999;18:185.
29. Lo RC, Buck DB, Herrmann J, Hamdan AD, Wyers M, Patel VI, et al. Risk factors and consequences of persistent type II endoleaks. J Vasc Surg. 2016;63(4):895–901. Epub 2016 Jan 12
30. Lalys F, Durrmann V, Duménil A, Göksu C, Cardon A, Clochard E, et al. Systematic review and meta-analysis of preoperative risk factors of type II endoleaks after endovascular aneurysm repair. Ann Vasc Surg. 2017;41:284.
31. Piazza M, Squizzato F, Miccoli T, Lepidi S, Menegolo M, Grego F, et al. Definition of type II endoleak risk based on preoperative anatomical characteristics. J Endovasc Ther. 2017;24(4):566.
32. Abularrage CJ, Crawford RS, Conrad MF, Lee H, Kwolek CJ, Brewster DC, et al. Preoperative variables predict persistent type 2 endoleak after endovascular aneurysm repair. J Vasc Surg. 2010;52(1):19–24.
33. Ueda T, Takaoka H, Petrovitch I, Rubin GD. Detection of broken sutures and metal-ring fractures in AneuRx stent-grafts by using three-dimensional CT angiography after endovascular abdominal aortic aneurysm repair: association with late endoleak development and device migration. Radiology. 2014;272(1):275.
34. Ward TJ, Cohen S, Fischman A, Kim E, Nowakowski FS, Ellozy SH, et al. Preoperative inferior mesenteric artery embolization before endovascular aneurysm repair: decreased incidence of type II endoleak and aneurysm sac enlargement with 24-month follow-up. J Vasc Interv Radiol. 2013;24(1):49–55.
35. Avgerinos ED, Dalainas I, Kakisis J, Moulakakis K, Giannakopoulos T, Liapis CD. Endograft accommodation on the aortic bifurcation: an overview of anatomical fixation and implications for long-term stent-graft stability. J Endovasc Ther. 2011;18(4):462–70.
36. Skibba AA, Evans JR, Greenfield DT, Yoon HR, Katras T, Ouriel K, et al. Management of late main-body aortic endograft component uncoupling and type IIIa endoleak encountered with the Endologix Powerlink and AFX platforms. J Vasc Surg. 2015;62(4):868–75.
37. Keith CJ Jr, Passman MA, Gaffud MJ, Novak Z, Pearce BJ, Matthews TC, et al. Comparison of outcomes following endovascular repair of abdominal aortic aneurysms based on size threshold. J Vasc Surg. 2013;58(6):1458–66.
38. Troutman DA, Chaudry M, Dougherty MJ, Calligaro KD. Endovascular aortic aneurysm repair surveillance may not be necessary for the first 3 years after an initially normal duplex postoperative study. J Vasc Surg. 2014;60(3):558–62.
39. Chung J, Kordzadeh A, Prionidis I, Panayiotopoulos Y, Browne T. Contrast-enhanced ultrasound (CEUS) versus computed tomography angiography (CTA) in detection of endoleaks in post-EVAR patients. Are delayed type II endoleaks being missed? A systematic review and meta-analysis. J Ultrasound. 2015;18(2):91.

40. White GH, May J, Waugh RC, Chaufour X, Yu W. Type III and type IV endoleak: toward a complete definition of blood flow in the sac after endoluminal AAA repair. J Endovasc Surg. 1998;5(4):305.
41. Fillinger M, Excluder Bifurcated Endoprosthesis Clinical Investigators. Three-dimensional analysis of enlarging aneurysms after endovascular abdominal aortic aneurysm repair in the Gore Excluder Pivotal clinical trial. J Vasc Surg. 2006;43:888.
42. Chaikof EL, Dalman RL, Eskandari MK, Jackson BM, Lee WA, Mansour MA, et al. The Society for Vascular Surgery practice guidelines on the care of patients with an abdominal aortic aneurysm. J Vasc Surg. 2018;67:2.
43. Zarins CK, Wolf YG, Lee WA, Hill BB, Olcott CIV, Harris EJ, et al. Will endovascular repair replace open surgery for abdominal aortic aneurysm repair? Ann Surg. 2000;232(4):501–7.
44. Heikkinen MA, Arko FR, Zarins CK. What is the significance of endoleaks and endotension. Surg Clin North Am. 2004;84(5):1337–52. vii
45. Cantisani V, Ricci P, Grazhdani H, Mapoli A, Fanelli F, Catalano C, et al. Prospective comparative analysis of colour-doppler ultrasound, contrast-enhanced ultrasound, computed tomography and magnetic resonance in detecting endoleak after endovascular abdominal aortic aneurysm repair. Eur J Vasc Endovasc Surg. 2011;41(2):186–92.
46. Stavropoulos SW, Charagundla SR. Imaging techniques for detection and management of endoleaks after endovascular aortic aneurysm repair. Radiology. 2007;243(3):641–55.
47. Guo Q, Zhao J, Huang B, Yuan D, Yang Y, Zeng G, et al. A systematic review of ultrasound or magnetic resonance imaging compared with computed tomography for endoleak detection and aneurysm diameter measurement after endovascular aneurysm repair. J Endovasc Ther. 2016;23(6):936.
48. Chaer RA, Gushchin A, Rhee R, Marone L, Cho JS, Leers S, et al. Duplex ultrasound as the sole long-term surveillance method post-endovascular aneurysm repair: a safe alternative for stable aneurysms. J Vasc Surg. 2009;49(4):845–9; discussion 849-50.
49. Harrison GJ, Oshin OA, Vallabhaneni SR, Brennan JA, Fisher RK, McWilliams RG. Surveillance after EVAR based on duplex ultrasound and abdominal radiography. Eur J Vasc Endovasc Surg. 2011;42(2):187–92.
50. Go MR, Barbato JE, Rhee RY, Makaroun MS. What is the clinical utility of a 6-month computed tomography in the follow-up of endovascular aneurysm repair patients? J Vasc Surg. 2008;47(6):1181–6. discussion 1186-7
51. Aoki A, Suezawa T, Sangawa K, Tago M. Effect of type II endoleaks and antiplatelet therapy on abdominal aortic aneurysm shrinkage after endovascular repair. J Vasc Surg. 2011;54:947.
52. Demehri S, Signorelli J, Kumamaru KK, Wake N, George E, Hanley M, et al. Volumetric quantification of type II endoleaks: an indicator for aneurysm sac growth following endovascular abdominal aortic aneurysm repair. Radiology. 2014;271(1):282.
53. Habets J, Zandvoort HJ, Reitsma JB, Bartels LW, Moll FL, Leiner T, et al. Magnetic resonance imaging is more sensitive than computed tomography angiography for the detection of endoleaks after endovascular abdominal aortic aneurysm repair: a systematic review. Eur J Vasc Endovasc Surg. 2013;45(4):340.
54. Mirza TA, Karthikesalingam A, Jackson D, Walsh SR, Holt PJ, Hayes PD, et al. Duplex ultrasound and contrast-enhanced ultrasound versus computed tomography for the detection of endoleak after EVAR: systematic review and bivariate meta-analysis. Eur J Vasc Endovasc Surg. 2010;39:418.
55. Karthikesalingam A, Al-Jundi W, Jackson D, Boyle JR, Beard JD, Holt PJ, et al. Systematic review and meta-analysis of duplex ultrasonography, contrast-enhanced ultrasonography or computed tomography for surveillance after endovascular aneurysm repair. Br J Surg. 2012;99(11):1514–23.
56. Kapetanios D, Kontopodis N, Mavridis D, McWilliams RG, Giannoukas AD, Antoniou GA. Meta-analysis of the accuracy of contrast-enhanced ultrasound for the detection of endoleak after endovascular aneurysm repair. J Vasc Surg. 2019;69(1):280.
57. Hoppe H, Segall JA, Liem TK, Landry GJ, Kaufman JA. Aortic aneurysm sac pressure measurements after endovascular repair using an implantable remote sensor: initial experience and short-term follow-up. Eur Radiol. 2008;18(5):957–65.

58. Harris PL, Vallabhaneni SR, Desgranges P, Becquemin JP, van Marrewijk C, Laheij RJ. Incidence and risk factors of late rupture, conversion, and death after endovascular repair of infrarenal aortic aneurysms: the EUROSTAR experience. European Collaborators on Stent/graft techniques for aortic aneurysm repair. J Vasc Surg. 2000;32(4):739.
59. Millen AM, Osman K, Antoniou GA, McWilliams RG, Brennan JA, Fisher RK. Outcomes of persistent intraoperative type Ia endoleak after standard endovascular aneurysm repair. J Vasc Surg. 2015;61(5):1185–91.
60. Faries PL, Cadot H, Agarwal G, Kent KC, Hollier LH, Marin ML. Management of endoleak after endovascular aneurysm repair: cuffs, coils, and conversion. J Vasc Surg. 2003;37(6):1155–61.
61. Bastos Gonçalves F, Verhagen HJ, Vasanthananthan K, Zandvoort HJ, Moll FL, van Herwaarden JA. Spontaneous delayed sealing in selected patients with a primary type-Ia endoleak after endovascular aneurysm repair. Eur J Vasc Endovasc Surg. 2014;48:53.
62. Rayt HS, Bown MJ, Lambert KV, Fishwisk NG, McCarthy MJ, London NJ, et al. Buttock claudication and erectile dysfunction after internal iliac artery embolization in patients prior to endovascular aortic aneurysm repair. Cardiovasc Intervent Radiol. 2008;31(4):728–34.
63. Ziegler P, Avgerinos ED, Umscheid T, Perdikides T, Erz K, Stelter WJ. Branched iliac bifurcation: 6 years experience with endovascular preservation of internal iliac artery flow. J Vasc Surg. 2007;46(2):204–10.
64. Moulakakis KG, Dalainas I, Mylonas S, Giannakopoulos TG, Avgerinos ED, Liapis CD. Conversion to open repair after endografting for abdominal aortic aneurysm: a review of causes, incidence, results, and surgical techniques of reconstruction. J Endovasc Ther. 2010;17(6):694.
65. Donas KP, Torsello G, Bisdas T, Osada N, Shonefeld E, Pitoulias GA. Early outcomes for fenestrated and chimney endografts in the treatment of pararenal aortic pathologies are not significantly different: a systematic review with pooled data analysis. J Endovasc Ther. 2012;19(6):723–8.
66. Kim NH, Kim WC, Jeon YS, Cho SG, Hong KC. Repair of type I endoleak by chimney technique after endovascular abdominal aortic aneurysm repair. Ann Surg Treat Res. 2014;86(5):274–7.
67. Katsargyris A, Yazar O, Oikonomou K, Bekkema F, Tielliu I, Verhoeven EL. Fenestrated stent-grafts for salvage of prior endovascular abdominal aortic aneurysm repair. Eur J Vasc Endovasc Surg. 2013;46(1):49–56.
68. de Vries JP, Ouriel K, Mehta M, Varnagy D, Moore WM Jr, Arko FR, et al. Analysis of EndoAnchors for endovascular aneurysm repair by indications for use. J Vasc Surg. 2014;60(6):1460–7.
69. Katsargyris A, Oikonomou K, Nagel S, Giannakopoulos T, Lg Verhoeven E. Endostaples: are they the solution to graft migration and type I endoleaks? J Cardiovasc Surg. 2015;56:363.
70. Karthikesalingam A, Hinchliffe RJ, Holt PJ, Boyle JR, Loftus IM, Thompson MM. Endovascular aneurysm repair with preservation of the internal iliac artery using the iliac branch graft device. Eur J Vasc Endovasc Surg. 2010;39(3):285–94.
71. Brown A, Saggu GK, Bown MJ, Sayers RD, Sidloff DA. Type II endoleaks: challenges and solutions. Vasc Health Risk Manag. 2016;12:53.
72. Quintas A, Alves G. Three-vessel chimney technique combined with endovascular aortic sealing device for the treatment of a type Ia endoleak. Eur J Vasc Endovasc Surg. 2017;53(3):379.
73. Aziz A, Menias CO, Sanchez LA, Picus D, Saad N, Rubin BG, et al. Outcomes of percutaneous endovascular intervention for type II endoleak with aneurysm expansion. J Vasc Surg. 2012;55(5):1263–7.
74. Sarac TP, Gibbons C, Vargas L, Liu J, Srivastava S, Bena J, et al. Long-term follow-up of type II endoleak embolization reveals the need for close surveillance. J Vasc Surg. 2012;55(1):33–40.

75. AbuRahma AF, Mousa AY, Campbell JE, Stone PA, Hass SM, Nanjundappa A, et al. The relationship of preoperative thrombus load and location to the development of type II endoleak and sac regression. J Vasc Surg. 2011;53:1534.
76. Sheehan MK, Ouriel K, Greenberg R, McCann R, Murphy M, Fillinger M, et al. Are type II endoleaks after endovascular aneurysm repair endograft dependent? J Vasc Surg. 2006;43:657.
77. van Marrewijk C, Buth J, Harris PL, Norgren L, Nevelsteen A, Wyatt MG. Significance of endoleaks after endovascular repair of abdominal aortic aneurysms: The EUROSTAR experience. J Vasc Surg. 2002;35(3):461.
78. Silverberg D, Baril DT, Ellozy SH, Carroccio A, Greyrose SE, Lookstein RA, et al. An 8-year experience with type II endoleaks: natural history suggests selective intervention is a safe approach. J Vasc Surg. 2006;44(3):453–9.
79. Lazarides MK, Georgiadis GS, Charalampidis DG, Antoniou GA, Georgakarakos EI, Trellopoulos G. Impact of long-term warfarin treatment on EVAR durability: a meta-analysis. J Endovasc Ther. 2014;21(1):148–53.
80. Uthoff H, Katzen BT, Gandhi R, Peña CS, Benenati JF, Geisbüsch P. Direct percutaneous sac injection for postoperative endoleak treatment after endovascular aortic aneurysm repair. J Vasc Surg. 2012;56(4):965–72.
81. Jones JE, Atkins MD, Brewster DC, Chung TK, Kwolek CJ, LaMuraglia GM, et al. Persistent type 2 endoleak after endovascular repair of abdominal aortic aneurysm is associated with adverse late outcomes. J Vasc Surg. 2007;46(1):1–8.
82. Schlösser FJ, Gusberg RJ, Dardik A, Lin PH, Verhagen HJ, Moll FL, et al. Aneurysm rupture after EVAR: can the ultimate failure be predicted? Eur J Vasc Endovasc Surg. 2009;37(1):15–22.
83. Baum RA, Carpenter JP, Stavropoulous SW, Fairman RM. Diagnosis and management of type 2 endoleaks after endovascular aneurysm repair. Tech Vasc Interv Radiol. 2001;4(4):222.
84. Massis K, Carson WG 3rd, Rozas A, Patel V, Zwiebel B. Treatment of type II endoleaks with ethylene-vinyl-alcohol copolymer (Onyx). Vasc Endovasc Surg. 2012;46(3):251–7.
85. Sheehan MK, Barbato J, Compton CN, Zajko A, Rhee R, Makaroun MS. Effectiveness of coiling in the treatment of endoleaks after endovascular repair. J Vasc Surg. 2004;40(3):430–4.
86. Mansueto G, Cenzi D, Scuro A, Gottin L, Griso A, Gumbs AA, et al. Treatment of type II endoleak with a transcatheter transcaval approach: results at 1-year follow-up. J Vasc Surg. 2007;45(6):1120–7.
87. Haq IU, Kelay A, Davis M, Brookes J, Mastracci TM, Constantinou J. Ten-year single-centre experience with type II endoleaks: intervention versus observation. Vasc Med. 2017;22(4):316.
88. Ferrari M, Sardella SG, Berchiolli R, Adami D, Vignali C, Napoli V, et al. Surgical treatment of persistent type 2 endoleaks, with increase of the aneurysm sac: indications and technical notes. Eur J Vasc Endovasc Surg. 2005;29:43.
89. Kolvenbach R, Pinter L, Raghunandan M, Cheshire N, Ramadan H, Dion YM. Laparoscopic remodeling of abdominal aortic aneurysms after endovascular exclusion: a technical description. J Vasc Surg. 2002;36:1267.
90. Mangialardi N, Ronchey S, Orrico M, Serrao E, Alberti V, Fazzini S, et al. Surgical conversion with graft salvage as a definitive treatment for persistent type II endoleak causing sac enlargement. J Vasc Surg. 2015;62:1437.
91. Eng ML, Brewer MB, Rowe VL, Weaver FA. Treatment options for late type III endoleaks after endovascular aneurysm repair. Ann Vasc Surg. 2015;29(3):594.
92. Cho JS, Dillavou ED, Rhee RY, Makaroun MS. Late abdominal aortic aneurysm enlargement after endovascular repair with the excluder device. J Vasc Surg. 2004;39:1236–42.
93. Wild JB, Dattani N, Stather P, Bown MJ, Sayers RD, Choke E. Effect of anticoagulation and antiplatelet therapy on incidence of endoleaks and sac size expansions after endovascular aneurysm repair. Ann Vasc Surg. 2014;28:554.

94. Johnson MS, Chiang J, Eldrup-Jorgensen J, Clark DE, Healey CT. Effect of chronic oral anticoagulation with warfarin on the durability and outcomes of endovascular aortic aneurysm repair. J Vasc Surg. 2013;58:319.
95. Bobadilla JL, Hoch JR, Leverson GE, Tefera G. The effect of warfarin therapy on endoleak development after endovascular aneurysm repair (EVAR) of the abdominal aorta. J Vasc Surg. 2010;52:267.
96. Parmer SS, Carpenter JP, Stavropoulos SW, Fairman RM, Pochettino A, Woo EY, et al. Endoleaks after endovascular repair of thoracic aortic aneurysms. J Vasc Surg. 2006;44:447.
97. Riambau V, Zipfel B, Coppi G, Czerny M, Tealdi DG, Ferro C, et al. Final operative and midterm results of the European experience in the RELAY Endovascular Registry for Thoracic Disease (RESTORE) study. J Vasc Surg. 2011;53:565.
98. Torsello GB, Torsello GF, Osada N, Teebken OE, Ratusinski CM, Nienaber CA. Midterm results from the TRAVIATA registry: treatment of thoracic aortic disease with the valiant stent graft. J Endovasc Ther. 2010;17:137.
99. Wheatley GH 3rd, Gurbuz AT, Rodriguez-Lopez JA, Ramaiah VG, Olsen D, Williams J, et al. Midterm outcome in 158 consecutive Gore TAG thoracic endoprostheses: single center experience. Ann Thorac Surg. 2006;81:1570.
100. Gleason TG. Endoleaks after endovascular aortic stent-grafting: impact, diagnosis, and management. Semin Thorac Cardiovasc Surg. 2009;21(4):363–72.
101. Lipsitz E, Michler RE, Neragi-Miandoab S. Hybrid arch debranching and proximal endograft extension to repair a type I endoleak after endovascular thoracic aneurysm repair. Ann Vasc Surg. 2014;28(3):740.
102. Neragi-Miandoab S, Bernik T. Endovascular repair of thoracic aortic aneurysms. Recent Pat Cardiovasc Drug Discov. 2009;4(3):211–21.
103. Neragi-Miandoab S, Tuchak J, Bakhos M, Schwartz JP. Open repair of a new aneurysm of the thoracoabdominal aorta after endovascular stent placement. J Thorac Cardiovasc Surg. 2006;132(1):157–8.
104. Belczak SQ, Silva ES, Klajner R, Puech-Leão P, De Luccia N. Type II endoleaks, left-arm complications, and need of revascularization after left subclavian artery coverage for thoracic aortic aneurysms endovascular repair: a systematic review. Ann Vasc Surg. 2017;41:294.
105. Greenberg RK, Deaton D, Sullivan T, Walker E, Lyden SP, Srivastava SD, et al. Variable sac behavior after endovascular repair of abdominal aortic aneurysm: analysis of core laboratory data. J Vasc Surg. 2004;39(1):95–101.
106. Mastracci TM, Greenberg RK, Eagleton MJ, Hernandez AV. Durability of branches in branched and fenestrated endografts. J Vasc Surg. 2013;57(4):926–33.
107. Lindblad B, Bin Jabr A, Holst J, Malina M. Chimney grafts in aortic stent grafting: hazardous or useful technique? Systematic review of current data. Eur J Vasc Endovasc Surg. 2015;50(6):722–31.
108. Mohan IV, Laheij RJ, Harris PL, EUROSTAR COLLABRATORS. Risk factors for endoleak and the evidence for stent-graft oversizing in patients undergoing endovascular aneurysm repair. Eur J Vasc Endovasc Surg. 2001;21(4):344.
109. Fabre D, Fadel E, Brenot P, Hamdi S, Gomez Caro A, Mussot S, et al. Type II endoleak prevention with coil embolization during endovascular aneurysm repair in high-risk patients. J Vasc Surg. 2015;62(1):1–7.
110. Gould DA, McWilliams R, Edwards RD, Martin J, White D, Joekes E, et al. Aortic side branch embolization before endovascular aneurysm repair: incidence of type II endoleak. J Vasc Interv Radiol. 2001;12(3):337–41.
111. Güntner O, Zeman F, Wohlgemuth WA, Heiss P, Jung EM, Wiggermann P, et al. Inferior mesenteric arterial type II endoleaks after endovascular repair of abdominal aortic aneurysm: are they predictable? Radiology. 2014;270(3):910–9.
112. Parry DJ, Kessel DO, Robertson I, Denton L, Patel JV, Berridge DC, et al. Type II endoleaks: predictable, preventable, and sometimes treatable? J Vasc Surg. 2002;36(1):105–10.

113. Mascoli C, Freyrie A, Gargiulo M, Gallitto E, Pini R, Faggioli G, et al. Selective intra-procedural AAA sac embolization during EVAR reduces the rate of type II endoleak. Eur J Vasc Endovasc Surg. 2016;51(5):632.
114. Simonte G, Parlani G, Farchioni L, Isernia G, Cieri E, Lenti M, et al. Lesson learned with the use of iliac branch devices: single centre 10 year experience in 157 consecutive procedures. Eur J Vasc Endovasc Surg. 2017;54(1):95. Epub 2017 May 7
115. Mehta M, Veith FJ, Ohki T, Cynamon J, Goldstein K, Suggs WD, et al. Unilateral and bilateral hypogastric artery interruption during aortoiliac aneurysm repair in 154 patients: a relatively innocuous procedure. J Vasc Surg. 2001;33(2 Suppl):S27–32.
116. Bosanquet DC, Wilcox C, Whitehurst L, Cox A, Williams IM, Twine CP, et al. Systematic review and meta-analysis of the effect of internal iliac artery exclusion for patients undergoing EVAR. Eur J Vasc Endovasc Surg. 2017;53(4):534.
117. Farahmand P, Becquemin JP, Desgranges P, Allaire E, Marzelle J, Roudot-Thoraval F. Is hypogastric artery embolization during endovascular aortoiliac aneurysm repair (EVAR) innocuous and useful? Eur J Vasc Endovasc Surg. 2008;35(4):429–35.
118. Posham R, Biederman D, Patel R, Kim E, Tabori N, Nowakowski SF, et al. Transradial approach for noncoronary interventions: a single-center review of safety and feasibility in the first 1,500 cases. J Vasc Interv Radiol. 2016;27(2):159–66.
119. Schueler A, Black SR, Shay N. Management of transradial access for coronary angiography. J Cardiovasc Nurs. 2013;28(5):468–72.
120. Shroff A, Siddiqui S, Burg A, Singla I. Identification and management of complications of transradial procedures. Curr Cardiol Rep. 2013;13:350.
121. Masuda N, Matsukage T, Ikari Y. Successful transradial intervention for two lesions with dual anomalous origins of coronary arteries. J Invasive Cardiol. 2011;13:E117–20.
122. Schiattarella GG, Magliulo F, Laurino FI, Bottino R, Giulio Bruno A, De Paulis M, et al. Transradial approach for the endovascular treatment of type I endoleak after aortic aneurysm repair: a case report. BMC Surg. 2013;13(Suppl 2):S47. https://doi.org/10.1186/1471-2482-13-S2-S47.
123. Fischman AF. Transradial Endoleak Angiography post EVAR for Aortic Aneurysm. Youtube.com. 2018. https://www.youtube.com/watch?v=R2PxlvsYt28. Accessed 01 Aug 2019.
124. Stern JR, Ellozy SH. Transradial delivery of a renal snorkel during complex endovascular aortic aneurysm repair. Vasc Endovasc Surg. 2017;51(7):513–6.
125. Fischman AF. Transradial Approach to Embolization of a Type I Endoleak of Abdominal Aortic Aneurysm Endograft. Youtube.com. 2016. https://www.youtube.com/watch?v=Dzft4hhipF8. Accessed 01 Aug 2019.

Chapter 12
Transradial Access for Peripheral Arterial Disease: Subclavian and Upper Arm Interventions

Shashidhara Murthy, Rahul S. Patel, and Aaron M. Fischman

Abbreviations

AVF	Arteriovenous fistula
DVT	Deep vein thrombosis
EVOH	Ethyl vinyl alcohol
n-BCA	n-Butyl cyanoacrylate
SVC	Superior vena cava

Subclavian and Upper Arm Interventions

Although arterial disease is diagnosed less often in the upper extremities, there are still a broad range of endovascular interventions that are routinely performed in the upper extremities and chest. Thoracic outlet syndrome, dialysis fistula formation, limb ischemia, and trauma are a few of the many reasons an intervention may be needed in the upper arms. 40% of all cases of extremity penetrating trauma involve the arm, and accessing the upper arm using the nearest access can be essential in controlling and fixing major upper extremity bleeds [1].

The radial artery is an ideal access point for upper arm interventions due to the proximity to the target area, reduced access-site related bleeding complications [2], reduced risk of groin complications in obese patients [3], and lack of arch manipulation. The use of the transradial approach also allows for immediate ambulation, which can help decrease the duration of hospital stays and reduce the risk of developing deep vein thrombosis (DVT). This chapter will outline the use of the transradial approach for five different interventions performed on the upper arm to show both the feasibility and safety of this approach.

S. Murthy · R. S. Patel (✉) · A. M. Fischman
Department of Diagnostic, Molecular and Interventional Radiology, Icahn School of Medicine at Mount Sinai, New York, NY, USA
e-mail: Shashidhara.Murthy@mountsinai.org; rahul.patel@mountsinai.org

A. M. Fischman et al. (eds.), *Transradial Access in Interventional Radiology*,
https://doi.org/10.1007/978-3-030-81678-0_12

Case 1

Left Subclavian Arteriovenous Malformation Causing Severe Left Upper Extremity Pain, Swelling, and Ulceration

Clinic Visit

80 M with a history of hypertension and hyperlipidemia who presented with severe left upper extremity pain, swelling, and erythema following pacer lead placement complicated by central venous stenosis, status-post angioplasty, found to have a left subclavian arteriovenous malformation on CT venogram. The patient underwent coil/ethyl vinyl alcohol (EVOH) embolization of subclavian artery branches supplying the AVF but returned with only a 50% reduction of left arm swelling with persistent left hand swelling and ulceration.

Procedure

1. Obtain radial access as described in Chap. 4. 3000 units of heparin, 200mcg of nitroglycerin, and 2.5 mg of verapamil are given through the arterial sheath with slow hemodilution.
2. A 4Fr angled Berenstein catheter was advanced through the left radial artery sheath into the left subclavian artery.
3. Upper extremity angiography was performed. Findings include:
   (a) Coils and EVOH from prior embolization are noted (A).
   (b) Multiple subclavian arterial feeders to the subclavian arteriovenous fistula are visualized (B).
4. A dominant superolateral feeding arterial branch was selected using a 4Fr diagnostic catheter.
5. Gentle contrast injection demonstrated brisk flow into the subclavian vein.
6. Further catheterization was performed by placing a 2.4Fr microcatheter through the diagnostic catheter.
7. Digital subtraction angiography was performed to evaluate the flow dynamics and volume of contrast required for embolization.
8. Embolization of this vessel was performed using 0.3 mL of n-Butyl cyanoacrylate (n-BCA) glue (1:7 ratio; glue/Lipiodol) under fluoroscopic guidance to ensure adequate embolization without reflux.
9. The microcatheter was then removed.
10. Digital subtraction angiography was performed in multiple projections demonstrating a significant decrease of flow into the subclavian vein through the subclavian arteriovenous fistula (C).
11. Remove the catheters, guidewire, and sheath from the wrist and apply a radial hemostasis band for 60 minutes.

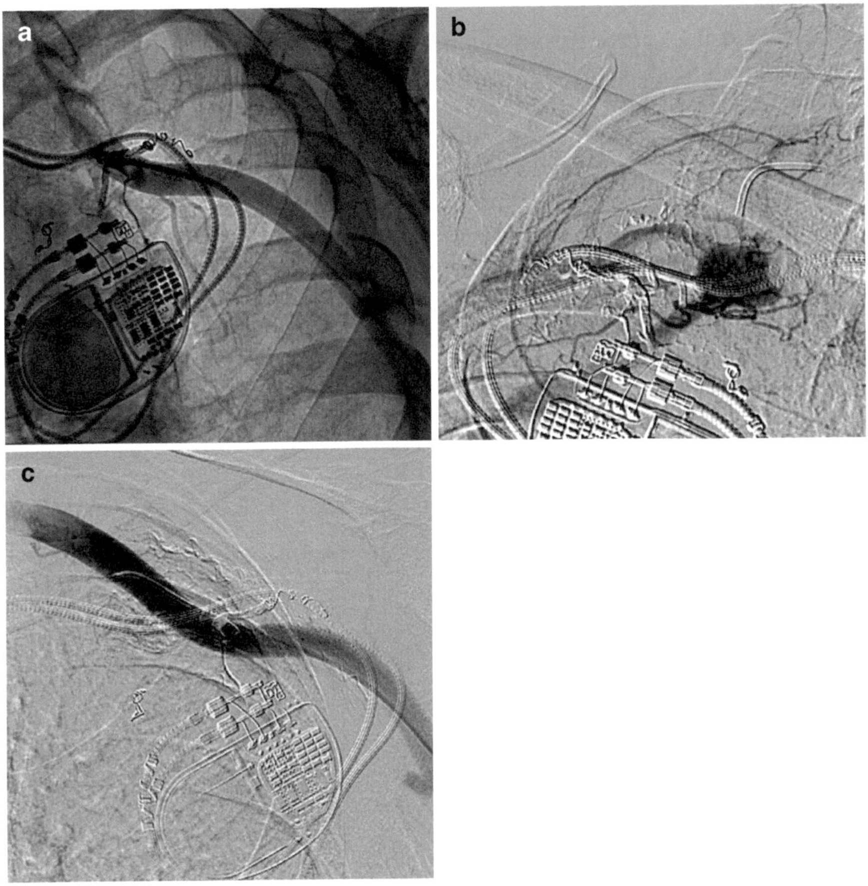

Case 2

Left Subclavian Artery Embolization in a Patient with Persistent Endoleak from Thoracic Stent Graft

Clinic Visit

59 M with a history of hypertension, diabetes, hyperlipidemia, stroke, and type B aortic dissection status-post thoracic endovascular aortic repair with CTA demonstrating a persistent endoleak. Angiogram demonstrated filling of the false lumen from the left subclavian artery.

Procedure

1. Obtain radial access as described in Chap. 4. 3000 units of heparin, 200mcg of nitroglycerin, and 2.5 mg of verapamil are given through the arterial sheath with slow hemodilution.
2. A 5Fr diagnostic catheter was advanced in the subclavian artery, and angiograms were performed in multiple obliquities to identify the origin of the left vertebral artery.
3. Angiogram demonstrated persistent filling into the false lumen of the thoracic aortic dissection, around the previously placed thoracic aortic artery stent graft (A).
4. The origin of the left subclavian artery was embolized using multiple 0.035 coils through the diagnostic catheter (B), and microcoils through a 2.4Fr microcatheter were used to fill the coil pack (C).
5. Microcatheter was removed and angiograms performed through the 5Fr diagnostic catheter demonstrated (D).

   (a) Brisk flow through the left vertebral artery.
   (b) No evidence of persistent flow through the origin of the left subclavian artery.

6. Remove the catheters, guidewire, and sheath from the wrist and apply a radial hemostasis band for 60 minutes.

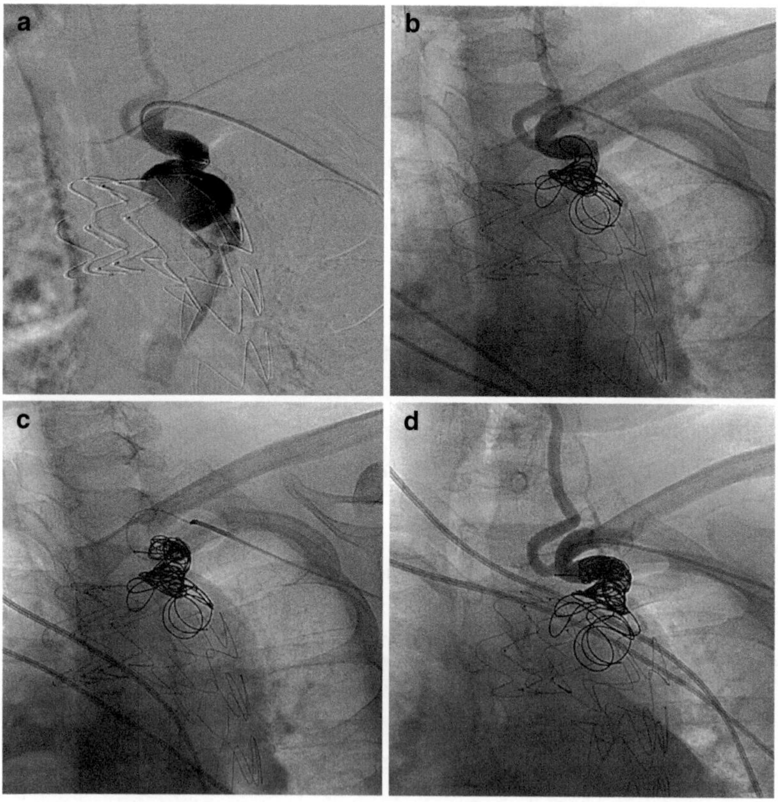

Case 3

Embolization of Right Brachial Artery Branches Supplying Metastatic Humeral Mass

Clinic Visit
60 M with a history of renal cell carcinoma status-post radical nephrectomy who presented with 3 weeks of right upper extremity weakness. CT showed a new metastatic bone lesion in the right humerus.

Procedure
1. Obtain right radial access as described in Chap. 4. 3000 units of heparin, 200mcg of nitroglycerin, and 2.5 mg of verapamil are given through the arterial sheath with slow hemodilution.
2. A 5Fr Sarah Radial catheter was advanced through the sheath into the right subclavian artery.
3. Arteriogram was performed from this location and showed a hypervascular mass with dominant feeding vessels from two deep brachial artery branches (A).
4. The 5Fr Sarah Radial catheter was exchanged for a Cobra Glidecath and a 2.4Fr microcatheter system.
5. Embolization was performed with ½ a vial of 300–500 micron embospheres of each brachial artery feeder.
6. Angiography was performed. Findings:

   (a) Decreased vascularity to the right humeral tumor mass (B and C).

7. Remove the catheters, guidewire, and sheath from the wrist and apply a radial hemostasis band for 60 minutes.

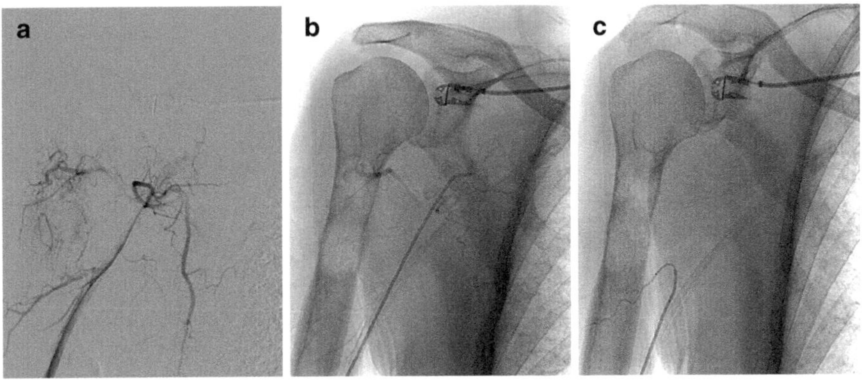

Case 4

Thrombosis of Left Arteriovenous Fistula in Dialysis Patient

Clinic Visit
75 M with a history of diabetes and end-stage renal disease on dialysis presented with decreased thrill of left arteriovenous fistula. Duplex imaging demonstrated venous thrombosis of the fistula requiring intervention.

Procedure

1. Obtain left radial access as described in Chap. 4. 3000 units of heparin, 200mcg of nitroglycerin, and 2.5 mg of verapamil are given through the arterial sheath with slow hemodilution after placement of a 5/6Fr Glideslender sheath.
2. A 5Fr Sarah Radial catheter was placed in the brachial artery and a fistulagram was performed. Findings:

   (a) Complete thrombosis of the arteriovenous fistula (A).

3. Using a 5Fr 100 cm angled glide catheter and a 0.035 angled Glidewire, the fistula was accessed and crossed to the level of the innominate vein (B).
4. A central venogram was performed demonstrating latency of the brachiocephalic vein and SVC.
5. Pulse spray thrombolysis was performed with 4 mg of tissue plasminogen activator (tPA) and 7000 units of heparin as the catheter was withdrawn from the level of the left innominate vein to the fistula anastomosis and left to dwell for 30 minutes.
6. The 5Fr glide catheter was exchanged for a 6 mm balloon to perform balloon maceration to the level of the innominate vein (C).
7. A Epic 10 × 40mm stent was placed in the venous outflow axillary vein due to persistent narrowing despite angioplasty (D).
8. A follow-up venogram was performed. Findings:

   (a) Patent arteriovenous fistula, anastomosis, and venous outflow (E).

9. Final fistula palpation demonstrated a palpable thrill.
10. Remove the catheters, guidewire, and sheath from the wrist and apply a radial hemostasis band for 60 minutes.

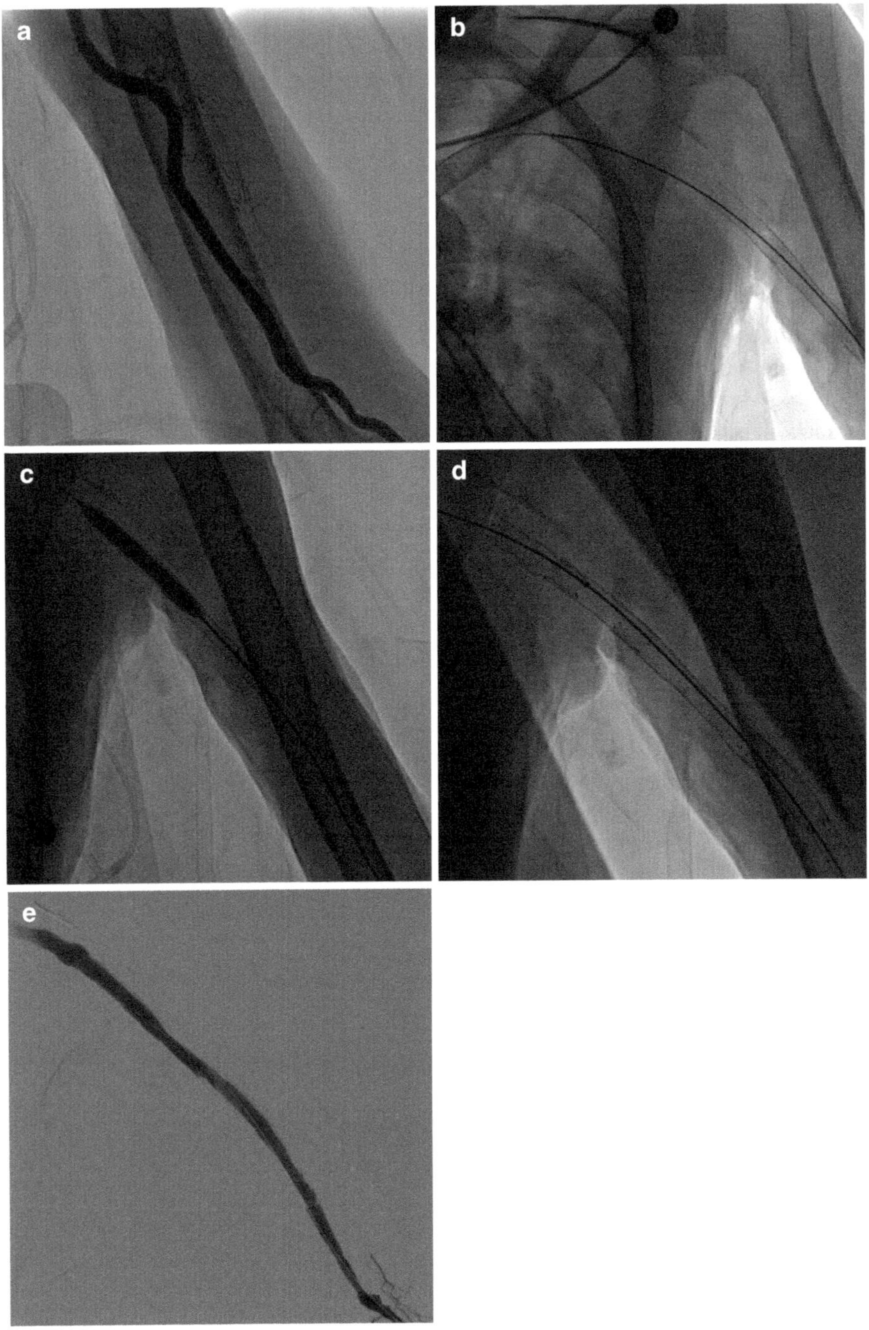
a
b
c
d
e

Case 5

Embolization of a Persistent Left Circumflex Humeral Artery Bleed

Clinic Visit

68 M with a history of alcoholic cirrhosis presented after a fall with anemia and left upper extremity swelling. Eight units of packed red blood cells were given over the course of 5 days; however, patient's hemoglobin and hematocrit continued to drop.

Procedure

1. Obtain radial access as described in Chap. 4. 3000 units of heparin, 200mcg of nitroglycerin, and 2.5 mg of verapamil are given through the arterial sheath with slow hemodilution.
2. A 5Fr MPA catheter was then used to navigate through the arm and into the left axillary artery, and angiography confirmed multiple foci of bleeding arising from vessels of the left circumflex humeral artery.
3. Ultimately, a branch of the left circumflex humeral artery was subselected using a 5Fr glide catheter and a 2.4Fr microcatheter (show pictures).
4. This branch was embolized using n-BCA in a 5:1 ratio. Glue cast seen in Fig. (B).
5. Angiogram was performed. Findings (C):

    (a) No evidence of early venous drainage or bleeding.
    (b) No evidence of non-target embolization.

6. Remove the catheters, guidewire, and sheath from the wrist and apply a radial hemostasis band for 60 minutes.

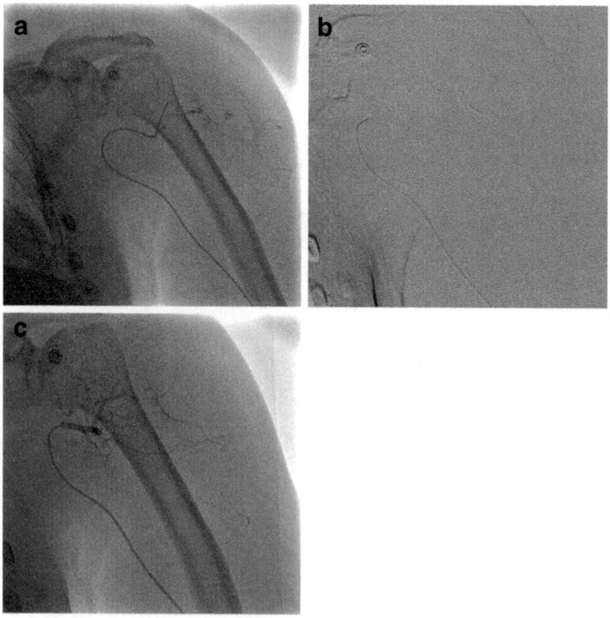

References

1. Kaufman JA, Lee MJ. Vascular and interventional radiology: the requisites. Philadelphia: Elsevier/Saunders; 2014.
2. Cox N, et al. Comparison of the risk of vascular complications associated with femoral and radial access coronary catheterization procedures in obese versus nonobese patients. Am J Cardiol. 2004;94(9):1174–7. https://doi.org/10.1016/j.amjcard.2004.07.088.
3. Yu J, Korabathina R, Coppola J, Staniloae C. Transradial approach to subclavian artery stenting. J Invasive Cardiol. 2010;22(5):204–6.

Chapter 13
Transradial Access in Uterine Artery Embolization

Ricki Korff, Shaun Honig, and Scott Nowakowski

Abbreviations

Cm	Centimeter
DAP	Dose area product
Fr	French
IR	Interventional radiology
UAE	Uterine artery embolization

Introduction

Before uterine artery embolization was first described in 1995 [1], patients with symptomatic uterine fibroids, adenomyosis, and post-partum bleeding who failed conservative management were traditionally treated with surgical options. In the 1990s, uterine artery embolization (UAE) began to be popularized as an alternative treatment option, particularly for patients who did not want to lose their uterus. Since then, comparisons between UAE and surgical treatments have demonstrated that the safety and efficacy of UAE is comparable to myomectomy [2–4], and that UAE patients recover faster with fewer major complications than hysterectomy patients, although they have a higher rate of re-intervention [5–9].

Like the vast majority of interventional radiology procedures, uterine artery embolization has traditionally been performed via unilateral femoral artery puncture. Some even perform bilateral femoral artery puncture to simultaneously embolize the uterine arteries and decrease fluoroscopy time in the young female UAE population [10]. Now, with the broad range of long catheters and wires available, transradial access is technically feasible and increasingly being used (case 1). Studies have demonstrated 100% technical success rates with transradial UAE [11,

R. Korff · S. Honig · S. Nowakowski (✉)
Department of Diagnostic, Molecular and Interventional Radiology, Icahn School of Medicine at Mount Sinai, New York, NY, USA
e-mail: scott.nowakowski@mountsinai.org

A. M. Fischman et al. (eds.), *Transradial Access in Interventional Radiology*,
https://doi.org/10.1007/978-3-030-81678-0_13

12]. Tools such as the Glidesheath Slender have allowed for intervention with the necessary sized tools while maintaining a smaller radial artery puncture site to reduce spasm and increase the technical ease of the procedure. Conventional catheter/guidewire combinations can readily access the bilateral uterine arteries. Catheter lengths are available to accommodate even taller patients, and successful transradial UAE in women up to 178 cm tall has been described in the literature [13]. Microcatheters can be used in a variety of situations including difficult anatomy, spasm, desire to bypass distal non-target vessels, and physician preference (case 2). Further development of longer, smaller diameter tools will improve the already low complication rate with transradial UAE.

In addition to treatment of fibroids and adenomyosis, radial access for UAE has also been performed in cases of post-partum and post-operative hemorrhage (case 3). Another advantage of radial access in post-operative patients includes access remote from the operative site.

Safety

Over the past several decades, there have been many developments in UAE which have improved the procedure's safety. With new fluoroscopy technology, DAP radiation exposure to our patients is reduced. In addition, new, longer microcatheters allow the operator to access vessels more distally and avoid nontarget embolization when necessary. Transradial access is the next innovation in improving patient safety in UAE. In the cardiology literature, procedures done via transradial access have demonstrated fewer access site complications than those done via transfemoral access. It has already been shown in the interventional oncology literature that transradial access is safe and feasible [14], and similar results have been found in UAE patient populations. Studies have demonstrated that in UAE, transradial access has zero to equivalently low complication rates compared to transfemoral access, without a difference in fluoroscopy times between the two access approaches [12, 13, 15].

The coronary artery intervention literature demonstrates that transradial access is not associated with an increased risk of clinically relevant procedure-related neurologic complications compared to the transfemoral approach [16]. This data suggests that neurologic complications associated with coronary artery interventions are not secondary to utilization of radial access. In addition, UAE patients are on average younger and healthier without coronary or peripheral vascular disease compared to the cohort evaluated in the coronary literature. Also, coronary interventions are performed upstream of all four great vessels, leading to a higher likelihood of atherosclerotic debris or clot causing a stroke; conversely, transradial UAE is performed downstream and remotely from the great vessels and passes only the origin of the left vertebral artery along its course. There have been no published cases of stroke after transradial UAE in the literature to date.

While the young and healthy UAE population has a lower risk of stroke with transradial procedures compared to patients undergoing transradial coronary artery or peripheral interventions, this population is at a greater risk for radial artery complications. There is a theoretical increased risk of upper extremity artery spasm in the UAE population, since female gender is an independent predictor of radial artery spasm [17]. In addition, women have a smaller mean radial artery diameter than men (2.59 vs 1.91 mm) [18], making radial artery occlusion more likely. Applying nitroglycerin paste pre-procedure and injecting a radial artery intraarterial medication solution at the start of the procedure allow for easier access and decreased risk of access site complication. Future research into methods for reducing radial artery spasm and occlusion like injection of subcutaneous nitroglycerin [19] and ulnar artery compression during radial artery hemostasis [20] have the potential to even further improve the safety of transradial UAE.

Pain Management and Patient Satisfaction

Pain control methods after UAE have evolved over the past several years. While some techniques like pre-procedure oxycodone have failed to demonstrate improved results [21], intraarterial lidocaine [22] and superior hypogastric nerve block [23] have demonstrated improvement in postoperative pain. A common peri-procedural pain-management regimen consists of intraarterial lidocaine during the procedure, 60 mg intravenous Toradol (1–2 doses) and 1000 mg intravenous Tylenol during the procedure, and NSAIDs such as ibuprofen or ketorolac with Percocet for breakthrough pain when patients are at home. It is also useful to emphasize the expected post-procedure cramping and pain when seeing patients in consult and again just prior to entering procedure room.

Transradial access is a cornerstone in the strategy to increase patient comfort after UAE. In oncology patients, it has already been demonstrated that patients prefer transradial access over transfemoral access [24]. In a small randomized trial, Basile showed a similar result in UAE patients, demonstrating that patient satisfaction and pain scores were better after transradial UAE than with transfemoral UAE [25]. In addition, patients who have had transfemoral access may have difficulty posturing and using the bathroom in the immediate post-procedure period. Transradial access obviates the concern for femoral complications in these situations. Lastly, transradial access during uterine artery embolization can play a role in increasing the frequency of same-day discharges [13].

Case Examples

Case 1: Uterine Artery Embolization Via Radial Approach for the Treatment of Symptomatic Uterine Fibroids

Clinic visit: 43F with PMH of obesity and hypertension presents to clinic with 2 years of worsening dysmenorrhea limiting her activities of daily living and quality of life, referred to the IR clinic by her OBGYN. MRI shows an enlarged uterus with multiple submucosal fibroids. Endometrial biopsy shows benign endometrium. Barbeau, B; BMI, 34.4; height, 5 feet, 4 inches.

1. Obtain left radial artery access.
2. Advance a 4Fr hydrophilic slender sheath over a wire, and inject a radial artery intraarterial medication solution of nitroglycerin 200 μg, verapamil 2.5 mg, and heparin 3000 units.
3. Use a 0.035″ wire and a 4Fr 125 cm Cordis Aqua Tempo vertebral catheter to navigate through the arm and catheterize the distal aorta.
4. Using the 0.035″ wire, advance the catheter into the right internal iliac artery and then into the right uterine artery.
5. Perform angiography to confirm appropriate positioning of the catheter prior to embolization (Fig. 13.1a).
6. Deliver 3 vials of 600 micron Terumo HydroPearl particles followed by 3 vials of 800 micron HydroPearl particles until near stasis is seen.
7. Pull back the 4Fr catheter to the common iliac bifurcation, and catheterize the left internal iliac artery followed by the left uterine artery.
8. Perform angiography to confirm appropriate positioning of the catheter prior to embolization (Fig. 13.1b).
9. Deliver 1 vial of 600 micron Terumo HydroPearl particles followed by 1 vial of 800 micron HydroPearl particles until near stasis is seen.
10. Remove the 4Fr catheter over a wire.
11. Place a TR band on the patient's left wrist for 1 hour.

Case 2: Uterine Artery Access Via Radial Approach for Uterine Artery Embolization Utilizing a Microcatheter

Clinic visit: 38F with no PMH presents to clinic with menorrhagia and bulk-related symptoms, referred to the IR clinic from her OBGYN. MRI shows a leiomyomatous uterus containing 7 intramural fibroids measuring up to 5 cm. Endometrial biopsy shows benign endometrium. Barbeau, A; BMI, 31; height, 5 feet, 7 inches.

1. Obtain left radial artery access.
2. Advance a 4Fr hydrophilic slender sheath over a wire, and inject a radial artery intraarterial medication solution of nitroglycerin 200 μg, verapamil 2.5 mg, and heparin 3000 units.
3. Use a 0.035″ wire and a 4Fr 125 cm Merit Metical Impress VERT catheter to navigate through the arm and catheterize the distal aorta.
4. Using the 0.035″ wire, advance the catheter into the right internal iliac artery and then into the right uterine artery.
5. Perform angiography to confirm appropriate positioning of the catheter prior to embolization.
6. Deliver 4 vials of 700 micron Embozene microspheres (Varian Medical Systems) until near stasis is seen.
7. Pull back the 4Fr catheter to the common iliac bifurcation, and catheterize the left internal iliac artery.

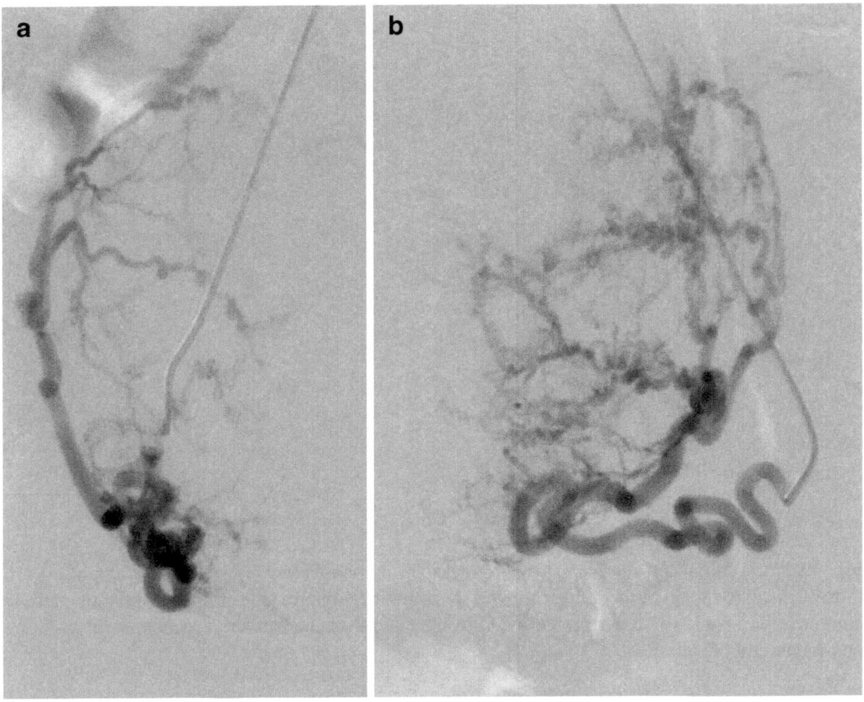

Fig. 13.1 Right (**a**) and left (**b**) uterine artery access via radial approach for uterine artery embolization in patient with symptomatic fibroids

8. After catheterizing the left uterine artery, angiography demonstrates a large cervicovaginal branch distal to the tip of the guide cathter (Fig. 13.2a).
9. Catheterize the left uterine artery with the microcatheter system distal to the cervicovaginal branch to avoid non-target embolization.
10. Perform angiography to confirm appropriate positioning of the microcatheter prior to embolization (Fig. 13.2b).
11. Deliver 1 vial of 700 micron Embozene microspheres (Varian Medical Systems) until near stasis is seen.
12. Remove the microcatheter system through the 4Fr guiding catheter.
13. Remove the 4Fr catheter over a wire.
14. Place a TR band on the patient's left wrist for 1 hour.

Case 3: Right Uterine Artery Access Via Radial Approach for Uterine Artery Embolization in an Unstable Patient with Post-myomectomy Bleeding

Inpatient consult: 37F who desires preservation of her fertility, status post myomectomy with postsurgical vaginal bleeding and hemoglobin drop of 3 g/dL over 5 hours, currently receiving her second unit of pRBCs. HR 116, BP 105/62, T 98.1F,

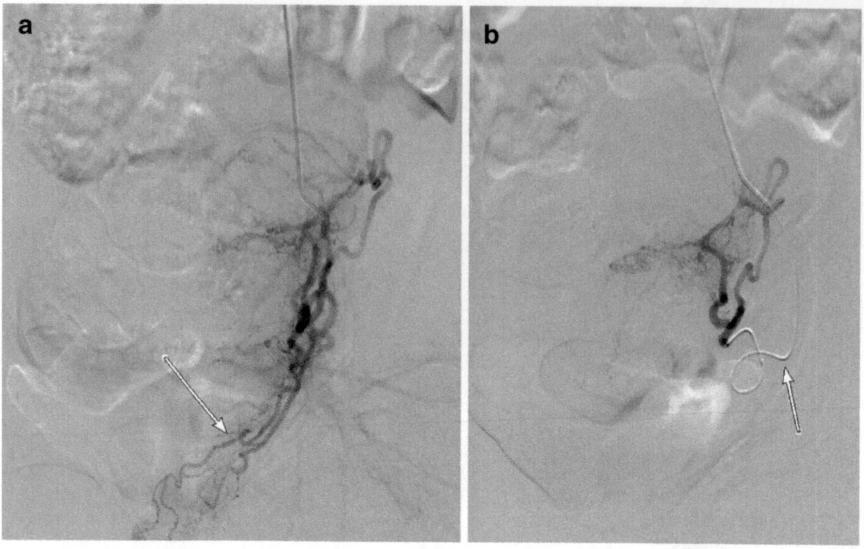

Fig. 13.2 (**a**) Initial left uterine artery angiography demonstrates a large cervicovaginal branch (arrow) distal to the tip of the guide catheter. (**b**) Utilizing a microcatheter system (arrow), particle embolization is able to be performed distal to the takeoff of the cervicovaginal branch, avoiding non-target embolization

O2 sat 97 on room air, respiratory rate 12. IR is consulted for urgent evaluation for potential embolization. Barbeau, A; BMI, 24; height, 5 feet, 5 inches.

1. Obtain left radial artery access.
2. Advance a 4Fr hydrophilic slender sheath over a wire, and inject a radial artery intraarterial medication solution of nitroglycerin 100 μg, verapamil 2.5 mg, and heparin 5000 units.
3. Use a 0.035″ wire and a 4Fr 120 cm Terumo Angle Glidecath to navigate through the arm and catheterize the distal aorta.
4. Using the 0.035″ wire, advance the catheter into the right internal iliac artery and then into the right uterine artery. Early right uterine artery arteriography reveals the right ovarian artery (Fig. 13.3a), as well as active arterial extravasation (Fig. 13.3b).
5. Advance a microcatheter system into the vessel with active extravasation and perform sub-selective arteriography to confirm that the microcatheter tip bypasses the origin of the right ovarian artery (Fig. 13.3c).
6. After flushing the microcatheter with D5, deliver n-butyl cyanoacrylate (NBCA) and lipiodol until near stasis is seen (Fig. 13.3d).
7. Remove the microcatheter system through the 4Fr guiding catheter. Then remove 4Fr catheter over a wire.
8. Place a TR band on the patient's left wrist for 1 hour.

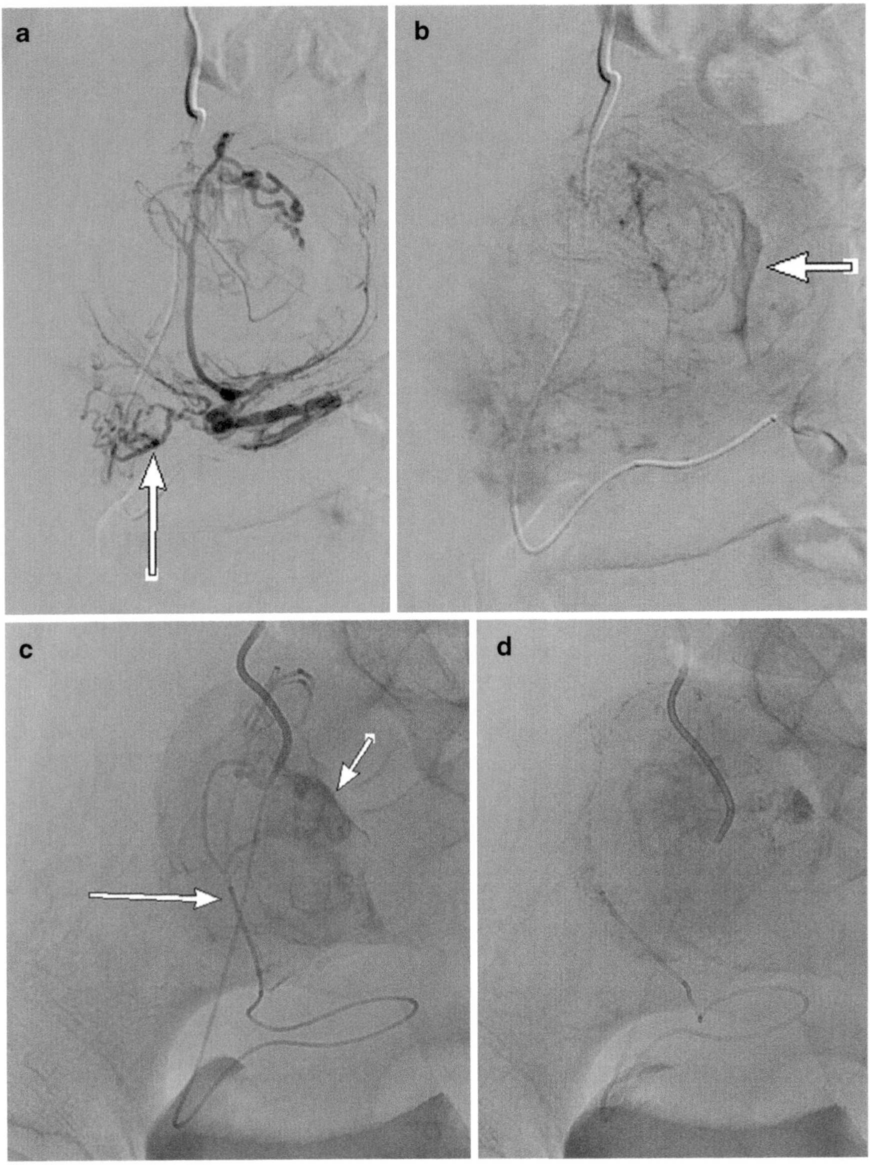

Fig. 13.3 (**a**) Early right uterine artery arteriography reveals the right ovarian artery (arrow). (**b**) Late phase of this run reveals active arterial extravasation (arrow). (**c**) Sub-selective arteriography demonstrates that the microcatheter tip (long arrow) was able to successfully bypass the origin of ovarian artery and sub-select the vessel with active extravasation (short arrow). (**d**) One-shot image without contrast injection reveals successful glue embolization of the right uterine artery without involvement of the right ovarian artery. Final arteriogram revealed no extravasation

Equipment List

Device type	Manufacturer	Product	Dimensions	Comments
Sheaths	Terumo Interventional Systems	Glidesheath slender	5Fr inner diameter, 2.14 mm outer diameter	
Guiding catheters	Cordis	Tempo AQUA Vertebral 135°	4Fr; 125 cm	
	Cordis	Multipurpose MPA 2	4Fr; 125 cm	
	Merit Medical	Impress VERT	4Fr; 125 cm	
	Terumo Interventional Systems	Angle GLIDECATH	4Fr; 120 cm, 150 cm	
Guidewires	Cook Medical	Bentson	0.035″; 180 cm	
Microcathteter systems	Terumo Interventional Systems	PROGREAT	2.7 Fr/2.8 Fr coaxial microcatheter system; 130 cm, 150 cm	Embolic compatibility: HydroPearl 800 ± 75 μm [16]
	Boston Scientific	Bern shape Direxion with Fathom guidewire	2.4 Fr; 130 cm, 155 cm	Embolic compatibility: Non-spherical embolics: up to 500 microns; Spherical embolics, up to 710 microns [26]
Embolic material [27]	Terumo Interventional Systems	HydroPearl microspheres		
	Varian Medical Systems	Embozene microspheres		
	Merit Medical	Embosphere		
	Merit Medical	Bearing nsPVA embolization particles		
	Boston Scientific	Bead Block		
	Boston Scientific	Contour embolization particles		

Technical Considerations

As part of the preoperative workup for transradial uterine artery embolization, the patient's height should be taken into account. A 125 cm diagnostic catheter is long enough to reach the pelvic vessels from a left radial artery approach in most patients. However, although there is no defined height cutoff over which uterine artery embolization is contraindicated, in our experience 125 cm catheters are difficult to navigate into the uterine artery in patients taller than 6 feet. Similarly, the group at Beth Israel Deaconess Medical Center reports experiencing difficulty cannulating the uterine arteries from a transradial approach in patients over 5 feet 10 inches [13]. In taller patients, using a microcatheter in combination with a 4 Fr catheter can be helpful when the length of a base catheter alone is inadequate.

Although there have been zero published cases in the literature, a feared theoretical complication of transradial endovascular arterial intervention is stroke, particularly when embolic material is being utilized. Once embolic material has been injected through a catheter, it is essential to re-insert a wire through the catheter before pulling the catheter back over the aortic arch in order to prevent residual embolic material from entering the cerebral vasculature.

In patients with tortuous or variant anatomy, there are tools available to allow for successful fibroid embolization from a radial artery approach. If a uterine artery with a sharp-angled takeoff is encountered and unable to be catheterized with a guiding catheter, a microcatheter can be used, such as a Boston Scientific Direxion or Terumo Progreat microcatheter. In addition, if an ovarian artery provides dominant supply to patient's fibroid uterus, it can often be easily selected with a Terumo Optitorque Sarah Radial diagnostic catheter via radial access.

References

1. Ravina JH, Herbreteau D, Ciraru-Vigneron N, et al. Arterial embolisation to treat uterine myomata. Lancet. 1995;346:671–2.
2. Siskin GP, Shlansky-Goldberg RD, Goodwin SC, et al. A prospective multicenter comparative study between myomectomy and uterine artery embolization with polyvinyl alcohol microspheres: long-term clinical outcomes in patients with symptomatic uterine fibroids. J Vasc Interv Radiol. 2006;17:1287–95.
3. Mara M, Maskova J, Fucikova Z, et al. Midterm clinical and first reproductive results of a randomized controlled trial comparing uterine fibroid embolization and myomectomy. Cardiovasc Intervent Radiol. 2008;31:73–85.
4. Manyonda IT, Bratby M, Horst JS, et al. Uterine artery embolization versus myomectomy: impact on quality of life--results of the FUME (Fibroids of the Uterus: Myomectomy versus Embolization) trial. Cardiovasc Intervent Radiol. 2012;35:530–6.
5. Pinto I, Chimeno P, Romo A, et al. Uterine fibroids: uterine artery embolization versus abdominal hysterectomy for treatment--a prospective, randomized, and controlled clinical trial. Radiology. 2003;226:425–31.
6. Edwards RD, Moss JG, Lumsden MA, et al. Uterine-artery embolization versus surgery for symptomatic uterine fibroids. N Engl J Med. 2007;356:360–70.
7. Moss JG, Cooper KG, Khaund A, et al. Randomised comparison of uterine artery embolisation (UAE) with surgical treatment in patients with symptomatic uterine fibroids (REST trial): 5-year results. BJOG. 2011;118:936–44.
8. Goodwin SC, Spies JB, Worthington-Kirsch R, et al. Uterine artery embolization for treatment of leiomyomata: long-term outcomes from the FIBROID registry. Obstet Gynecol. 2008;111:22–33.

9. Hirst A, Dutton S, Wu O, et al. A multi-centre retrospective cohort study comparing the efficacy, safety and cost-effectiveness of hysterectomy and uterine artery embolisation for the treatment of symptomatic uterine fibroids. The HOPEFUL study. Health Technol Assess. 2008;12:1–248, iii.
10. Costantino M, Lee J, McCullough M, et al. Bilateral versus unilateral femoral access for uterine artery embolization: results of a randomized comparative trial. J Vasc Interv Radiol. 2010;21:829–35; quiz 835.
11. Resnick NJ, Kim E, Patel RS, et al. Uterine artery embolization using a transradial approach: initial experience and technique. J Vasc Interv Radiol. 2014;25:443–7.
12. Gjoreski A, Gjoreski J, Nancheva A. Uterine fibroid embolization via transradial versus transfemoral arterial access: technical results. Open Access Maced J Med Sci. 2019;7:579–82.
13. Nakhaei M, Mojtahedi A, Faintuch S, et al. Transradial and transfemoral uterine fibroid embolization comparative study: technical and clinical outcomes. J Vasc Interv Radiol. 2020;31:123–9.
14. Bishay VL, Biederman DM, Ward TJ, et al. Transradial approach for hepatic radioembolization: initial results and technique. AJR Am J Roentgenol. 2016;207:1112–21.
15. Mortensen C, Chung J, Liu D, et al. Prospective study on total fluoroscopic time in patients undergoing uterine artery embolization: comparing transradial and transfemoral approaches. Cardiovasc Intervent Radiol. 2019;42:441–7.
16. Terumo Medical Corporation. Progreat microcatheters. https://www.terumois.com/products/catheters/progreat.html, 2020.
17. Gorgulu S, Norgaz T, Karaahmet T, et al. Incidence and predictors of radial artery spasm at the beginning of a transradial coronary procedure. J Interv Cardiol. 2013;26:208–13.
18. Kotowycz MA, Johnston KW, Ivanov J, et al. Predictors of radial artery size in patients undergoing cardiac catheterization: insights from the Good Radial Artery Size Prediction (GRASP) study. Can J Cardiol. 2014;30:211–6.
19. Chen Y, Ke Z, Xiao J, et al. Subcutaneous injection of nitroglycerin at the radial artery puncture site reduces the risk of early radial artery occlusion after transradial coronary catheterization: a randomized, placebo-controlled clinical trial. Circ Cardiovasc Interv. 2018;11:e006571.
20. Pancholy SB, Bernat I, Bertrand OF, et al. Prevention of radial artery occlusion after transradial catheterization: the PROPHET-II randomized trial. JACC Cardiovasc Interv. 2016;9:1992–9.
21. Konstantatos AH, Kavnoudias H, Stegeman JR, et al. A randomized, double-blind, placebo-controlled study of preemptive oral oxycodone with morphine patient-controlled anesthesia for postoperative pain management in patients undergoing uterine artery embolization for symptomatic uterine fibroids. Cardiovasc Intervent Radiol. 2014;37:1191–7.
22. Noel-Lamy M, Tan KT, Simons ME, et al. Intraarterial lidocaine for pain control in uterine artery embolization: a prospective, randomized study. J Vasc Interv Radiol. 2017;28:16–22.
23. Yoon J, Valenti D, Muchantef K, et al. Superior hypogastric nerve block as post-uterine artery embolization analgesia: a randomized and double-blind clinical trial. Radiology. 2018;289:248–54.
24. Liu LB, Cedillo MA, Bishay V, et al. Patient experience and preference in transradial versus transfemoral access during transarterial radioembolization: a randomized single-center trial. J Vasc Interv Radiol. 2019;30:414–20.
25. Basile A, Rebonato A, Failla G, et al. Early post-procedural patients compliance and VAS after UAE through transradial versus transfemoral approach: preliminary results. Radiol Med. 2018;123:885–9.
26. Boston Scientific Corporation. Direxion and direxion HI-FLO torqueable microcatheters. https://www.bostonscientific.com/en-US/products/embolization/Direxion_and_Direxion_HI-FLO_Microcatheters.html, 2020.
27. Kaufman C. Currently available embolics for uterine fibroid embolization. Endovascular Today. https://evtoday.com/articles/2020-apr/currently-available-embolics-for-uterine-fibroid-embolization, 2020.

Chapter 14
Prostate Artery Embolization

Jason Gruener and Ardeshir R. Rastinehad

Introduction

Surgical techniques including prostatectomy and TURP have long been the traditional interventions for prostatic pathology, most commonly BPH, a condition which affects at least 50% of men above age 50 and 80% of men above age 70 [1], representing a significant source of morbidity and medical cost. Besides effects on quality of life, BPH can lead to complications such as urinary retention requiring catheterization, urinary tract infection, bladder stones/diverticula, and renal insufficiency.

Prostate artery embolization (PAE) was first described in several case series as early as the 1970s to treat hematuria originating from the prostate [2–5]. In 2000, DeMeritt et al. first reported significant improvement in lower urinary tract symptoms (LUTS) and decrease in prostate size following unilateral PAE in a patient who originally presented with refractory hematuria and acute urinary retention [6].

In 2010, Carnevale et al. reported the first two successful human cases of PAE performed specifically to treat urinary retention in the setting of BPH [7]. Over the past decade, an increasing number of case series, retrospective studies, prospective randomized clinical trials, and meta-analyses have been published not only evaluating the safety and technical feasibility of PAE but also comparing PAE with alternative BPH treatments. For example, a recent review of several notable PAE trials and meta-analyses found that PAE was an effective treatment for BPH with technical success ranging from 75% to 92.6% and clinical success ranging from 76.3% to

J. Gruener (✉)
Department of Diagnostic, Molecular and Interventional Radiology,
Icahn School of Medicine at Mount Sinai, New York, NY, USA
e-mail: jason.gruener@icahn.mssm.edu

A. R. Rastinehad
Department of Urology, Lenox Hill Hospital, Northwell Health, New York, NY, USA

A. M. Fischman et al. (eds.), *Transradial Access in Interventional Radiology*,
https://doi.org/10.1007/978-3-030-81678-0_14

93.3% [8]. Average International Prostate Symptom Score (IPSS) reduction at short-term follow-up ranged from 9.2 to 14.6 with standard technique PAE. Major adverse events were uncommon.

Radial artery access to perform PAE was first reported in a 2015 case series by Isaacson et al. [9]. 19 consecutive transradial PAE procedures at a single institution were retrospectively reviewed. Technical success was 100% and no major complications were reported. There were three minor access related complications in this series – two patients developed small forearm hematomas and one developed left forearm pain. The higher-than-expected rate of access related complications was attributed to the learning curve operators faced during their early experience with transradial access. A subsequent retrospective study in 2017 compared transradial or transulnar access versus transfemoral access for PAE [10]. There was no difference in technical success or adverse events, including those related to arterial access. Procedure time and fluoroscopy time were lower in the transradial/transulnar group.

The advantages of radial access specifically in the PAE population have not been well studied. However, many of the advantages documented for other patient populations undergoing transarterial procedures likely apply (Table 14.1) [11–15]. Additional potential benefits specific to PAE patients include decreased time to urination (due to the patient being able to stand immediately following the procedure) and increased technical success in certain patients due to more favorable angles when catheterizing the internal iliac and prostatic arteries from above.

In summary, current evidence suggests that in appropriately selected men with moderate to severe LUTS and BPH, transradial PAE is a reasonable treatment option [16]. PAE is minimally invasive with a high rate of 5-year clinical success, lack of need for hospitalization or Foley catheterization, and a favorable side effect profile. PAE may be particularly beneficial in patients who are unwilling or unable to undergo surgery, patients who do not desire a transurethral procedure, patients on anticoagulation, and patients seeking to preserve sexual function. PAE may also be especially beneficial in patients with very large prostates (>80 cm^3) [17–22], who may not be good candidates for TURP or minimally invasive transurethral therapies and might otherwise require open prostatectomy. PAE remains an effective treatment option for prostatic-origin hematuria [23, 24].

Table 14.1 Possible advantages of transradial access for PAE

Increased patient satisfaction
Patient perception as less invasive than transfemoral access
Decreased major vascular complications
Decreased post-procedure pain
Shorter time to ambulation
Shorter time to post-procedure urination
Shorter time to discharge
Decreased cost
Improved technical success in patients with challenging anatomy from a transfemoral approach

Disadvantages of PAE include treatment failure in a minority of patients at 1- and 5-year follow-up leading to repeat intervention. PAE is technically challenging and may not be feasible in some patients with severe atherosclerosis or tortuous vascular anatomy. PAE may be less effective in patients with small prostates <40 cm^3 [21]. Finally, unlike most BPH treatments, PAE requires ionizing radiation and intravenous contrast, precluding patients with severe renal insufficiency.

As for all patients, potential PAE candidates who present with LUTS require a comprehensive clinical evaluation in accordance with current guidelines. Alternative diagnoses (including prostate cancer) should be assessed for, and additional BPH treatment options (including medical therapy and transurethral therapies) should be discussed prior to scheduling the procedure. Though critical, details of this clinical workup are beyond the scope of this chapter.

Equipment List

- Fluoroscopy system with high resolution display screen and cone beam CT capability.
- Arm board for the patient's left arm.
- Standard sterile angiographic table including gown, gloves, towels, drape, gauze, ultrasound probe cover, connective tubing, 10 and 20 cc syringes, saline, heparinized saline, iodinated contrast (iopamidol; Isovue 300, Bracco, Milan, Italy).
- 1% Lidocaine.
- Micropuncture access kit.
- 4/5F hydrophilic radial access sheath.
- Medication solution of 3000 U heparin, 2.5 mg verapamil, and 200 μg nitroglycerin hemodiluted in 20 mL and injected slowly through the sheath sidearm immediately following access.
- Diagnostic catheter to catheterize the internal iliac arteries: 130 cm 5F glide-tip Berenstein (Penumbra; Alameda, CA) or 125 cm 5F vertebral (Cordis; Miami, FL).
- 180 cm 0.035″ Bentson guidewire.
- Angled tip microcatheters (1.7–2.4F depending on prostate artery diameter; at least 150 cm length) and microwires (0.014″ or 0.018″).
- Tuohy-Borst adapter.
- 3 cc and 1 cc Medallion syringes (Merit Medical, South Jordan, UT).
- Embolic particles: Embospheres (Merit Medical, South Jordan, UT) or Embozene Color-Advanced Microspheres (Boston Scientific, Marlborough, MA) or HydroPearl Microspheres (Terumo Corporation, Tokyo, Japan). We use 100–300 μm particles, as smaller particles are associated with greater IPSS score reduction following PAE at 1 year follow-up [25].
- Inflatable hemostatic arterial closure band (TR Band; Terumo Corporation, Tokyo, Japan).

- Optional: Microcoils 2–4 mm diameter × 4 cm (Boston Scientific Interlock, Terumo CX, or Penumbra microcoils, Alameda, CA).
- Optional: 150 cm balloon occlusion microcatheter (Sniper; Embolx, Los Altos, CA).
- Optional: automated vessel tracking software (EmboGuide; Philips Healthcare; Best, Netherlands) to facilitate prostate artery identification.

Procedural Overview and Technical Considerations

1. Pre-Procedure Setup

A fluoroscopy suite with cone beam CT capability should be chosen. The patient is positioned supine with his left arm directly at his side, supinated on an arm-board (Fig. 14.1); this setup allows for deft catheter and guidewire manipulation in a similar manner to PAE performed from a transfemoral approach. In this setup, a sterile table is placed at the operator's back. Alternatively, the patient's left arm may be positioned in 90 degree abduction, which can facilitate subsequent positioning for cone beam CT; the sterile table is then placed parallel to the abducted arm (Fig. 14.2). Periprocedural antibiotics, analgesia, and sedation are given.

2. Radial Access Considerations

The left radial artery is accessed in the typical manner, as described earlier in the text. Depending on patient anatomy, a variety of wires and catheters are often necessary (Fig. 14.3) for PAE; they must provide stability to traverse the curve of the

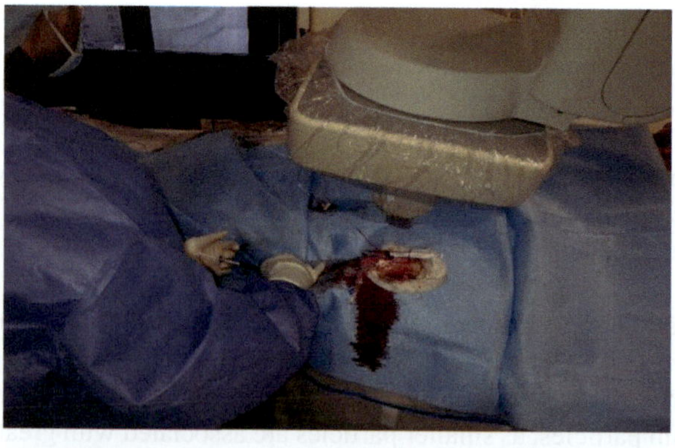

Fig. 14.1 Transradial PAE procedure. The left arm is located directly at the patient's side allowing for patient positioning similar to transfemoral access. A standard transfemoral angiographic drape is used. Note the presence of a 5F hydrophilic sheath in the radial artery with a side flush attached. A 155 cm microcatheter inserted into the left prostatic artery is nearly hubbed with approximately 15 cm of length external to the patient. The operator injects embolic particles through a 1 mL syringe under fluoroscopic guidance. Procedure table (not pictured) is at the operator's back

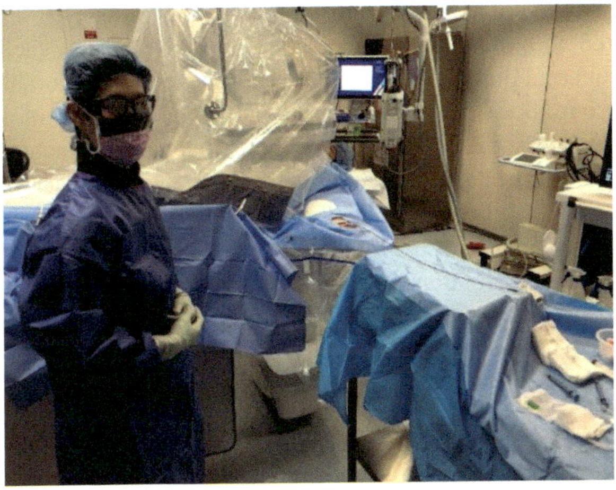

Fig. 14.2 Transradial PAE procedure with alternative table setup. The left arm is abducted 90° on an arm board in line with the procedure table. This position allows for easy positioning for cone beam CT imaging

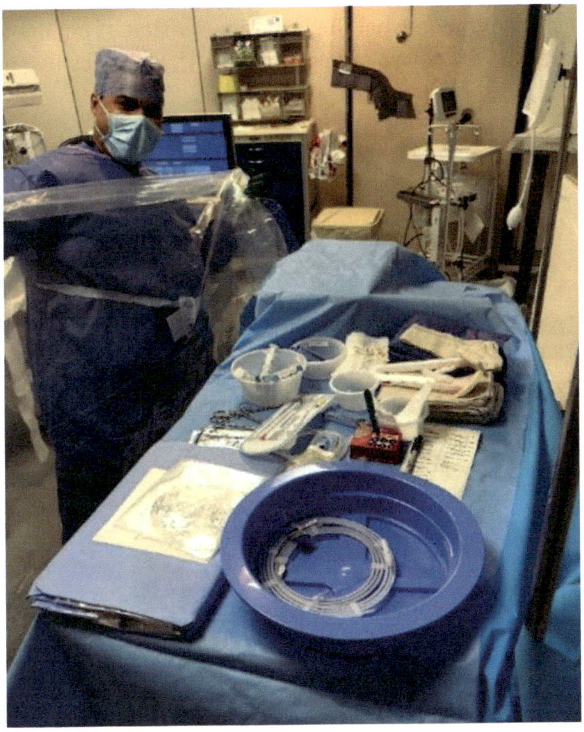

Fig. 14.3 Table setup for transradial PAE. The standard tools for transradial access, including micropuncture kit and 5F hydrophilic radial sheath, should be available. A variety of microwires and angled-tip microcatheters (minimum length 150 cm) should be close at hand; depending on the diameter and origin of the prostatic arteries, different catheters may be needed for successful cannulation. Notice the left front corner has a bumped up area to allow for a parallel working level to the radial puncture

thoracic inlet and be long enough to reach the prostatic arteries from the left wrist. When compared with transfemoral access, transradial PAE may facilitate catheterization of the internal iliac and prostatic arteries due to more favorable angles when approaching from above; this advantage is particularly helpful in patients with a more acutely angled aortic bifurcation, tortuous iliac arterial anatomy, and atherosclerotic disease, as is frequently encountered in older male patients with BPH. Given current catheter availability, transradial access for PAE may be challenging in tall patients due to insufficient catheter length. The tallest reported patient who underwent technically successful transradial PAE was 76 inches [9]. If necessary, a "high" radial artery access 5–10 cm proximal to the styloid process can be attempted; however, it is advisable to counsel tall patients on the increased risk of conversion to transfemoral access.

3. Identification and Selection of the Prostatic Arteries

The variable anatomy of the internal iliac and prostatic arteries makes PAE challenging for new operators. Understanding this anatomy is fundamental to performing technically and clinically successful embolization, reducing procedure time/radiation dose, and avoiding complications, particularly non-target embolization. Prostatic arteries are found bilaterally and most commonly (but not exclusively) arise from branches of the internal iliac anterior division. A common classification scheme, known as the Carnevale system (Fig. 14.4), describes five primary origins

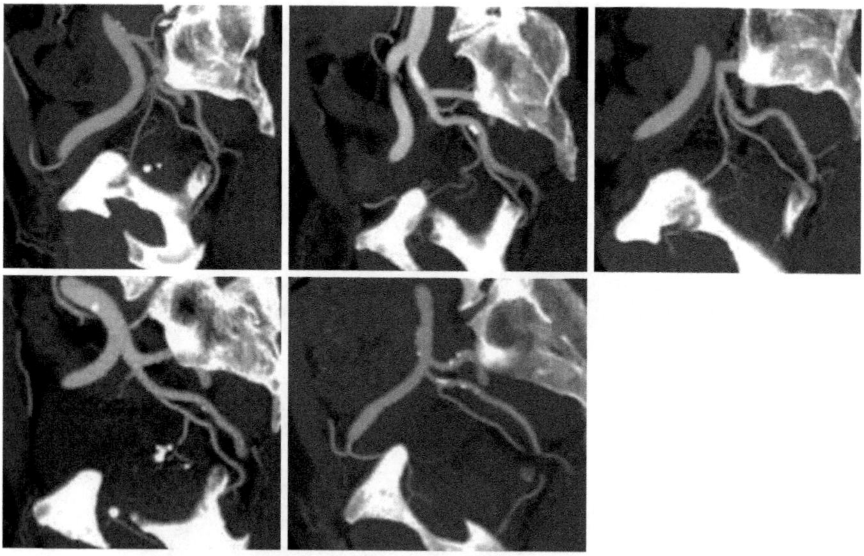

Fig. 14.4 Pelvic CTA from five different patients demonstrating the Carnevale classification [26] of prostatic artery origin (type I–V left to right). Type I – common trunk with superior vesical artery from internal iliac anterior division. Type II – separate origin inferior to the superior vesical artery. Type III – obturator artery origin. Type IV – Internal pudendal artery origin. Type V – other (in this case origin from replaced obturator off the external iliac artery). (Reprinted by permission from Springer Nature, Maclean et al., Copyright, April 2018 [27])

of the prostatic artery [26], with the most common origin being type IV (internal pudendal artery, 31.1%).

The 5F diagnostic catheter is advanced over the Bentson wire into the proximal left internal iliac artery. Digital subtraction angiography with 30–40° ipsilateral anterior oblique and 10° cranial angulation generally delineates the internal iliac branching pattern to best advantage. Different tube angulation can be selected based on preoperative vascular imaging findings. If available, automated vessel tracking software (in combination with cone beam CT) is sometimes helpful to identify the prostatic arteries (EmboGuide; Philips Healthcare; Best, Netherlands); use of this software has been associated with a lower PAE radiation dose [28]. If the prostatic artery is not identified on initial angiography of the internal iliac anterior division, angiography of the posterior division and external iliac arteries should be performed. Rarely, atherosclerosis may preclude identification of the prostatic artery despite a comprehensive search [26].

Once the prostate artery is identified, a microcatheter and hydrophilic microwire are advanced into the artery under fluoroscopic guidance. The prostatic arteries are tortuous and small in diameter, making catheterization challenging; multiple microwires or catheters may be required in difficult cases. We have successfully used microcatheters ranging from 1.7 to 2.4F depending on prostate artery diameter; however the length must be at least 150 cm and an angled tip may assist in cannulating the origin. The prostatic artery commonly divides into anteromedial and posterolateral pedicles which course cranially and caudally, respectively [29]. While both branches should ideally be embolized, the anteromedial pedicle primarily supplies the central gland and is the more important target for embolization; the posterolateral pedicle supplies mostly the peripheral zone and capsule.

Prostate artery angiography is performed to determine the appropriate catheter position for embolization and identify potential extra-prostatic anastomoses which might result in non-target embolization. Anastomoses to other pelvic arteries are common (Fig. 14.5) and may include vessels supplying the bladder, penis, rectum, and seminal vesicles [30]. Cone beam CT is advisable prior to embolization to confirm appropriate catheter position [31]. To best predict the flow dynamics during embolization, the injection rate during prostate angiography and cone beam CT should match the anticipated injection rate during embolization. Depending on the flow patterns identified, various techniques may be employed to prevent non-target embolization, including coil embolization of non-target branches [32], vasodilator injection [33], and balloon occlusion [34, 35].

Setting up for cone beam CT requires attention to patient positioning to avoid dislodgement of wires and catheters. If using the "left arm adduction" position for radial access, the left arm should be tucked against the patient's side and all wires/catheters secured to prevent contact with the image intensifier as the C-arm rotates around the patient. This risk is minimized with cone beam CT systems that use an open trajectory. Alternatively, if using the "90-degree abduction position," the arm board should have already been placed in a position that allows for the clearance for the spin.

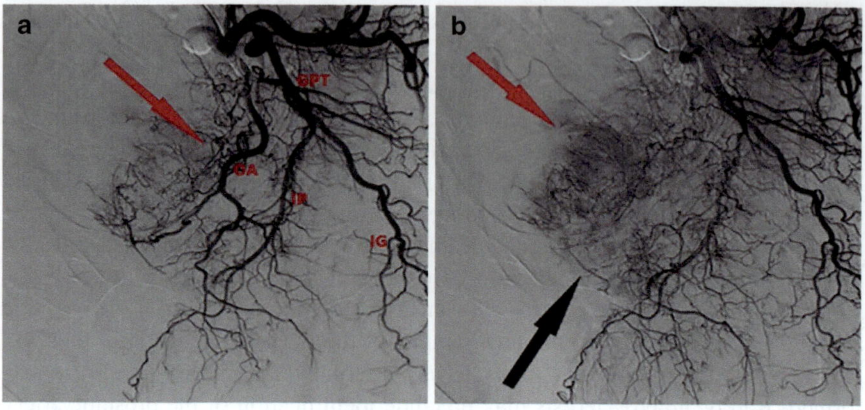

Fig. 14.5 (**a**) Left internal iliac artery angiogram performed from left radial approach, 30° ipsilateral oblique and 10° cranial angulation. Note the anatomy of the branches of anterior division. OA obturator artery, GPT inferior gluteal-pudendal trunk, IP internal pudendal artery, IG inferior gluteal artery. Red arrow – prostatic artery arising from the obturator artery. (**b**) More delayed phase left internal iliac angiogram from the same injection demonstrates contrast opacification of the left hemiprostate (red arrow). A small vessel is visible (black arrow) extending from the inferior left hemiprostate toward the internal pudendal artery representing a prostatic anastomosis

4. Embolization

Once microcatheter position is satisfactory and non-target branches have been accounted for, embolization is performed with particles. Technical success and safety with use of polyvinyl alcohol particles (PVA), trisacryl gelatin microspheres, and Polyzene-coated hydrogel microspheres of various shapes and sizes has been reported [36–38]. We prefer 100–300 μm particles, as smaller particle size is associated with greater IPSS score reduction following PAE at 1 year follow-up [25].

The desired embolization endpoint is near-stasis of blood flow when a suspension of particles in 50% dilute contrast is injected into the prostatic artery through the microcatheter under fluoroscopic guidance. Slow injection with a 1 mL syringe prevents early proximal occlusion and facilitates distal penetration of particles. Over-embolization beyond the point of stasis may result in reflux leading to non-target embolization. Post-procedure angiography is performed to identify accessory prostatic branches requiring embolization.

Although not yet widely practiced, our early experience suggests supplemental deployment of coils in the main prostatic artery following injection of particles leads to more complete embolization, more rapid relief of symptoms, and faster Foley catheter removal in patients with urinary retention. Detachable coils measuring 2–4 mm in diameter are generally appropriate. The primary disadvantage of coil deployment is loss of future access to the prostatic artery in the event LUTS recur and repeat PAE is desired.

The microcatheter is flushed and then removed, and the diagnostic 5F catheter is retracted into the abdominal aorta; the procedure is then repeated from the opposite side. Generally, a lower volume of embolic is required to reach near-stasis on the contralateral pelvic side due to the presence of left-right intraprostatic anastomoses [30].

5. Closure and Post-Procedure Care

After removal of all guidewires and catheters, the left radial artery is closed using an inflatable hemostatic band, as described in previous chapters. Once sedation wears off, patients may eat, ambulate, and void in the usual standing position. Non-steroidal anti-inflammatories (NSAIDs) and opiates may be given for pain relief, although post-procedural pain is typically absent or mild. Once patients void with post-void residual (PVR) <200 mL (or similar to their pre-procedure PVR) and the hemostatic band is removed, they may be discharged home. Discharge is usually 1–2 hours post-procedure, earlier than transfemoral PAE even with the use of a femoral artery closure device.

Prior to discharge, patients should be reminded of possible side effects including hematuria, dysuria, bladder spasm, hematospermia, and post-embolization syndrome resulting in fever and pelvic pain [39]. Most of these effects are mild and self-limited, typically resolving within 5 days. Patients should be counseled to call if they notice more serious adverse effects, such as tissue ulceration.

Patients are discharged with NSAIDs as needed for pain relief. They may also be given a proton pump inhibitor in the event of post-embolization syndrome and phenazopyridine for post-procedure dysuria. Some operators continue oral antibiotics for 1 week. Given the adverse effects associated with antibiotics and the relatively low rate of PAE-associated UTI, we do not routinely continue antibiotics unless the patient has UTI risk factors, in which case the patient may be discharged with trimethoprim-sulfamethoxazole. BPH medications may be stopped immediately following the procedure depending on the patient's clinical scenario, but by 1 month, the patient should be off his alpha blocker therapy.

A standard follow-up schedule calls for office visits at 1 month, 3 months, 6 months, and 12 months post-procedure [40]. Beyond 1 year, we prefer to see patients every 6 months. At all visits, the patient's symptoms are reassessed with the IPSS questionnaire. Patients should be asked about persistent side effects related to the procedure.

Although patient satisfaction following PAE is high, some patients may nevertheless require repeat interventions due to persistent or recurrent LUTS. In a study of 317 patients undergoing PAE, Carnevale et al. reported that 72 (23%) experienced recurrent LUTS at a median follow-up time of 72 months [41]. Treatment options in the setting of PAE failure may include resumption of BPH medications, minimally invasive transurethral therapies, TURP, open prostatectomy, and repeat PAE. Collaboration with a urologist can be helpful in this setting to determine optimal therapy.

Case Example

A 70-year-old male presented with LUTS and hematuria due to BPH for 1 month despite alfuzosin and dutasteride therapy. He endorsed nocturia (2 episodes nightly), urinary frequency (every 15 minutes), weak stream, and intermittent dysuria. IPSS score was 21. He recently was treated for a urinary tract infection and had an episode of urinary retention temporarily requiring a Foley catheter. PVR was increased

(177 mL) and peak urinary flow was decreased (8.2 mL/s). Prostate specific antigen (PSA) was elevated to 17.9 ng/mL, but stable over many years, and the patient had a history of multiple negative prostate biopsies. Prostate MRI revealed a gland volume of 173 mL without suspicious lesions. After discussion of treatment options in the setting of a massively enlarged gland, the patient opted for transradial PAE, which was technically successful. The patient noted improvement in his symptoms at short-term follow-up. Images from the procedure are shown in Fig. 14.6.

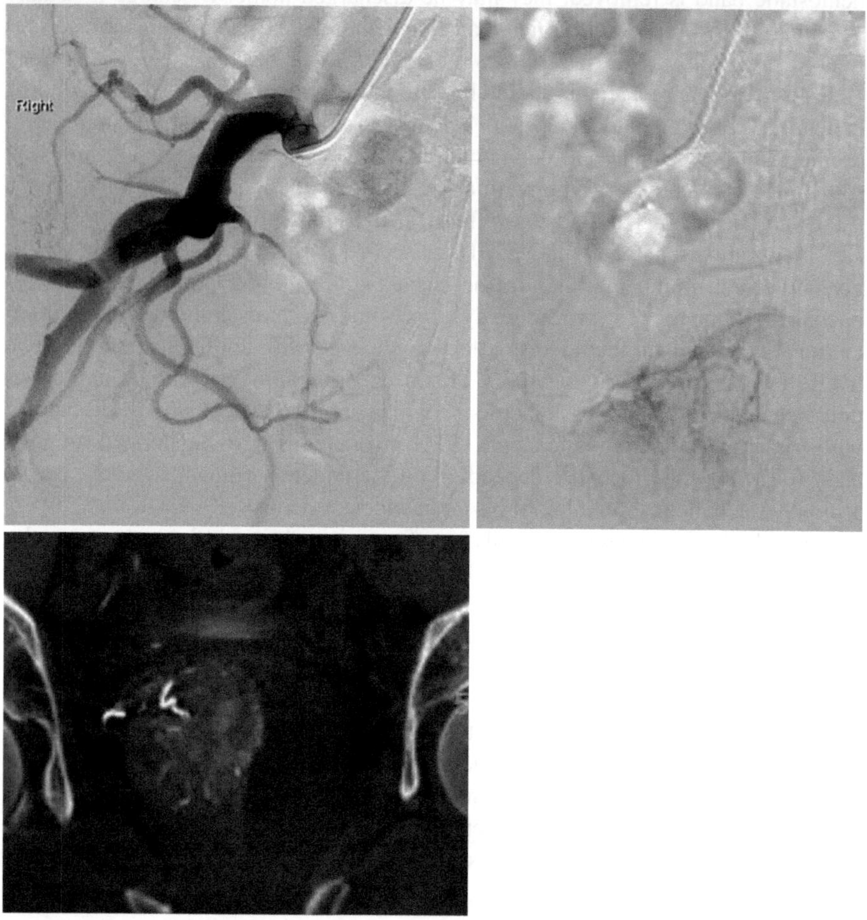

Fig. 14.6 Intra-procedural cone beam CT during PAE performed via transradial access. Top left: Digital subtraction angiography of right internal iliac artery anterior division (30° ipsilateral oblique, 10° cranial angulation). The right prostatic artery (arrow) arises off a common trunk from the anterior division with the inferior vesical artery. Top right: A microcatheter has been advanced into the prostatic artery. Delayed phase angiography demonstrates opacification of the right hemiprostate. Bottom: Contrast enhanced cone beam CT was performed from the same catheter position as on top right. Coronal image confirms complete opacification of the right hemiprostate without non-target opacification. Bilateral PAE was successfully performed with 100–300 μm particles and 2–3 mm diameter microcoils

References

1. Egan KB. The epidemiology of benign prostatic hyperplasia associated with lower urinary tract symptoms: prevalence and incident rates. Urol Clin North Am. 2016;43(3):289–97.
2. Mitchell ME, Waltman AC, Athanasoulis CA, Kerr WS, Dretler SP. Control of massive prostatic bleeding with angiographic techniques. J Urol. 1976;115(6):692–5.
3. Bischoff W, Goerttler U. Successful intra-arterial embolization of bleeding carcinoma of the prostate (author's transl). Urologe A. 1977;16(2):99–102.
4. Appleton DS, Sibley GN, Doyle PT. Internal iliac artery embolisation for the control of severe bladder and prostate haemorrhage. Br J Urol. 1988;61(1):45–7.
5. Li BC. Internal iliac artery embolization for the control of severe bladder and prostate haemorrhage. Zhonghua Wai Ke Za Zhi. 1990;28(4):220–1, 253.
6. DeMeritt JS, Elmasri FF, Esposito MP, Rosenberg GS. Relief of benign prostatic hyperplasia-related bladder outlet obstruction after transarterial polyvinyl alcohol prostate embolization. J Vasc Interv Radiol. 2000;11(6):767–70.
7. Carnevale FC, Antunes AA, da Motta Leal Filho JM, de Oliveira Cerri LM, Baroni RH, Marcelino AS, et al. Prostatic artery embolization as a primary treatment for benign prostatic hyperplasia: preliminary results in two patients. Cardiovasc Intervent Radiol. 2010;33(2):355–61.
8. Patel TV, Yu H, Isaacson AJ. Preclinical and clinical evidence for prostate artery embolization. In: Isaacson AJ, Bagla S, Raynor MC, Yu H, editors. Prostate artery embolization. Cham: Springer Nature; 2019. p. 71–82.
9. Isaacson AJ, Fischman AM, Burke CT. Technical feasibility of prostatic artery embolization from a transradial approach. AJR Am J Roentgenol. 2016;206(2):442–4.
10. Bhatia S, Harward SH, Sinha VK, Narayanan G. Prostate artery embolization via transradial or transulnar versus transfemoral arterial access: technical results. J Vasc Interv Radiol. 2017;28(6):898–905.
11. Liu LB, Cedillo MA, Bishay V, Ranade M, Patel RS, Kim E, et al. Patient experience and preference in transradial versus transfemoral access during transarterial radioembolization: a randomized single-center trial. J Vasc Interv Radiol. 2019;30(3):414–20.
12. Yamada R, Bracewell S, Bassaco B, Camacho J, Anderson MB, Conrad A, et al. Transradial versus transfemoral arterial access in liver cancer embolization: randomized trial to assess patient satisfaction. J Vasc Interv Radiol. 2018;29(1):38–43.
13. Iezzi R, Pompili M, Posa A, Annicchiarico E, Garcovich M, Merlino B, et al. Transradial versus transfemoral access for hepatic chemoembolization: intrapatient prospective single-center study. J Vasc Interv Radiol. 2017;28(9):1234–9.
14. Valgimigli M, Gagnor A, Calabró P, Frigoli E, Leonardi S, Zaro T, et al. Radial versus femoral access in patients with acute coronary syndromes undergoing invasive management: a randomised multicentre trial. Lancet. 2015;385(9986):2465–76.
15. Mamas MA, Tosh J, Hulme W, Hoskins N, Bungey G, Ludman P, et al. Health economic analysis of access site practice in England during changes in practice: insights from the British Cardiovascular Interventional Society. Circ Cardiovasc Qual Outcomes. 2018;11(5):e004482.
16. McWilliams JP, Bilhim TA, Carnevale FC, Bhatia S, Isaacson AJ, Bagla S, et al. Society of interventional radiology multisociety consensus position statement on prostatic artery embolization for treatment of lower urinary tract symptoms attributed to benign prostatic hyperplasia: from the Society of Interventional Radiology, the Cardiovascular and Interventional Radiological Society of Europe, Société Française de Radiologie, and the British Society of Interventional Radiology: endorsed by the Asia Pacific Society of Cardiovascular and Interventional Radiology, Canadian Association for Interventional Radiology, Chinese College of Interventionalists, Interventional Radiology Society of Australasia, Japanese Society of Interventional Radiology, and Korean Society of Interventional Radiology. J Vasc Interv Radiol. 2019;30(5):627–37.e1.

17. Bhatia S, Sinha VK, Kava BR, Gomez C, Harward S, Punnen S, et al. Efficacy of prostatic artery embolization for catheter-dependent patients with large prostate sizes and high comorbidity scores. J Vasc Interv Radiol. 2018;29(1):78–84.e1.
18. Bhatia S, Sinha VK, Harward S, Gomez C, Kava BR, Parekh DJ. Prostate artery embolization in patients with prostate volumes of 80 mL or more: a single-institution retrospective experience of 93 patients. J Vasc Interv Radiol. 2018;29(10):1392–8.
19. Wang MQ, Guo LP, Zhang GD, Yuan K, Li K, Duan F, et al. Prostatic arterial embolization for the treatment of lower urinary tract symptoms due to large (>80 mL) benign prostatic hyperplasia: results of midterm follow-up from Chinese population. BMC Urol. 2015;15:33.
20. Kurbatov D, Russo GI, Lepetukhin A, Dubsky S, Sitkin I, Morgia G, et al. Prostatic artery embolization for prostate volume greater than 80 cm3: results from a single-center prospective study. Urology. 2014;84(2):400–4.
21. Zhang JL, Wang MQ, Duan F, Yuan B. A comparative study of prostatic artery embolization in the treatment of benign prostatic hyperplasia with different prostatic volume. Zhonghua Yi Xue Za Zhi. 2019;99(31):2435–9.
22. Mathevosian S, Plotnik AN, McWilliams JP. Prostate artery embolization for giant prostatic enlargement: short-term efficacy and safety. J Vasc Interv Radiol. https://doi.org/10.1016/j.jvir.2019.06.021.
23. Rastinehad AR, Caplin DM, Ost MC, VanderBrink BA, Lobko I, Badlani GH, et al. Selective arterial prostatic embolization (SAPE) for refractory hematuria of prostatic origin. Urology. 2008;71(2):181–4.
24. Pereira K, Halpern JA, McClure TD, Lewis NA, Kably I, Bhatia S, et al. Role of prostate artery embolization in the management of refractory haematuria of prostatic origin. BJU Int. 2016;118(3):359–65.
25. Geevarghese R, Harding J, Parsons N, Hutchinson C, Parsons C. The relationship of embolic particle size to patient outcomes in prostate artery embolisation for benign prostatic hyperplasia: a systematic review and meta-regression. Clin Radiol. 2020;75(5):366–74.
26. de Assis AM, Moreira AM, de Paula Rodrigues VC, Harward SH, Antunes AA, Srougi M, et al. Pelvic arterial anatomy relevant to prostatic artery embolisation and proposal for angiographic classification. Cardiovasc Intervent Radiol. 2015;38(4):855–61.
27. Maclean D, Maher B, Harris M, Dyer J, Modi S, Hacking N, et al. Planning prostate artery embolisation: is it essential to perform a pre-procedural CTA. Cardiovasc Intervent Radiol. 2018;41(4):628–32.
28. Schott P, Katoh M, Fischer N, Freyhardt P. Radiation dose in prostatic artery embolization using cone-beam CT and 3D roadmap software. J Vasc Interv Radiol. 2019;30(9):1452–8.
29. Bilhim T, Tinto HR, Fernandes L, Martins Pisco J. Radiological anatomy of prostatic arteries. Tech Vasc Interv Radiol. 2012;15(4):276–85.
30. Bilhim T, Pisco JM, Rio Tinto H, Fernandes L, Pinheiro LC, Furtado A, et al. Prostatic arterial supply: anatomic and imaging findings relevant for selective arterial embolization. J Vasc Interv Radiol. 2012;23(11):1403–15.
31. Bagla S, Rholl KS, Sterling KM, van Breda A, Papadouris D, Cooper JM, et al. Utility of cone-beam CT imaging in prostatic artery embolization. J Vasc Interv Radiol. 2013;24(11):1603–7.
32. Bhatia S, Sinha V, Bordegaray M, Kably I, Harward S, Narayanan G. Role of coil embolization during prostatic artery embolization: incidence, indications, and safety profile. J Vasc Interv Radiol. 2017;28(5):656–64.e3.
33. Yu SCH, Cho C, Hung E, Wang D, Chiu P, Yee CH, et al. Case-control study of intra-arterial verapamil for intraprostatic anastomoses to extraprostatic arteries in prostatic artery embolization for benign prostatic hypertrophy. J Vasc Interv Radiol. 2017;28(8):1167–76.
34. Ayyagari R, Powell T, Staib L, Chapiro J, Schoenberger S, Devito R, et al. Case-control comparison of conventional end-hole versus balloon-occlusion microcatheter prostatic artery embolization for treatment of symptomatic benign prostatic hyperplasia. J Vasc Interv Radiol. 2019;30(9):1459–70.

35. Bilhim T, Costa NV, Torres D, Pisco J, Carmo S, Oliveira AG. Randomized clinical trial of balloon-occlusion versus conventional microcatheter prostatic artery embolization for benign prostatic hyperplasia. J Vasc Interv Radiol. https://doi.org/10.1016/j.jvir.2019.06.019.
36. Torres D, Costa NV, Pisco J, Pinheiro LC, Oliveira AG, Bilhim T. Prostatic artery embolization for benign prostatic hyperplasia: prospective randomized trial of 100-300 μm versus 300-500 μm versus 100- to 300-μm + 300- to 500-μm embospheres. J Vasc Interv Radiol. 2019;30(5):638–44.
37. Bilhim T, Pisco J, Campos Pinheiro L, Rio Tinto H, Fernandes L, Pereira JA, et al. Does polyvinyl alcohol particle size change the outcome of prostatic arterial embolization for benign prostatic hyperplasia? Results from a single-center randomized prospective study. J Vasc Interv Radiol. 2013;24(11):1595–602.e1.
38. Franiel T, Aschenbach R, Trupp S, Lehmann T, von Rundstedt FC, Grimm MO, et al. Prostatic artery embolization with 250-μm spherical polyzene-coated hydrogel microspheres for lower urinary tract symptoms with follow-up MR imaging. J Vasc Interv Radiol. 2018;29(8):1127–37.
39. Moreira AM, de Assis AM, Carnevale FC, Antunes AA, Srougi M, Cerri GGA. Review of adverse events related to prostatic artery embolization for treatment of bladder outlet obstruction due to BPH. Cardiovasc Intervent Radiol. 2017;40(10):1490–500.
40. Mouli S, Hohlastos E, Salem R. Prostate artery embolization. Semin Intervent Radiol. 2019;36(2):142–8.
41. Carnevale FC, Moreira AM, de Assis AM, Antunes AA, Cristina de Paula Rodrigues V, Srougi M, et al. Prostatic artery embolization for the treatment of lower urinary tract symptoms due to benign prostatic hyperplasia: 10 years' experience. Radiology. 2020;296(2):444–51.

Chapter 15
Hemodialysis Access Interventions

Timothy Carlon and Joseph J. Titano

Introduction

Hemodialysis access issues are a leading cause of morbidity and hospitalization in end stage renal disease patients, and current guidelines recommend vigilant care in maintaining adequate dialysis access in all chronic kidney disease stage V patients [1]. As a result, intervention is frequently needed on both an elective and urgent basis to maintain patent and fully functional dialysis circuits. Dialysis grafts and fistulas present a unique anatomic challenge for percutaneous intervention. Access approach needs to take into account the type of dialysis shunt, the site of the abnormality, and the nature of the malfunction. A standard approach is to access the dialysis circuit outflow directly via antegrade, retrograde, or a combined approach. Less commonly, antegrade access of the inflow artery is utilized although this approach can make post-procedure hemostasis difficult and access site complications have the potential to injure both the dialysis shunt and the vessels supplying the hand. Retrograde radial artery access – distal to the arteriovenous anastomosis – has been described for all major percutaneous dialysis access interventions and offers several unique advantages.

First, all parts of the circuit can be evaluated and treated from the same access. This is particularly valuable when the cause of abnormality is not known prior to angiographic evaluation as the source of failure can occur at the anastomosis, outflow, central veins, or occasionally the inflow artery. Radial access allows in-line work at any part of the shunt in most cases. Second, the fistula or graft itself does not need to be punctured or directly compressed to achieve hemostasis, so the process of obtaining hemostasis is unlikely to cause thrombosis of the dialysis shunt. Third, reflux angiography with outflow compression is not necessary to evaluate the anastomosis or inflow artery. This reduces the risk of clot reflux into the arteries

T. Carlon (✉) · J. J. Titano
Department of Diagnostic, Molecular and Interventional Radiology,
Icahn School of Medicine at Mount Sinai, New York, NY, USA

A. M. Fischman et al. (eds.), *Transradial Access in Interventional Radiology*,
https://doi.org/10.1007/978-3-030-81678-0_15

when evaluating a thrombosed circuit and also theoretically increases the distance between the operator and the fluoroscopy equipment, reducing radiation exposure.

The primary limitation to radial access is sheath size, which constrains the equipment that can be introduced for intervention. As a result, treatment of central lesions may not be feasible without an additional antegrade access. Additional disadvantages include complications of radial artery access such as spasm, dissection, or occlusion. As long as the integrity of the ulnar artery and palmar arch is confirmed, such complications should not result in hand ischemia.

Generally, dialysis interventions can be divided into two categories: (1) access dysfunction, which can mean primary failure to mature or difficulty completing adequate dialysis sessions with a previously functional graft, and (2) access failure, typically due to acute thrombosis. While technique is similar and both can be treated via transradial access, they present unique challenges and reported results vary.

Dysfunction (Case 1) and Non-maturation (Cases 2 and 3)

Failure to mature is seen is as many as 30% of autogenous fistulas, and endovascular intervention can be an effective therapy in these cases, particularly when the cause is a focal stenosis [2, 3]. Often the culprit lesion is located at the arteriovenous anastomosis either alone or in combination with additional outflow stenosis [4]. These lesions are uniquely amenable to retrograde transradial access as it both allows excellent visualization of the lesion and eliminates the need to pass wires in a "u-turn" around the anastomosis. As a result, patient and operator positioning are simplified. Liang et al. also note that the radial approach is beneficial when the anastomosis is completely obliterated as the outflow vessel is both small and likely thrombosed, increasing the difficulty of a traditional transvenous approach [5].

Success is defined using the SIR reporting standards. Anatomic success is defined as <30% residual stenosis, and clinical success as at least one complete dialysis session via the access following intervention. Primary patency is access patency following the initial intervention until any additional thrombosis or intervention. Secondary patency is patency following any additional interventions [6].

In the limited primary studies, anatomic success rates between 61% and 100% have been reported, and clinical success rates range from 84% and 100%. Primary patency rates at 12 months have ranged from 33% to 64% and secondary patency from 63% to 90% [2, 7–13]. While no studies to date have directly compared efficacy, these numbers are consistent with those reported for standard percutaneous methods [5, 11].

Acute Circuit Thrombosis (Case 4)

Acute thrombosis of a fistula or graft interrupts a patient's normal dialysis schedule and can often result in emergency intervention or hospitalization [1]. These cases can be challenging, and when approaching them, the choice of access site should take into account minimization of procedure time and procedure-related complications, working in-line at site of intervention, and limiting disruption of a regular dialysis schedule. By working from a transradial access, the entire length of the outflow can be addressed in-line and from a single access. Furthermore, thrombus is unlikely to be pushed into the arterial circulation as reflux angiography is not required. Finally, there is no need to compress the outflow, risking repeat thrombosis, in order to achieve hemostasis.

Of note, a 7 Fr sheath may be necessary for mechanical or aspiration thrombectomy, larger than what is typically used for radial access [14]. However, larger sheaths are occasionally required for coronary interventions, and limited data suggests their safety for transradial intervention [15, 16]. In addition, there are sheaths presently available with the outer diameter of a traditional 6 Fr sheath that accommodate 7 Fr catheters and devices.

In the limited primary studies, anatomic success rates between 46% and 100% have been reported, and clinical success rates between 79% and 100%. Primary patency rates at 12 months have ranged from 40% to 52% [8–11, 13, 14, 17–19].

Our Technique

The procedure at our institutions is as follows. A Barbeau type A, B, or C waveform is documented prior to transradial access. Percutaneous access is then obtained under real-time ultrasound guidance using an echogenic 21 gauge needle and a 5, 6, or 7 Fr hydrophilic Glidesheath (Terumo, Tokyo, Japan) depending on the intended intervention. A radial access cocktail of 3000 U of heparin, 0.2 mg of nitroglycerin, and 2.5 mg of verapamil is administered slowly through the arterial sheath following hemodilution.

If the anastomosis is sufficiently distal as in the case of a radiocephalic fistula, then the initial angiography can be performed directly via the sheath without accessing the anastomosis. Otherwise a 4 or 5 Fr catheter is advanced over a 0.035″ wire to the level of the inflow artery, and angiography is performed. Following angiography, the anastomosis is crossed with a hydrophilic wire. For distal radiocephalic shunts, it is necessary to retract the access sheath such that the anastomosis can be accessed readily; the access sheath should be fixed in place with a transparent film dressing. If angioplasty of the inflow artery is necessary, it is typically performed prior to crossing the anastomosis.

For thrombosed fistulas and grafts, we administer 4–8 mg of alteplase directly into the thrombosed segment depending on the thrombus burden, and additional balloon maceration or mechanical thrombectomy is performed as necessary. Balloons up to 10 mm diameter can be introduced through a 6 Fr sheath, so central stenosis can be treated in most cases (Case 4).

A TR band (Terumo, Tokyo, Japan) is used for sheath removal and compression of the access site. If the presence of the fistula prevents appropriate positioning of the TR band, manual compression is used following sheath removal and a compressive dressing is applied. The fistula is not compressed at any point while obtaining hemostasis.

Practical Tips

1. Access – No consensus on patient eligibility for radial access of hemodialysis circuits exists, and numerous criteria have been referenced in the literature. Several authors relied on a normal Allen's test plus a palpable radial artery to identify suitable vessels [8, 10, 11]. Radial artery diameter larger than 2 mm without further evaluation has been proposed as an alternative criterion for transradial access [7]. Others have noted the presence of the anastomosis within 2 cm of the radial styloid as a contraindication because it limits sheath placement [2, 20]. As discussed in Chap. 2, at our institution, we perform a Barbeau test prior to all radial access and choose an alternative access site if a type D waveform is observed. Otherwise, we have no absolute contraindications.
2. Adjunctive medication – After obtaining access, numerous radial access cocktails consisting of heparin, nitroglycerin, and/or verapamil have been described, with some groups varying their approach based on the indication. For example, Wang and Yang administered heparin only for occluded fistulas, and Wu et al. gave nitroglycerin only if spasm was encountered [13, 19].
3. Crossing an occluded anastomosis – For radiocephalic fistulas with a juxta-anastomotic stenosis, a buddy wire technique as described by Kawarada et al. may be helpful for crossing the lesion. A 0.025″ guidewire is left in the radial artery, while a second 0.014″ guidewire is passed alongside it and into the cephalic vein [9].
4. Closure – At the conclusion of the case, radial access obviates the need for direct compression of the fistula. Distal arterial access also makes compression easier relative to more proximal access where the vessels are deeper. Most operators use manual compression alone to achieve hemostasis, with as little as two minutes of compression being described as adequate in one report [19]. While we typically compress radial punctures with a TR Band when feasible, the location of the fistula may preclude appropriate placement of this device. A compressive dressing can be used following manual compression to ensure hemostasis.

Conclusion

Radial access is well-suited for evaluation of and intervention upon upper extremity dialysis circuits. It offers particular advantages in two situations: (1) intervention on a juxta-anastomotic stenosis, especially in the setting of multiple outflow vein stenoses, and (2) evaluation of a dysfunctional or thrombosed fistula when pre-procedural evaluation does not definitively localize the abnormality. In addition to general radial access risks including vasospasm and hand ischemia, the smaller sheaths required for radial access also constrain balloon size, limiting intervention options in the setting of a central stenosis and for some upper-arm grafts.

Summary of Primary Evidence

Citation	Dialysis access	Abnormality	Cases (patients)	Key reported outcomes	Complications
Kawarada [9]	Mature radiocephalic AVF	Dysfunction or occlusion	11 (11)	Anatomic success – 100% Clinical success – 100% Primary patency – 64% (6 months)	None reported
Wang [13]	Mature radiocephalic AVF	Dysfunction or occlusion	50 (49)	Anatomic success – 91% Clinical success – 93%	None reported
Lin [11]	Upper-arm AVF or AVG	Dysfunction or occlusion	165 (101)	Anatomic success – 90% Clinical success – 84%	7 (4.2%) distal embolism 9 (5.5%) localized extravasation
Wu [19]	Upper-arm AVG	Occlusion	101 (63)	Anatomic success – 87% Clinical success – 79%	8 (7.9%) arterial embolization 3 (3%) axillary vein extravasation
Chen [8]	Mature AVF	Dysfunction or occlusion	154 (131)	Anatomic success – 61% (46% when occluded) Clinical success – 84% Primary patency – 52% (12 months) Secondary patency – 90% (12 months)	1 (0.6%) venous extravasation
Hsieh [17]	Mature radiocephalic AVF	Occlusion	54 (54)	Anatomic success – 92% Clinical success – 92% Primary patency – 40% (12 months)	2 (3.7%) venous extravasation

Citation	Dialysis access	Abnormality	Cases (patients)	Key reported outcomes	Complications
Jeon [18]	Upper extremity AVG	Occlusion	7 (5)	Anatomic success – 100% Clinical success – 100% Primary patency – 60% (4 months) Secondary patency – 100% (4 months)	None reported
Wu [14]	Mature radiocephalic AVF	Occlusion	48 (48)	Anatomic success – 96% Clinical success – 96% Primary patency – 44% (12 months) Secondary patency – 89% (12 months)	2 (4%) venous extravasation
Hsieh [2]	Immature radiocephalic AVF	Non-maturation	51 (51)	Anatomic success – 96% Clinical success – 94% Primary patency – 51% (6 months) Secondary patency – 90% (6 months)	6 (12%) venous extravasation
Le [10]	AVF or AVG	Dysfunction or occlusion	55 (40)	Anatomic success – 88% Clinical success – 84% Secondary patency – 83% (12 months)	1 (1.8%) ruptured pseudoaneurysm
Rahmatzadeh [12]	Upper-arm AVF or AVG	Dysfunction	30 (30)	Anatomic success – 100% Clinical success – 100% Primary patency – 33% (12 months) Secondary patency – 63% (12 months)	None reported

Citation	Dialysis access	Abnormality	Cases (patients)	Key reported outcomes	Complications
Alsheekh [7]	Immature AVF	Non-maturation	44 (27)	Patency of fistula and radial artery – 100% (1 week)	25 (57%) outflow vein wall injury 4 (9%) venous extravasation 3 (6.8%) AVF spasm 3 (6.8%) intimal flap formation 2 (4.5%) puncture site hematoma

Cases

Case 1: 66-year-old male with a mature radiocephalic fistula having issues with low flow and clotting while on dialysis resulting in hospitalization for multiple missed sessions. Initial fistulogram (A) performed via the sheath revealed a juxta-anastomotic stenosis (black arrowhead) and an additional outflow vein stenosis (white arrowhead). Angioplasty was performed first of the radial artery (B) and then of the anastomosis and cephalic vein (C). Completion fistulogram demonstrated technical success (D). The patient was able to complete a full dialysis session via the fistula on the same day and was discharged the following morning.

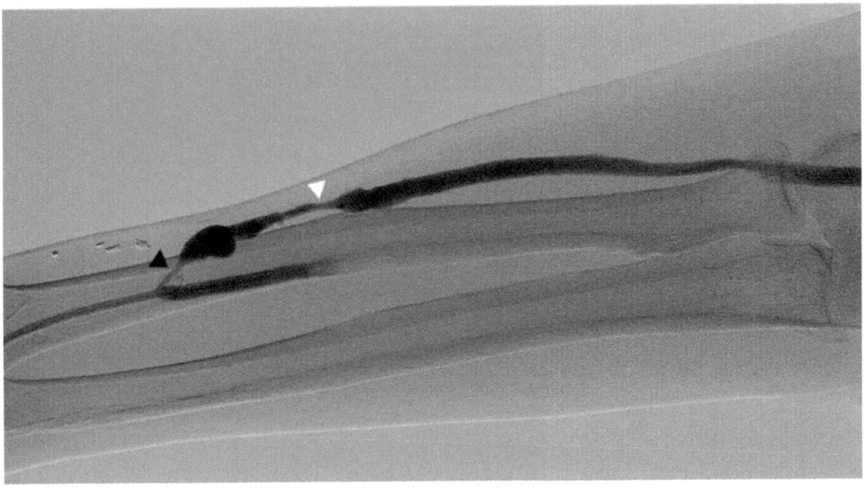

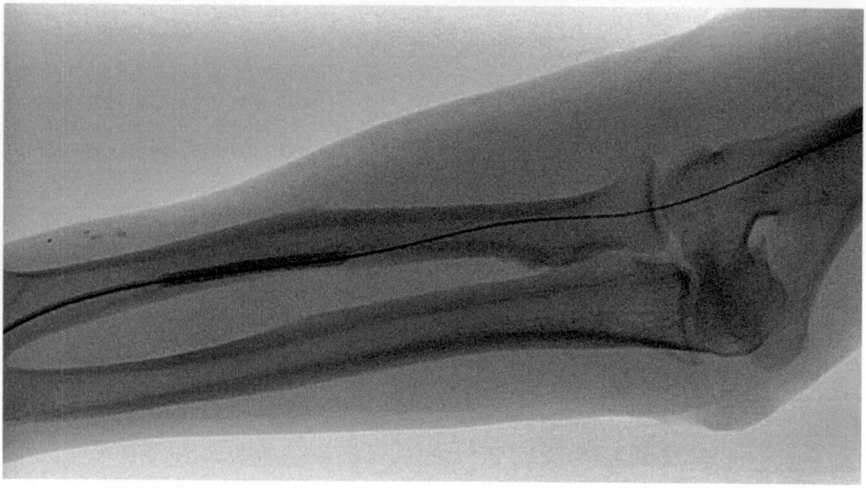

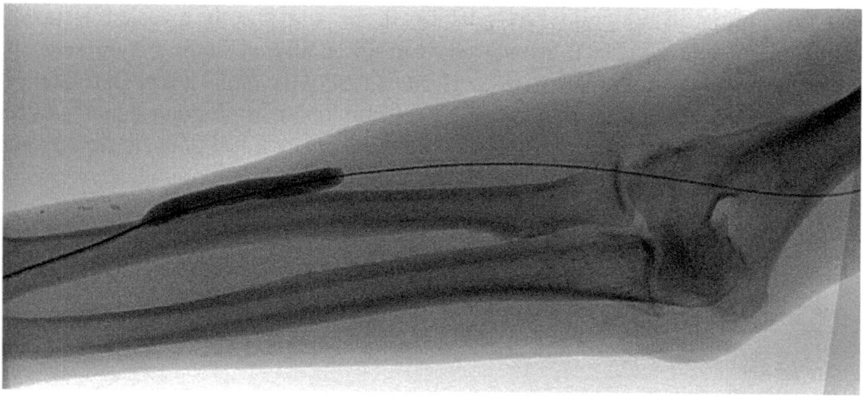

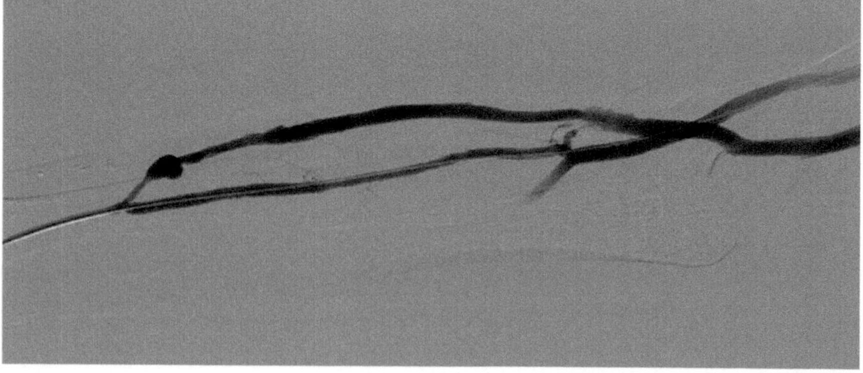

Case 2: 72-year-old male receiving hemodialysis via a tunneled catheter for the past 2 years. His radiocephalic fistula was non-maturing at 10 weeks after creation. Initial fistulogram performed via a catheter in the brachial artery demonstrated a diminutive radial artery and a juxta-anastomotic stenosis (A). The entire length of the radial artery was angioplastied (B), followed by the cephalic vein (C). Completion fistulogram performed via the sheath demonstrates improvement in the juxta-anastomotic stenosis (D). The patient initiated hemodialysis via the fistula 3 weeks after the intervention, and his tunneled catheter was removed 6 weeks following intervention.

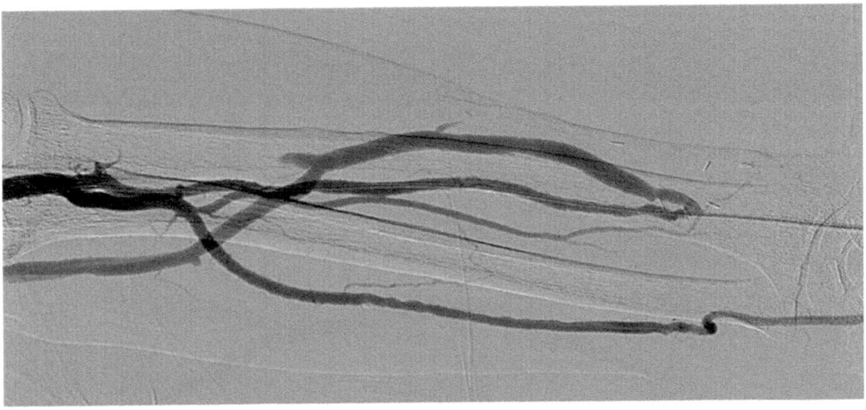

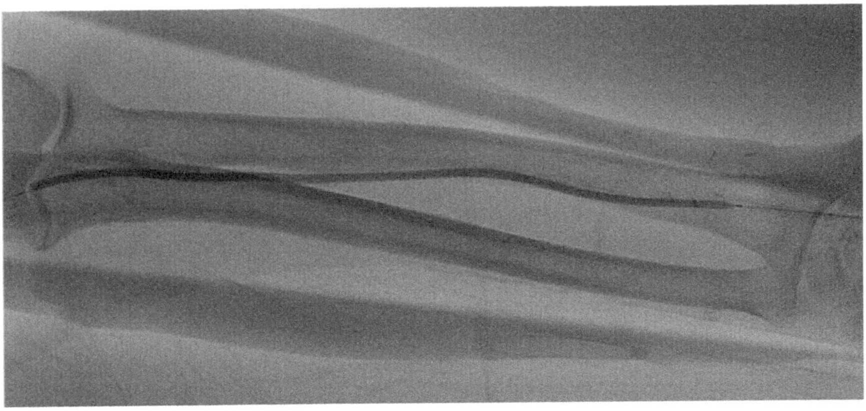

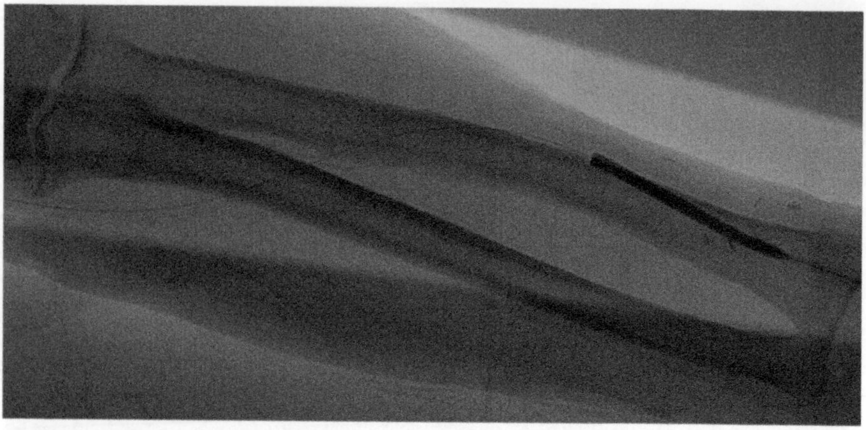

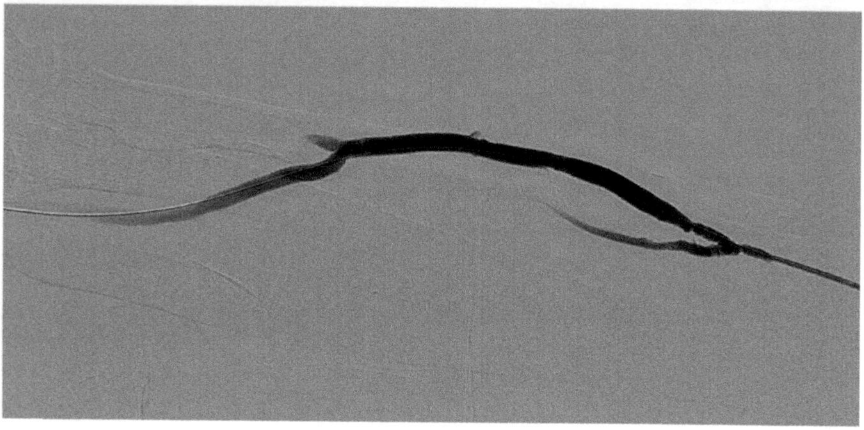

Case 3: 51-year-old male with a radiocephalic fistula created 6 months prior and never used. The patient had undergone one prior intervention for non-maturation. Initial fistulogram (A) demonstrated a single juxta-anastomotic stenosis, which improved following angioplasty (B and C). Doppler ultrasound 3 weeks post-procedure showed flows of 880 mL/min, increased from 362 mL/min pre-operatively.

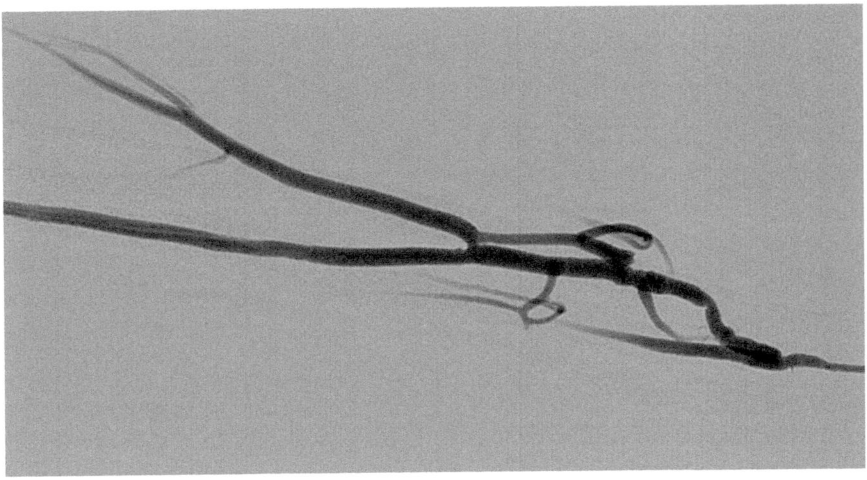

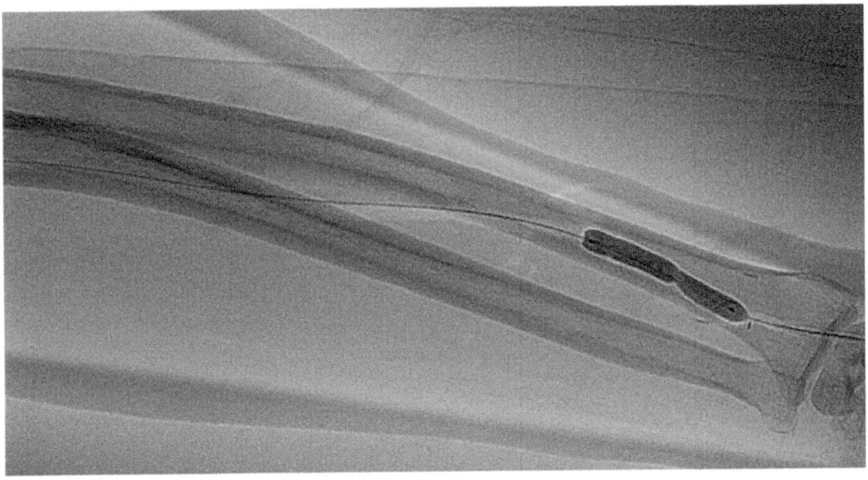

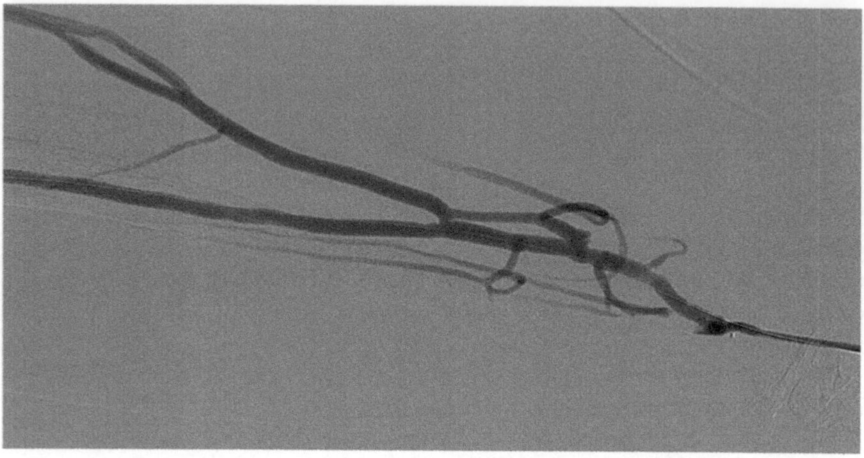

Case 4: 68-year-old female admitted with acute failure of a right upper arm graft. On initial evaluation, there was thrombus within both the graft and the outflow vein as well as extensive central venous collateralization (A). Following infusion of 4 mg TPA and mechanical thrombectomy with AngioJet, the graft was patent, but central occlusion persisted (B). Via the same 6 Fr radial sheath, two 12 mm central stents were placed and post-dilated with a 10 mm balloon (C). On completion fistulogram, the graft was patent (D), and the central venous collaterals were no longer visualized (E).

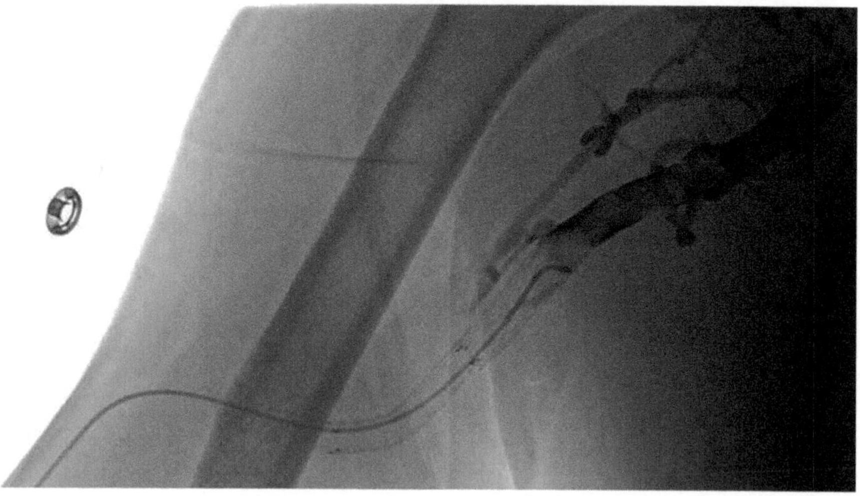

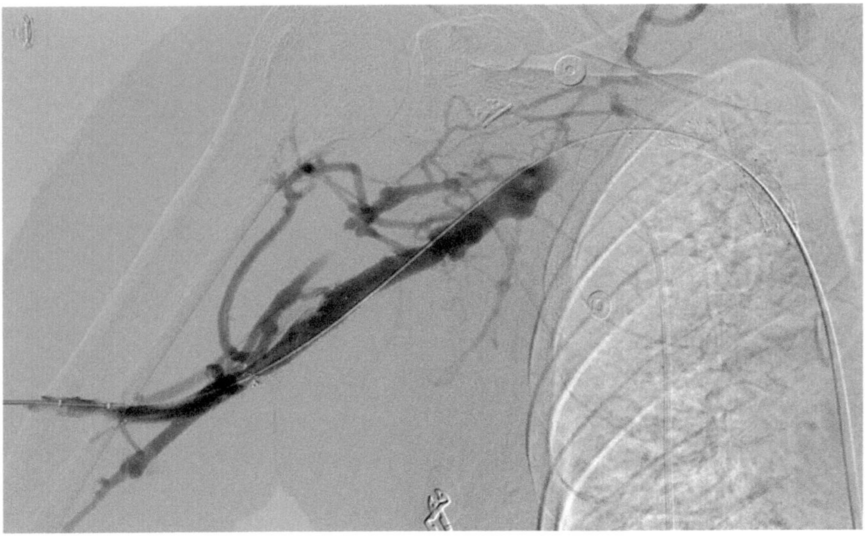

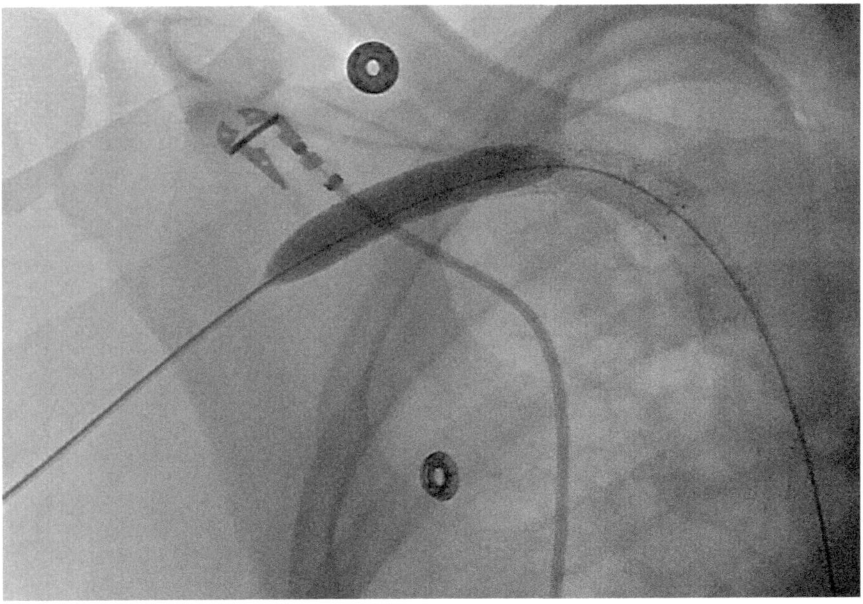

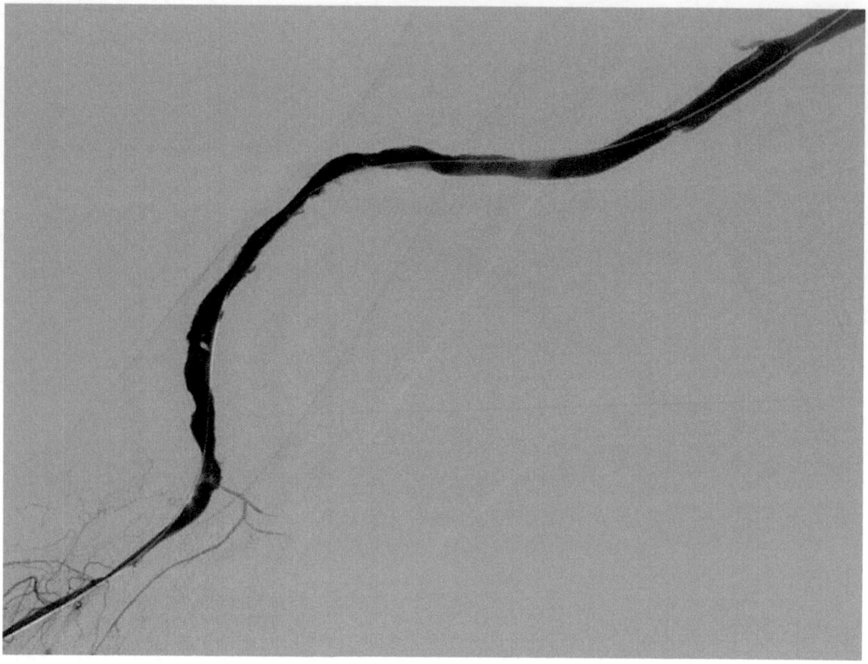

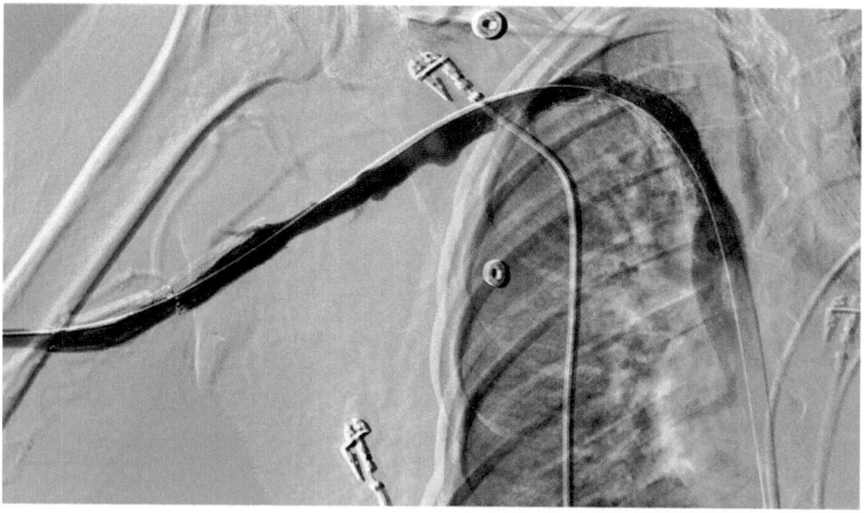

Bibliography

1. Vascular Access 2006 Work Group. Clinical practice guidelines for vascular access. Am J Kidney Dis. 2006;48(Suppl 1):S176–247.
2. Hsieh M-Y, Lin L, Tsai K-C, Wu C-C. Radial artery approach to salvage nonmaturing radiocephalic arteriovenous fistulas. Cardiovasc Intervent Radiol. 2013;36:957–63.
3. Miller PE, Tolwani A, Luscy CP, Deierhoi MH, Bailey R, Redden DT, Allon M. Predictors of adequacy of arteriovenous fistulas in hemodialysis patients. Kidney Int. 1999;56:275–80.
4. Beathard GA, Arnold P, Jackson J, Litchfield T, Physician Operators Forum of RMS Lifeline. Aggressive treatment of early fistula failure. Kidney Int. 2003;64:1487–94.
5. Liang H-L, Fu J-H, Wang P-C, Chen MC-Y, Wang C-C, Lin Y-H, Pan H-B. Endovascular salvage of immature autogenous hemodialysis fistulas. Cardiovasc Intervent Radiol. 2014;37:671–8.
6. Gray RJ, Sacks D, Martin LG, Trerotola SO. Reporting standards for percutaneous interventions in dialysis access. J Vasc Interv Radiol. 1999;10:1405–15.
7. Alsheekh A, Hingorani A, Aurshina A, Kibrik P, Chait J, Ascher E. Early results of duplex-guided transradial artery fistuloplasties. Ann Vasc Surg. 2019. https://doi.org/10.1016/j.avsg.2019.02.036.
8. Chen S-M, Hang C-L, Yip H-K, Fang C-Y, Wu C-J, Yang C-H, Hsieh Y-K, Guo GB-F. Outcomes of interventions via a transradial approach for dysfunctional Brescia-Cimino fistulas. Cardiovasc Intervent Radiol. 2009;32:952–9.
9. Kawarada O, Yokoi Y, Nakata S, Morioka N, Takemoto K. Transradial intervention for native fistula failure. Catheter Cardiovasc Interv. 2006;68:513–20.
10. Le L, Brooks A, Donovan M, Smith TA, Sternbergh WC 3rd, Bazan HA. Transradial approach for percutaneous intervention of malfunctioning arteriovenous accesses. J Vasc Surg. 2015;61:747–53.
11. Lin Y-S, Lin P-C, Hsu J-T, Chang S-T, Yang T-Y, Cheng H-W, Chung C-M. Feasibility of trans-radial approach in percutaneous intervention for upper arm dialysis access. Semin Dial. 2008;21:567–74.
12. Rahmatzadeh M, Vijayan V, Ritter CJ, Hockley J, Leong BD, Sandford M, Mwipatayi BP. Transradial approach for challenging vascular access interventions. Vascular. 2015;23:374–81.
13. Wang H-J, Yang Y-F. Percutaneous treatment of dysfunctional Brescia-Cimino fistulae through a radial arterial approach. Am J Kidney Dis. 2006;48:652–8.
14. Wu C-C, Wen S-C, Chen M-K, Yang C-W, Pu S-Y, Tsai K-C, Chen C-J, Chao C-H. Radial artery approach for endovascular salvage of occluded autogenous radial-cephalic fistulae. Nephrol Dial Transplant. 2009;24:2497–502.
15. Aminian A, Iglesias JF, Van Mieghem C, Zuffi A, Ferrara A, Manih R, Dolatabadi D, Lalmand J, Saito S. First prospective multicenter experience with the 7 French Glidesheath slender for complex transradial coronary interventions. Catheter Cardiovasc Interv. 2017;89:1014–20.
16. Tumscitz C, Pirani L, Tebaldi M, Campo G, Biscaglia S. Seven French radial artery access for PCI: a prospective single-center experience. Int J Cardiol. 2014;176:1074–5.
17. Hsieh L-C, Wang H-J, Chen Y-P, Lin J-J, Lee H, Lo P-H. Radial arterial approach with adjunctive urokinase for treating occluded autogenous radial-cephalic fistulas. Cardiovasc Intervent Radiol. 2009;32:1202–8.
18. Jeon UB, Kim CW, Chung SW. Percutaneous treatment of thrombosed prosthetic brachial-basilic access by the transradial approach. J Vasc Surg. 2009;49:1057–9.
19. Wu L-S, Lin Y-S, Chung C-M, Hsu J-T, Chang S-T, Yang T-Y, Chen H-W, Kuo C-T, Lin P-C. Percutaneous trans-radial intervention for acute thrombosis of upper arm grafts: an outpatient-based, effective, and feasible option. Acta Cardiologica Sinica. 2008;24:86–91.
20. Lai C-C, Fang H-C, Lin C-H, Mar G-Y, Tseng C-J, Liu C-P. Distal radial artery pressures predict angiographic result and short-term patency outcome in hemodialysis patients with juxta-anastomotic inflow stenosis of radiocephalic fistula undergoing transradial angioplasty. Ther Apher Dial. 2013;17:311–8.

Bibliography

1. Vascular Access 2006 Work Group. Clinical practice guidelines for vascular access. Am J Kidney Dis. 2006;48(Suppl 1):S176–247.
2. Hsieh M-Y, Lin L, Tsai K-C, Wu C-C. Radial artery approach to salvage nonmaturing radiocephalic arteriovenous fistulas. Cardiovasc Intervent Radiol. 2013;36:957–63.
3. Miller PE, Tolwani A, Luscy CP, Deierhoi MH, Bailey R, Redden DT, Allon M. Predictors of adequacy of arteriovenous fistulas in hemodialysis patients. Kidney Int. 1999;56(1):275–80.
4. Beathard GA, Arnold P, Jackson J, Litchfield T; Physician Operators Forum of RMS Lifeline. Aggressive treatment of early fistula failure. Kidney Int. 2003;64:1487–94.
5. Chan H-L, Liu J-R, Wang P-C, Chen M-Y, Wang X-C, Lin C-H, Lin H-B. Endovascular salvage of nonmaturing fistulas in hemodialysis patients. Cardiovasc Intervent Radiol. 2011;...

Chapter 16
Carotid and Vertebral Intervention

Reade De Leacy, Devin V. Bageac, Brett Marinelli, Sayan Manna, and J. Mocco

Abbreviations

CAS	Carotid artery stenting
CEA	Carotid endarterectomy
CT	Computed tomography
CTA	Computed tomography angiogram
DSA	Digital subtraction angiography
DWI	Diffusion weighted imaging
FMD	Fibromuscular dysplasia
ICA	Internal carotid artery
MRI	Magnetic resonance imaging
PA	Posteroanterior
PTA	Percutaneous transluminal angioplasty
TF	Transfemoral
TR	Transradial
VA	Vertebral artery
VAS	Vertebral artery stenting

Introduction

Carotid artery stenting (CAS) has steadily grown in popularity since the early 2000s, as a series of randomized trials have shown that the procedure confers long-term benefits similar to carotid endarterectomy (CEA) in appropriately selected patients [2, 9, 10, 13]. Vertebral artery stenting (VAS), though less well supported than CAS, is also performed in patients meeting select criteria. Over the past decade, evidence has grown to support the use of the transradial (TR) approach. Benefits of

R. De Leacy (✉) · D. V. Bageac · B. Marinelli · S. Manna · J. Mocco
Departments of Neurosurgery and Diagnostic, Molecular and Interventional Radiology, Icahn School of Medicine at Mount Sinai, New York, NY, USA
e-mail: reade.deleacy@mountsinai.org; devin.bageac@mountsinai.org; brett.marinelli@mountsinai.org; sayan.manna@icahn.mssm.edu; j.mocco@mountsinai.org

A. M. Fischman et al. (eds.), *Transradial Access in Interventional Radiology*,
https://doi.org/10.1007/978-3-030-81678-0_16

this approach include fewer access site complications and, in select cases, avoidance of tortuous anatomy when navigating to the target lesion. This chapter aims to guide the reader through the utilization of TR access in carotid and vertebral artery interventions first by explaining the basics of arch navigation and relevant equipment, followed by four illustrative cases.

Recent studies have demonstrated that, compared to transfemoral (TF) access, transradial CAS has similar rates of procedural success, and similar or fewer access-site complications, myocardial infarctions, and strokes [6, 11, 14]. Depending on proceduralist experience, fluoroscopy time and total procedure time may also be shorter [6, 11, 14]. Table 16.1 briefly summarizes results of notable case series evaluating the safety and efficacy of transradial CAS. Through multiple case series, transfemoral VAS has demonstrated similar safety outcomes [4, 6, 8, 12, 16]. The four cases presented in this chapter offer examples of how the TR approach might be used to access the vertebral and common carotid arteries for intervention.

Before deciding on a TR approach for supra-aortic neuro-interventions, the anatomy of the aortic arch should be thoroughly examined on pre-procedural cross-sectional imaging.

Due to branch vessel angulation, types II, III, and the bovine variant are challenging to access from a TF approach and have been associated with increased fluoroscopy time, contrast dose, stroke risk, and procedural failure [1, 15]. TR access allows for negotiation of these complex configurations, particularly the bovine variant (see "Left ICA Primary Stenting"), in which inferior support for sheaths can be provided by the initial horizontal segment of the left common carotid artery [5].

Table 16.1 Results of transradial CAS in selected cohort studies

Author	Year published	Sample size (n)	Mean age (years)	Procedural success rate	Complications
Folmar et al.	2007	42	71	83%	Stroke (1)
Pinter et al.	2007	20	72	90%	Symptomatic radial artery occlusion (1); severe pain at access site (1)
Patel et al.	2009	20	65	80%	Transient ischemic attack (1)
Etxegoien et al.	2012	382	68	91%	Stroke (4); radial artery occlusion (1); death (1)
Lee et al.	2016	33	69	100%	Transient ischemic attack (1)
Mendiz et al.	2016	101	71	100%	Stroke (2), transient ischemic attack (1)
Gao et al.	2018	28	72	100%	Temporary bradycardia (3)
Iwata et al.	2019	26	72	100%	Transient ischemic attack (1)
Ruzsa et al.	2014	130	66	90%	Symptomatic radial artery occlusion (2), asymptomatic radial artery occlusion (8), forearm hematoma (2)

Due to the asymmetry of the aortic arch, the technique and laterality of the TR approach varies widely based upon patient anatomy and the vessel to be treated. Many clinicians prefer a default right radial approach due to a combination of convention (carried over from its use in coronary interventions) and support provided when cannulating common carotid ostia at acute angles [3, 11]. For vertebral interventions in common arch variants, an ipsilateral TR approach is utilized for straightforward access through the subclavian artery. These procedures can be performed from the patient's right side via left distal TR access, with the left hand resting comfortably near the patient's right hip.

Procedural failure with transradial CAS or VAS is due either to failed navigation of the catheter to the target vessel, or inadequate support in maintaining the position of the catheter system. For right-sided lesions, failure rates increase with steeper angulation between the right subclavian and right common carotid [7]. On the left, non-bovine arches have been shown to increase failure rates due to poor inferior support for catheter systems [5]. The cases presented here are intended to elucidate some of the techniques involved in avoiding these issues, in order to facilitate the use of TR access in these procedures.

Top Five Tips

1. Thorough evaluation of cross-sectional imaging evaluation of the neck and arch prior to any intervention.
2. Local injection of dilute perivascular nitroglycerine (50mcg) at the radial artery access site can aid in local vasodilation prior to micropuncture and initial glide sheath access.
3. Upsize to a 0.088″ sheath over a long exchange wire anchored at the subclavian artery.
4. Pair long (≥125 cm) selecting catheters coaxially with a long 0.088″ sheath to access the right or left common carotid arteries.
5. When advancing guide sheath to optimal location within the common carotid artery, maximize support using 0.038″ or stiff 0.035″ glidewire (≥180 cm) with wire tip positioned distally within either the occipital or internal maxillary artery.

Equipment List

With the exception of the stents themselves, the basic equipment lists are similar for TR CAS and VAS. These can be categorized according to the phase of the procedure during which they are employed.

- Access
  - Micropuncture access set and a 5/6-Fr slender sheath
  - 0.088″ guiding sheath or long reinforced 6Fr sheath

- Planning
  - ≥125 cm 5-Fr selecting catheter (e.g., Simmons or Berenstein select)
  - Exchange length 0.035″ Bentson or Amplatz wire
  - Selection of glidewires (≥180 cm 0.038″ and 0.035″ stiff)
- Intervention
  - Selection of balloon expandable stents for ostial disease or self-expanding nitinol stents for common carotid or internal carotid lesions
  - Embolic protection device
  - Selection of monorail PTA catheters in various lengths and balloon sizes
  - Selection of 0.014″ neurovascular micro-guidewires
- Closure
  - Radial puncture compression device

Arch Navigation

The fundamental techniques of arch navigation for supra-aortic vessel selection are common to all of the procedures discussed in this chapter, as well as those presented in Chap. 17. In the majority of cases, TR access allows for direct catheterization of the ipsilateral vertebral artery (VA). The same is true less frequently for right common carotid artery (CCA) or bovine origins that branch at shallow angles with respect to the catheter approach.

In most cases of TR access, the left and right CCAs can be selected using a Simmons 2 catheter after forming its shape in the ascending aorta. This can be achieved by advancing the guidewire into the descending aorta, and coaxially advancing the Simmons 2 such that the genu is located just distal to the origin of the innominate artery. The wire is then withdrawn proximal to the genu. The system is pinned and advanced as a unit such that the shape is formed with the elbow of the catheter in the inferior ascending aorta. Right innominate and left carotid arteries can then be selected.

In order to facilitate access to the left subclavian artery from a right TR approach, it is often advantageous to form shape of the Simmons 2 in the descending aorta, using the stepwise approach illustrated in Fig. 16.1. First, the catheter is navigated into the descending aorta and positioned with the genu of the catheter distal to the apex of the arch. Second, the guidewire is withdrawn proximal to the genu, and the catheter is rotated such that a loop forms distal to the wire. Third, the wire is then gently advanced, pushing the loop distally. As the loop is pushed, the natural curve of catheter causes the tip to invert, and the Simmons 2 shape is formed.

Though variations in technique may be required to accommodate individual patient anatomy, these basic techniques allow for successful supra-aortic vessel selection in the majority of cases, and serve as the basis upon which TR angiographic procedures in these territories are performed.

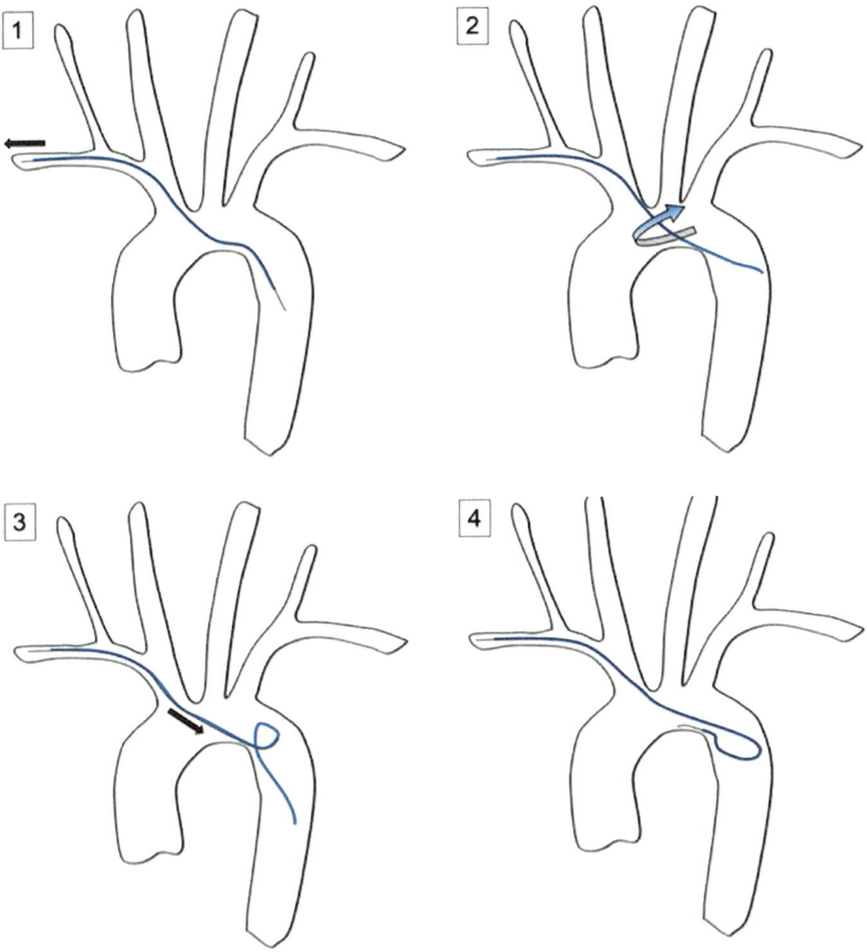

Fig. 16.1 Basic steps of Simmons 2 shape formation in the descending aorta

Right Vertebral Artery Origin Angioplasty and Stenting

Case Description

In order to illustrate a standard case of right vertebral artery stenting, consider the case of a 56-year-old man with history of hyperlipidemia and stroke who presented to clinic with intermittent episodes of left homonymous hemianopsia and left-sided weakness. MRI revealed ischemic changes compatible with watershed hypoperfusion in the right cerebrum and vertebrobasilar insufficiency. Cerebral angiography demonstrated extensive vascular disease including chronic occlusion of the right ICA and left VA, as well as severe stenosis of the dominant right vertebral artery. He underwent vertebral artery angioplasty and stenting. Special attention will be paid to the process of TR access, which will be referred back to in subsequent cases.

Procedure

Access Cardiopulmonary monitoring was placed, monitored anesthesia care was initiated, and a time-out was performed. The right wrist and both groins were prepped and draped in the usual sterile fashion. Using ultrasound guidance, the radial artery was localized and local anesthesia (1% Lidocaine) was infiltrated subdermally. Under continued ultrasound, a single wall puncture of the radial artery is performed at the level of the radial epiphysis on the volar radial surface.

Using modified Seldinger technique, a 5/6-Fr slender sheath was gently inserted into the radial artery and maintained on a heparinized flush. A radial artery access cocktail consisting of 3000 U heparin, 200 ug nitroglycerin, and 2.5 mg verapamil was mixed with 10 cc of the patient's blood and slowly infused through the sheath over 5–10 minutes to induce vasodilation. Throughout this infusion, the patient's vital signs were closely monitored for hypotension. Roadmapping of the radial artery was performed to evaluate for anatomic variations that may complicate catheter navigation.

Planning A 6-Fr guide catheter was carefully advanced over a 0.35″ Bentson guidewire through the right radial, brachial, axillary, and subclavian arteries. Weight-based dosing of intravenous heparin was administered. Angiography of the right subclavian artery demonstrated >80% stenosis at the origin of the right vertebral artery with evidence of flow limitation (Fig. 16.2a). Cerebral angiography revealed no abnormalities.

Intervention A 0.014″ microguidewire was used to traverse the stenosis at the origin of the right vertebral artery under fluoroscopic and roadmap guidance. A 5 mm × 12 mm balloon mounted stent was positioned at the level of maximal stenosis (Fig. 16.2b), and the balloon was carefully inflated to nominal pressures (Fig. 16.2c). The balloon was deflated, withdrawn, and reinflated at the proximal margin of the stent to flare it outward at the vessel ostium (Fig. 16.2d). Angiography demonstrated immediate marked improvement in vessel caliber and arterial flow through the right vertebral artery (Fig. 16.2e). Repeat cerebral angiography revealed no vessel occlusions. The catheters were removed, followed by the radial sheath, and hemostasis achieved with a compressive band. His neurologic exam remained unchanged from his pre-procedure baseline.

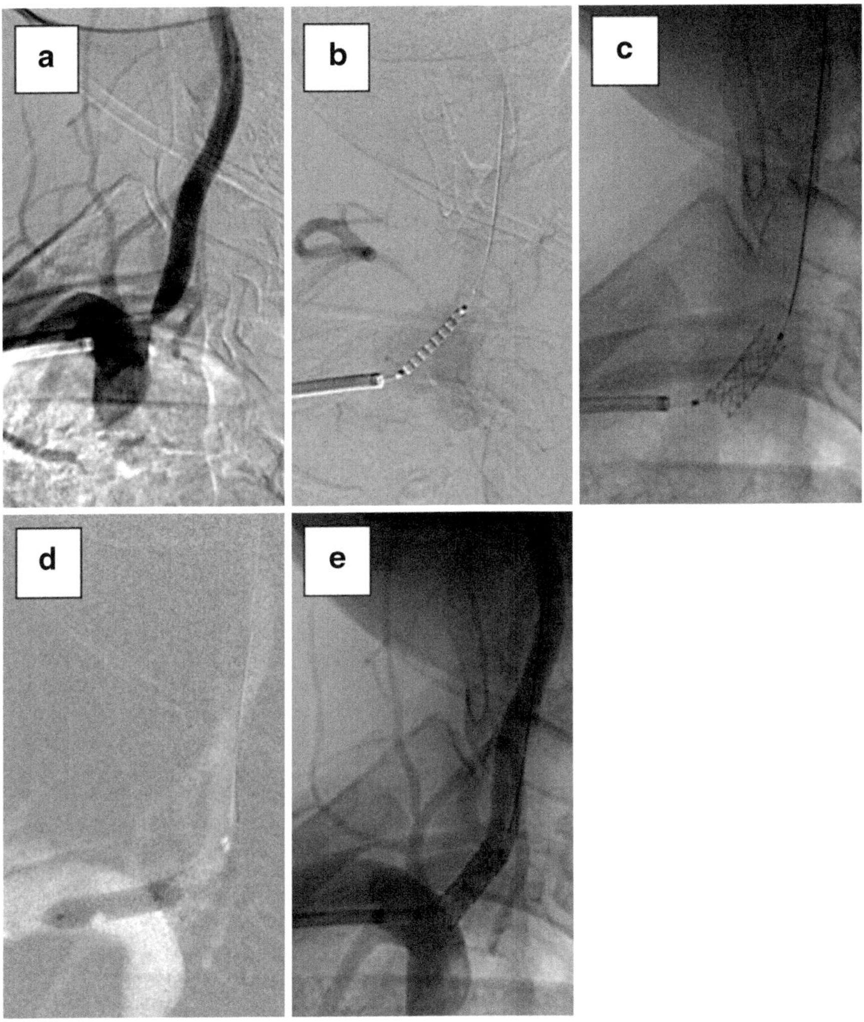

Fig. 16.2 (**a**) Arterial phase digital subtraction angiography (DSA), subclavian injection, working view demonstrates right vertebral ostial stenosis. (**b**) DSA taken after crossing the lesion with balloon mounted stent. (**c**) Unsubtracted radiograph following balloon inflation. (**d**) Roadmap shows second balloon inflation at the level of the ostia. (**e**) Final arterial phase angiogram, subclavian injection, working view shows resolution of stenosis

Right ICA Angioplasty and Stenting

Case Description

An 84 year-old man with a history of hypertension, hyperlipidemia, myocardial infarction, and intermittent left upper extremity numbness for 1 month presents to the ED with acute onset left facial droop and intermittent dysarthria. CTA of the head and neck shows >85% stenosis of the proximal right internal carotid artery. Diffusion weighted magnetic resonance imaging demonstrated multiple foci of restricted diffusion in the right frontal lobe compatible with embolic stroke (Fig. 16.3a). He is indicated for CAS.

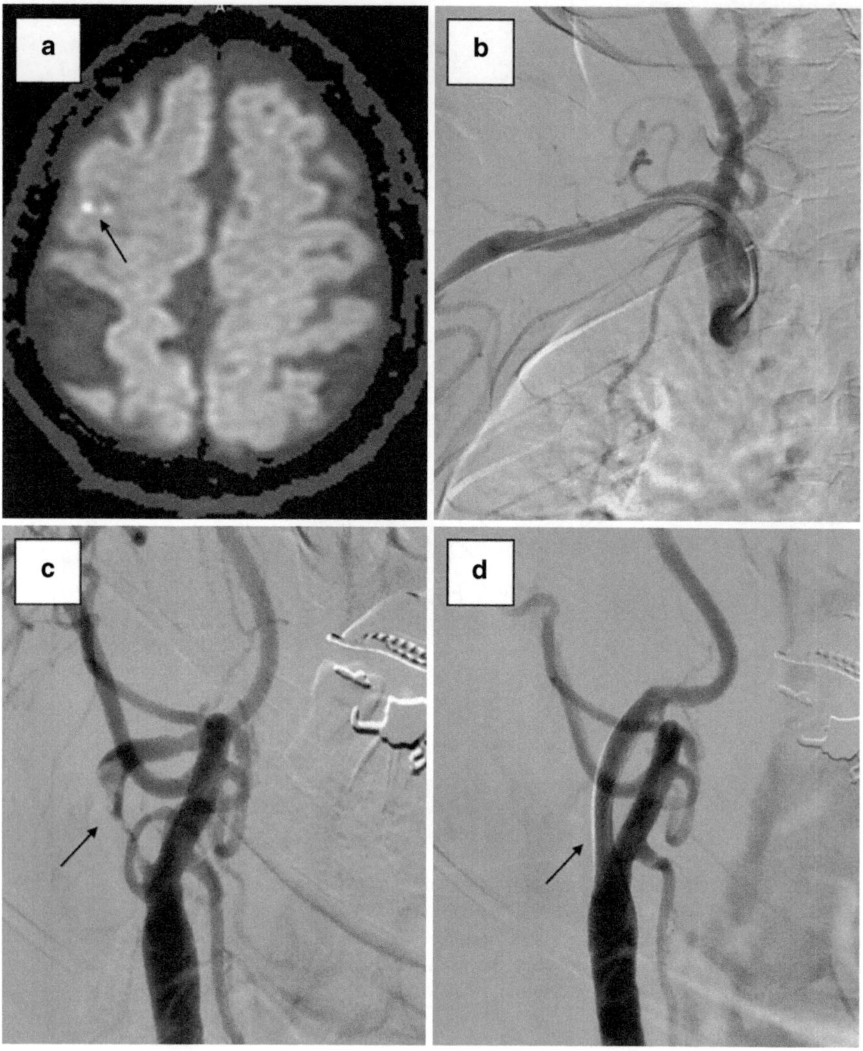

Fig. 16.3 (**a**) Diffusion weighted imaging (DWI) showing small area of restricted diffusion (arrow). (**b**) Arterial phase DSA, subclavian injection, PA view demonstrating steep takeoff the right CCA. (**c**) Arterial phase DSA, CCA injection, working view demonstrating critical right ICA stenosis (arrow). (**d**) Final arterial phase angiogram, right CCA injection, working view shows resolution of stenosis (arrow)

Procedure

Access Standard monitoring, prep, and right-sided TR access was performed as described in "Procedure".

Planning The access sheath was exchanged over a Bentson wire for a navigable 0.088″ long sheath. An angiographic run of the right subclavian artery was performed, demonstrating a steep takeoff of the right CCA. A 120 cm long 5-Fr Simmons 2 catheter was inserted over a 0.038″ guidewire, shaped in the ascending aorta following the technique described in "Arch Navigation", and used brought back through the innominate artery to catheterize the right CCA (Fig. 16.3b). The 0.088″ sheath was advanced over the selecting catheter and positioned in the right common carotid artery. Baseline cervical and cerebral angiography performed depicting critical right ICA origin stenosis (Fig. 16.3c) and right hemispheric hypoperfusion (not shown). Stent and balloon sizing was determined from baseline cervical angiogram.

Intervention Weight-based dosing of intravenous heparin was administered. The lesion was crossed with 0.014″ neurovascular microguidewire and embolic protection device deployed using appropriate technique. A 8 × 29 mm self-expanding nitinol stent was deployed across the area of stenosis, and angioplastied to nominal pressure with a 4 × 30 mm monorail percutaneous transluminal angioplasty (PTA) catheter. Distal embolic protection system recaptured using appropriate technique. Post-intervention cervical and cerebral angiography demonstrated appropriate stent placement, resolution of baseline stenosis (Fig. 16.3d), no intracranial branch occlusions, and improved cerebral perfusion (not shown). The long sheath was removed, and hemostasis achieved with a compressive band.

Left ICA Primary Stenting

Case Description

The following case serves to illustrate the usefulness of TR access when approaching left ICA pathology through a bovine arch. A 67-year-old woman with a history of hypertension, hyperlipidemia, diabetes, prior stroke, and bilateral severe symptomatic carotid artery stenosis presents for consultation. She underwent right CEA 1 month prior and suffered a significant period of nausea and vomiting postoperatively. She recovered, but required treatment of the left-sided lesion. Given her adverse reaction to prior CEA, she is considered high risk for a second operation. She elects to undergo left CAS, and a right TR approach was selected due to the presence of a bovine arch (Fig. 16.4a).

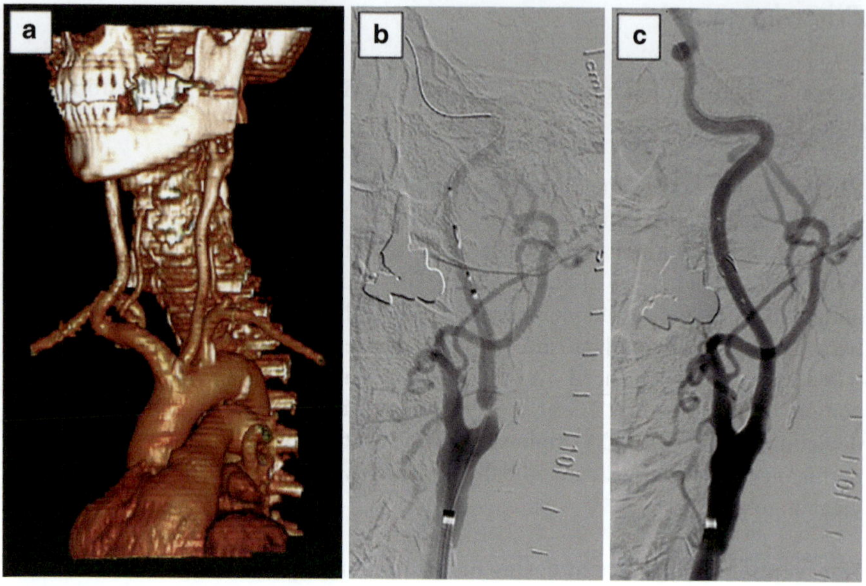

Fig. 16.4 (**a**) 3D reconstruction of the patient's computed tomography angiogram (CTA) demonstrates a bovine arch. (**b**) Arterial phase DSA, left CCA injection, working view shows critical stenosis at the ICA origin. (**c**) Final arterial phase DSA, working view, CCA injection shows resolution of stenosis after primary stenting

Procedure

Access Standard monitoring, prep, and right-sided TR access was performed as described in "Procedure".

Planning The access sheath was exchanged over a Bentson wire for a navigable 0.088″ long sheath. A 120 cm long 5-Fr Simmons Select catheter was inserted over a 0.038″ guidewire to facilitate cannulation of the left CCA, emerging from the right innominate artery. The 0.088″ sheath was advanced over the selecting catheter and positioned in the left CCA. DSA of the left ICA revealed critical stenosis. Cerebral angiogram revealed no abnormalities.

Intervention Weight-based dosing of intravenous heparin was administered. A 4 mm embolic protection device was advanced across the area of stenosis over a microguidewire and deployed (Fig. 16.4b). A 8 × 29 mm self-expanding nitinol was deployed across the area of stenosis, which resulted in resolution of the abnormality without the need for angioplasty (Fig. 16.4c). The distal embolic protection system was carefully recaptured. Post-intervention cervical and cerebral angiography demonstrated excellent placement of the stent with no significant residual stenosis and no sign of thromboembolic event. The catheters were removed, followed by the long sheath, and hemostasis achieved with a compressive band.

Left Vertebral Artery Origin Angioplasty and Stent

Case Description

In this final case, TR access is utilized when TF access fails to result in adequate inferior support for the catheter system. A 64-year-old man with history of multiple posterior circulation infarctions over the prior 5 months presented for evaluation. Magnetic resonance angiography revealed complete occlusion of the right VA and critical stenosis of the left VA origin. He elects to undergo diagnostic angiogram and possible stenting of the stenotic left VA.

Procedure

Access A transfemoral approach was initially attempted and abandoned due to inability to obtain a stable platform for intervention (Fig. 16.5a). Subsequently, standard TRA of the left radial artery was performed as described in "Procedure".

Planning Supplemental heparin was administered to total 5000 U, and the access sheath was exchanged over a Bentson wire for a 100 cm long 5-Fr sheath. Angiograms of neck and brain were performed, revealing normal cerebral vasculature, and left vertebral ostial stenosis >80% (Fig. 16.5b).

Intervention The ostial lesion was crossed with by a 5-Fr angle taper catheter and a 0.014″ straight tip guidewire (Fig. 16.5b). Predilation was performed using a 2 mm × 20 mm monorail PTA catheter (Fig. 16.5c), and a 4 mm × 12 mm balloon mounted stent was subsequently deployed and expanded to nominal diameter (Fig. 16.5d). Post-deployment angiogram demonstrated no residual stenosis. Intracranial angiography shows no branch occlusions and improved cerebral perfusion. The microguidewire and guide sheath were removed, and hemostasis was achieved with a compressive band. The right femoral sheath was also removed, and the arteriotomy was closed with an extraluminal closure device.

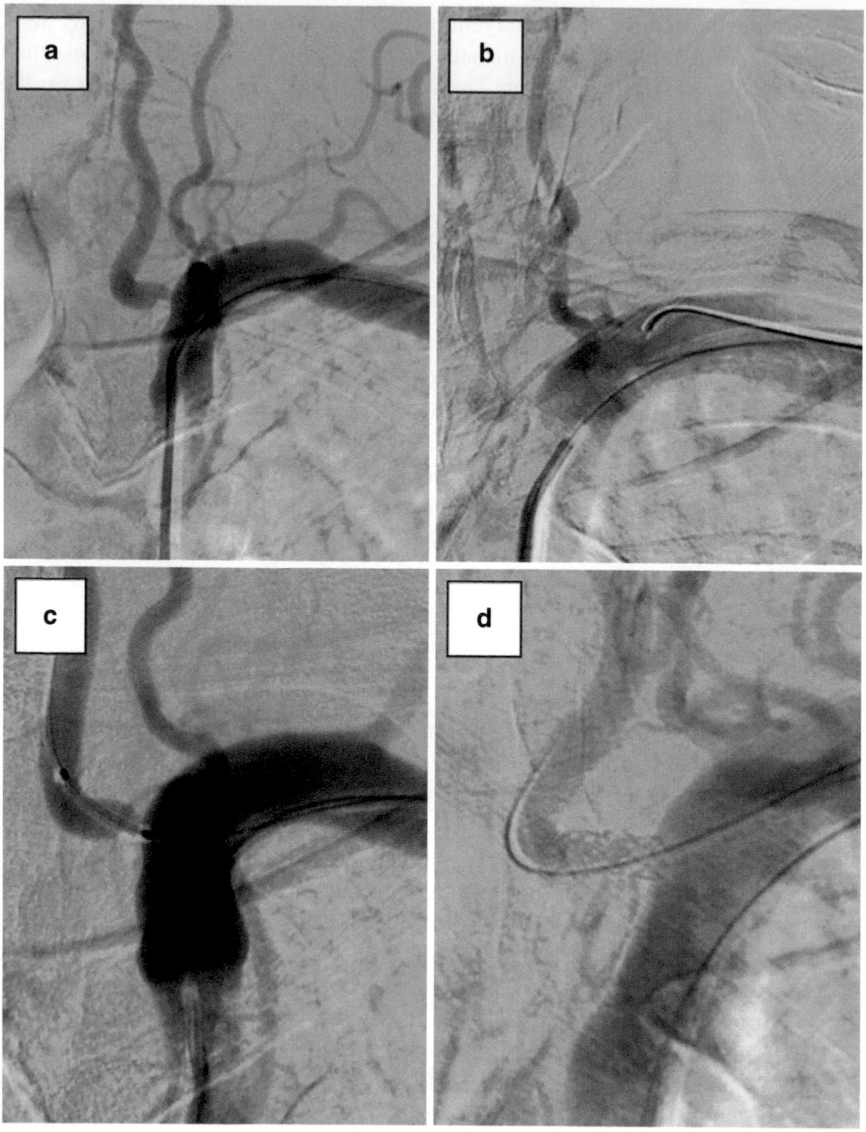

Fig. 16.5 (**a**) Arterial phase DSA, left subclavian injection, working view shows initial attempt at TF approach to the lesion (arrow). (**b**) Arterial phase DSA, left subclavian injection, working view demonstrates >80% stenosis at the vertebral artery origin. Note the transfemoral catheter still in place. (**c**) Arterial phase DSA, left subclavian injection, working view shows the lesion crossed by the stent. (**d**) Final arterial phase DSA, left subclavian injection, working view shows resolution of stenosis

References

1. Bendszus M, Koltzenburg M, Burger R, Warmuth-Metz M, Hofmann E, Solymosi L. Silent embolism in diagnostic cerebral angiography and neurointerventional procedures: a prospective study. Lancet. 1999;354(9190):1594–7.
2. Bonati LH, Dobson J, Featherstone RL, Ederle J, van der Worp HB, de Borst GJ, Mali WP, et al. Long-term outcomes after stenting versus endarterectomy for treatment of symptomatic carotid stenosis: The International Carotid Stenting Study (ICSS) randomised trial. Lancet. 2015;385(9967):529–38.
3. Etxegoien N, Rhyne D, Kedev S, Sachar R, Mann T. The transradial approach for carotid artery stenting. Catheter Cardiovasc Interv. 2012;80(7):1081–7.
4. Fessler RD, Wakhloo AK, Lanzino G, Guterman LR, Hopkins LN. Transradial approach for vertebral artery stenting: technical case report. Neurosurgery. 2000;46(6):1524–7. discussion 1527–28
5. Folmar J, Sachar R, Mann T. Transradial approach for carotid artery stenting: a feasibility study. Catheter Cardiovasc Interv. 2007;69(3):355–61.
6. Gao F, Lo WJ, Sun X, Ma N, Mo D, Xu X, Miao Z. Selective use of transradial access for endovascular treatment of severe intracranial vertebrobasilar artery stenosis. Clin Neurol Neurosurg. 2015;134(July):116–21.
7. Jaroenngarmsamer, T., K. D. Bhatia, H. Kortman, E. Orru T. Krings. 2019. Procedural success with radial access for carotid artery stenting: systematic review and meta-analysis. J Neurointerv Surg. 2019/06/16. https://doi.org/10.1136/neurintsurg-2019-014994.
8. Maciejewski D, Pieniazek P, Tekieli L, Paluszek P, Dzierwa K, Trystula M, Wojcik-Pedziwiatr M, Podolec P. Transradial approach for carotid artery stenting in a patient with severe peripheral arterial disease. Postepy Kardiol Interwencyjnej. 2014;10(1):47–9.
9. Mantese VA, Timaran CH, Chiu D, Begg RJ, Brott TG. The Carotid Revascularization Endarterectomy versus Stenting Trial (CREST): stenting versus carotid endarterectomy for carotid disease. Stroke. 2010;41(10 Suppl):S31–4.
10. Mas JL, Trinquart L, Leys D, Albucher JF, Rousseau H, Viguier A, Bossavy JP, et al. Endarterectomy Versus Angioplasty in patients with symptomatic severe carotid stenosis (EVA-3S) trial: results up to 4 years from a randomised, multicentre trial. Lancet Neurol. 2008;7(10):885–92.
11. Mendiz OA, Fava C, Lev G, Caponi G, Valdivieso L. Transradial versus transfemoral carotid artery stenting: a 16-year single-center experience. J Interv Cardiol. 2016;29(6):588–93.
12. Patel T, Shah S, Malhotra H, Radadia R, Shah L, Shah S. Transradial approach for stenting of vertebrobasilar stenosis: a feasibility study. Catheter Cardiovasc Interv. 2009;74(6):925–31.
13. Ringleb PA, Allenberg J, Bruckmann H, Eckstein HH, Fraedrich G, Hartmann M, Hennerici M, et al. 30 day results from the SPACE trial of stent-protected angioplasty versus carotid endarterectomy in symptomatic patients: a randomised non-inferiority trial. Lancet. 2006;368(9543):1239–47.
14. Ruzsa Z, Nemes B, Pinter L, Berta B, Toth K, Teleki B, Nardai S, et al. A randomised comparison of transradial and transfemoral approach for carotid artery stenting: RADCAR (RADial Access for CARotid Artery Stenting) study. EuroIntervention. 2014;10(3):381–91.
15. Shen S, Jiang X, Dong H, Peng M, Wang Z, Che W, Zou Y, Yang Y. Effect of aortic arch type on technical indicators in patients undergoing carotid artery stenting. J Int Med Res. 2019;47(2):682–8.
16. Yip H-K, Youssef AA, Chang W-N, Lu C-H, Yang C-H, Chen S-M, Chiung-Jen W. Feasibility and safety of transradial arterial approach for simultaneous right and left vertebral artery angiographic studies and stenting. Cardiovasc Intervent Radiol. 2007;30(5):840–6.

Chapter 17
Endovascular Neurosurgery and Stroke Intervention

Reade De Leacy, Devin V. Bageac, Jennifer M. Watchmaker, Sayan Manna, and J. Mocco

Abbreviations

AVM	Arteriovenous malformation
CCA	Common carotid artery
CT	Computed tomography
CTA	Computed tomography angiogram
dAVF	Dural arteriovenous fistula
DMSO	Dimethylsulfoxide
DSA	Digital subtraction angiography
ECA	External carotid artery
ICA	Internal carotid artery
MCA	Middle cerebral artery
MRI	Magnetic resonance imaging
PA	Postero-anterior
PCA	Posterior cerebral artery
SAH	Subarachnoid hemorrhage
TFA	Transfemoral
TR	Transradial
VA	Vertebral artery

Introduction

After rising in popularity throughout the 1990s, transradial (TR) access for neuroangiography began to cross over into clinical practice during the early 2000s. Since that time, case series have been published supporting its safety, cost

R. De Leacy (✉) · D. V. Bageac · J. M. Watchmaker · S. Manna · J. Mocco
Departments of Neurosurgery and Diagnostic, Molecular and Interventional Radiology, Icahn School of Medicine at Mount Sinai, New York, NY, USA
e-mail: reade.deleacy@mountsinai.org; devin.bageac@mountsinai.org; jennifer.watchmaker@mountsinai.org; sayan.manna@icahn.mssm.edu; j.mocco@mountsinai.org

A. M. Fischman et al. (eds.), *Transradial Access in Interventional Radiology*,
https://doi.org/10.1007/978-3-030-81678-0_17

effectiveness, and shorter recovery times rendering it preferable to transfemoral (TF) access in certain anatomic contexts [1–7]. This chapter is designed to act as a guide through five illustrative cases utilizing TR access in endovascular neurosurgery and stroke intervention.

Section "Neuroangiography" details an example of a standard elective diagnostic angiogram for treatment planning. Though not discussed further in this chapter, it should be also noted that TR access offers major advantages during intraoperative angiography by allowing the patient to be in comfortable position in the lateral or prone position without the use of long femoral sheaths [8, 9].

More recently, advancements in guide and access catheter technology have permitted TR access to be employed to a broad range of intracranial interventions. The safety and feasibility of TR access for cerebral aneurysm treatment has been described in a number of large case series [3, 10–13]. The in "Stent Assisted Coiling of Unruptured Right MCA Wide-neck Bifurcation Aneurysm", the patient described in "Neuroangiography" returns 2 months later to undergo TR stent-assisted coiling of a wide-neck MCA bifurcation aneurysm. Continuing the theme of aneurysm treatment, "LICA Blister Aneurysm Embolization with Flow Diversion" describes TR intervention on a subarachnoid hemorrhage patient with an enlarging left internal carotid artery (ICA) blister aneurysm using a flow diverting stent.

Retroperitoneal hematoma, a rare but serious complication of TF access, carries an estimated mortality risk between 4% and 12% and is associated with prolonged hospital admissions [14]. TR access obviates this unnecessary risk. "Right Occipital AVM embolization with Onyx" describes a patient with a previously ruptured occipital arteriovenous malformation (AVM) who experienced a severe access associated retroperitoneal hematoma following a TF catheter angiogram. Subsequent interventions proceeded via TR and ulnar access without complication.

In select cases of stroke intervention, particularly posterior circulation occlusions such as the one illustrated in "Direct Aspiration Thrombectomy of Distal Basilar Occlusion", TR access can provide increased guide catheter stability and ease of navigation. The TR approach can allow the interventionalist to circumvent proximal great vessel tortuosity, and may also be advantageous when facing severe aortoiliac disease or ectasia, Stanford type A and B aortic dissections, and prior aortic root/arch reconstructions [15–17].

Top Five Tips and Tricks

1. Ultrasound for access or radial artery over the volar radial surface or within the snuff box. Never access proximal to brachioradialis insertion due to risk of deep forearm space hematoma/compartment syndrome.
2. Obtain a roadmap of forearm vasculature to evaluate for anatomic variants.
3. At the time of writing, for 6-vessel diagnostic angiography, navigation of the aortic arch and branches is best achieved with hydrophilic Simmons 2 or Simmons 3 catheters.

4. For access of the left vertebral artery, form the diagnostic Simmons catheter, with the elbow of the catheter within the descending arch/thoracic aorta.
5. For interventional case, pair a 125 cm diagnostic catheter, coaxially within your chosen guiding catheter rather than utilizing a long exchange technique.

Neuroangiography

Case Description

In order to illustrate standard technique for the safe performance of TR neuroangiography, we first present the case of a 49-year-old female with a history of multinodular goiter, who was found to have an unruptured 7 mm right middle cerebral artery (MCA) aneurysm on workup for thyroid surgery. She underwent cerebral angiography performed for treatment planning. 3D computed tomography angiography (CTA) reconstruction demonstrating arch and great vessel anatomy is included in Fig. 17.1. A basic equipment list for this procedure includes:

- Access
  - Micropuncture access set and a 4/5-Fr slender sheath
- Angiography
  - 5-Fr Simmons 2 for Simmons 3 catheter
  - Bentson and 0.035″ guidewires
- Closure
  - Radial puncture compression device

Procedure

Access Cardiopulmonary monitoring was placed, monitored anesthesia care was initiated, and a time-out was performed. The right wrist and both groins were prepped and draped in the usual sterile fashion. Using ultrasound guidance, the radial artery was localized, and local anesthesia (1% Lidocaine) was infiltrated subdermally. Under continued ultrasound, a single wall puncture of the radial artery is performed at the level of the radial epiphysis on the volar radial surface.

Using modified Seldinger technique, a 4/5-Fr slender sheath was gently inserted into the radial artery and maintained on a heparinized flush. A radial artery access cocktail consisting of 3000 U heparin, 200 ug nitroglycerin, and 2.5 mg verapamil

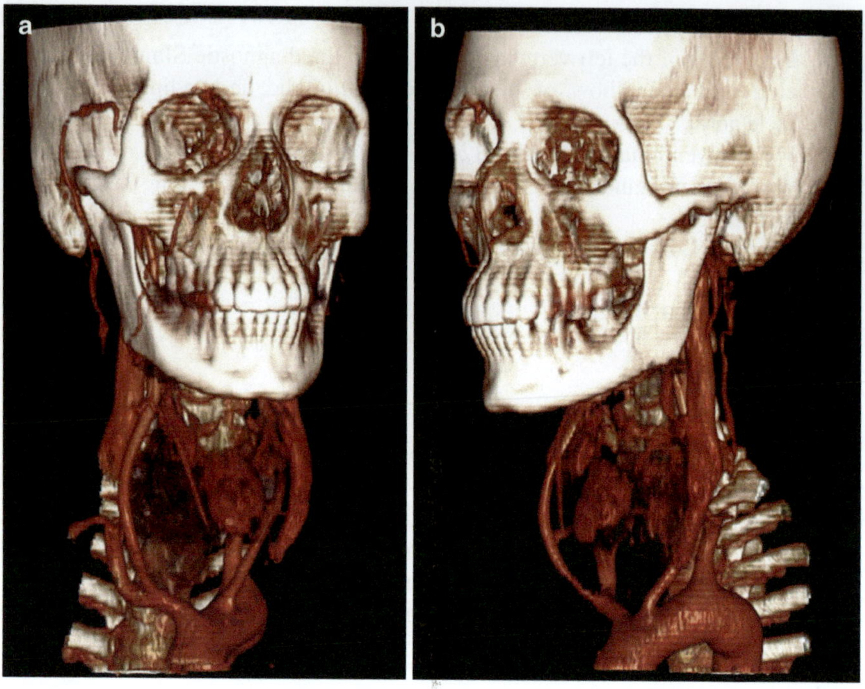

Fig. 17.1 Preprocedural CTA, 3D reconstruction in two views demonstrates Type 2 arch. The course of the right CCA is deviated laterally due to a large multinodular goiter

was mixed with 10 cc of the patient's blood and slowly infused through the sheath over 5–10 minutes to induce vasodilation. Throughout this infusion, the patient's vital signs were closely monitored for hypotension. Roadmapping of the radial artery revealed a proximal brachial bifurcation, a normal anatomic variant (Fig. 17.2a).

Angiography Using coaxial technique, a 5-Fr Simmons 2 catheter was advanced into the right subclavian artery over the Bentson wire, and roadmapping was performed. Following techniques described in section "Equipment List", and with the aid of the roadmapping (Fig. 17.2b), fluoroscopy, and careful guidewire manipulation when necessary, bilateral common ceratoid arteries (CCAs), internal carotid arteries (ICAs), external carotid arteries (ECAs), and vertebral arteries (VAs) were selectively catheterized. Digital subtraction angiography (DSA) was performed upon each successive selective catheterization. Right ICA injection revealed a wide-neck MCA bifurcation aneurysm, arising primarily from the superior division and projecting laterally (Fig. 17.2c). 3D rotational angiography better characterized the extent of superior division involvement, as well as a multilobular morphology

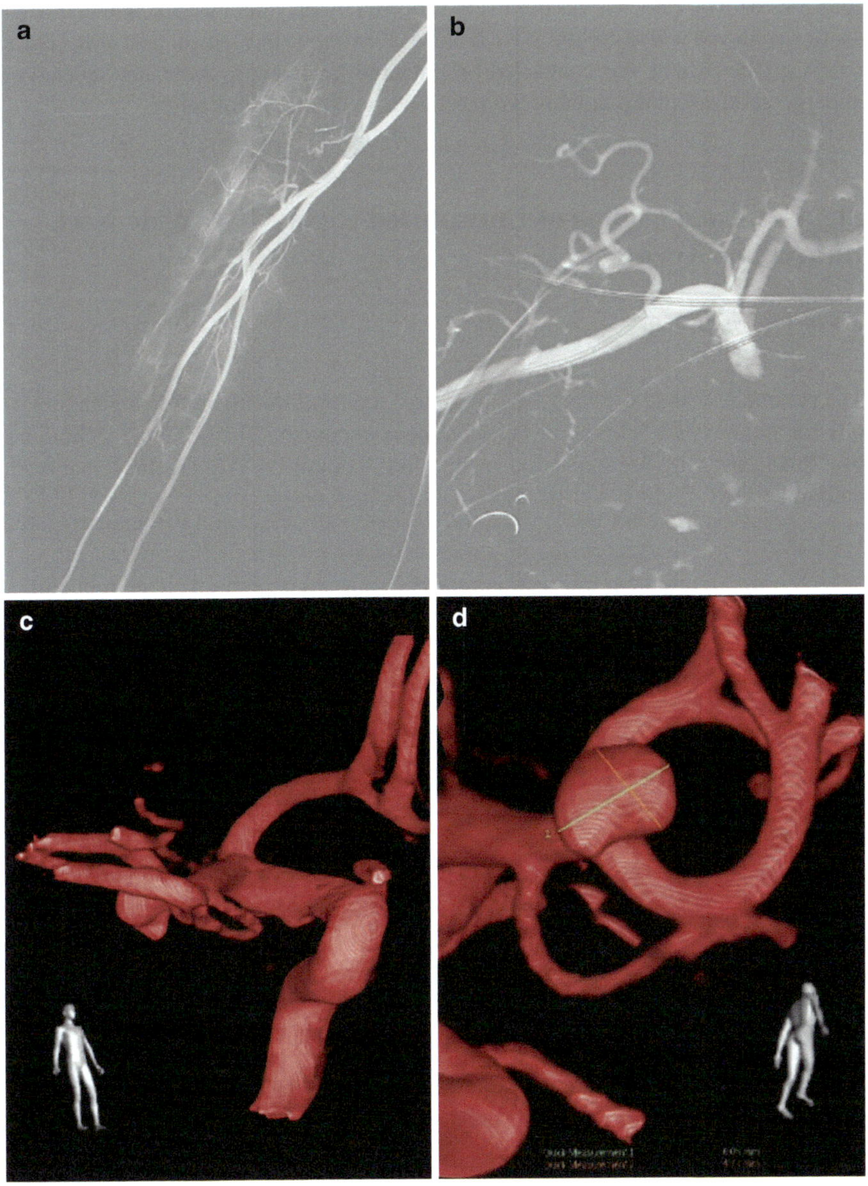

Fig. 17.2 (**a**) Roadmap of the radial artery demonstrating a proximal brachial bifurcation. (**b**) Sample roadmap of the right CCA shows catheter loop formed in the ascending aorta. (**c**) Arterial phase DSA, right ICA injection, postero-anterior (PA) view shows a wide-neck MCA bifurcation aneurysm. (**d**) Reconstructed 3D rotational angiogram orientated as displayed by figure inset

(Fig. 17.2d). The catheter was removed, followed by the radial sheath, and hemostasis was achieved with a compressive band. Following an uneventful post-procedural recovery, the patient was counseled on potential treatment options, and elected to undergo endovascular treatment with stent-assisted coil embolization.

Stent-Assisted Coiling of Unruptured Right MCA Wide-Neck Bifurcation Aneurysm

Case Description

The patient described in "Neuroangiography" returns 2 months following angiography for stent-assisted coiling of her wide-neck aneurysm. The principal techniques of TR angiography are expanded in this first example of TR cerebral aneurysm embolization, for which a basic equipment list includes:

- Access
  - Micropuncture access set and a 5/6-Fr slender sheath
  - 0.070″ or 0.071″ navigable guiding catheter
- Planning
  - >125 cm 5-Fr selecting catheter (e.g., Simmons or Berenstein select)
  - 150 cm Bentson guidewire
  - 0.035″ or 0.038″ stiff guidewire
- Intervention
  - Variable, and may include endovascular coils, coil-assist stents or balloon microcatheters, flow-diverting stents, and intrasaccular devices
  - Intermediate catheter for distal pathology
- Closure
  - Radial puncture compression device

In this case, endovascular coils were used in conjunction with an open-celled stent bridging the wide neck of the aneurysm.

Procedure

Access Standard monitoring, prep, and TR access of the right radial artery was performed following the technique described in "Case Description". As opposed to the 4/5-Fr sheath sufficient for diagnostic angiography, a 5/6-Fr slender glide sheath was placed to facilitate the larger interventional catheter system. The procedure was performed under general anesthesia.

Planning Using coaxial technique, a 6-Fr guide catheter was advanced into the right subclavian artery over a Bentson wire. A long (125 cm) 5-Fr Simmons 2 catheter was passed coaxially through guide, shaped within the aortic arch, and used to select the right CCA. The guiding catheter was then advanced further to the skull base. In order to determine the appropriate stent size, 3D rotational angiography was performed, and the diameters of parent and distal vessels were recorded (Fig. 17.3a).

Intervention Working projections were obtained from 3D acquisition, and heparin was administered to achieve and activated clotting time (ACT) target of 2–2.5 above baseline. The first (stenting) microcatheter was advanced under guidance to the intracranial circulation over a 0.014″ microguidewire, and the superior M2 MCA division was selected. Superselective angiography confirmed free flow of contrast (Fig. 17.3b). Using similar technique, a second (coiling) microcatheter was positioned within the aneurysm sac. To prevent dome perforation by the tip of the coiling microcatheter during stent deployment, a single loop of framing coil was placed within the aneurysm sac. Next, a 3.0 × 15 mm open-cell stent was deployed via the first catheter from the superior M2 branch into the distal M1, bridging the aneurysm neck and jailing the coiling microcatheter (Fig. 17.3c). After successful jailing was confirmed, coils were sequentially placed and deployed within the aneurysm sac under guidance using standard technique. Final angiographic evaluation in working projections demonstrated trace contrast filling coil interstices consistent with modified Raymond-Roy Class IIIA result, and final standard projection angiography showed no branch occlusions (Fig. 17.4). The catheters were removed, followed by the radial sheath, and hemostasis achieved with a compressive band.

LICA Blister Aneurysm Embolization with Flow Diversion

Case Description

In select cases, cerebral aneurysm may be treated by the placement of a flow diverting stent. This can also be accomplished transradially, as demonstrated in this case of a 46-year-old female who presented with severe onset of headache, nausea, and vomiting. CT head (Fig. 17.5a) demonstrated left carotid cistern and left sylvian fissure subarachnoid hemorrhage (SAH), corresponding to a modified Fischer Grade 1. Initial angiography showed possible supraclinoid left ICA blister. Repeat DSA 1 week later confirmed a subtle ICA blister aneurysm of the dorsal ICA approximately $\frac{2}{3}$ the distance between the ophthalmic origin and ICA terminus, which had grown slightly (Fig. 17.5b). She presents for endovascular treatment with

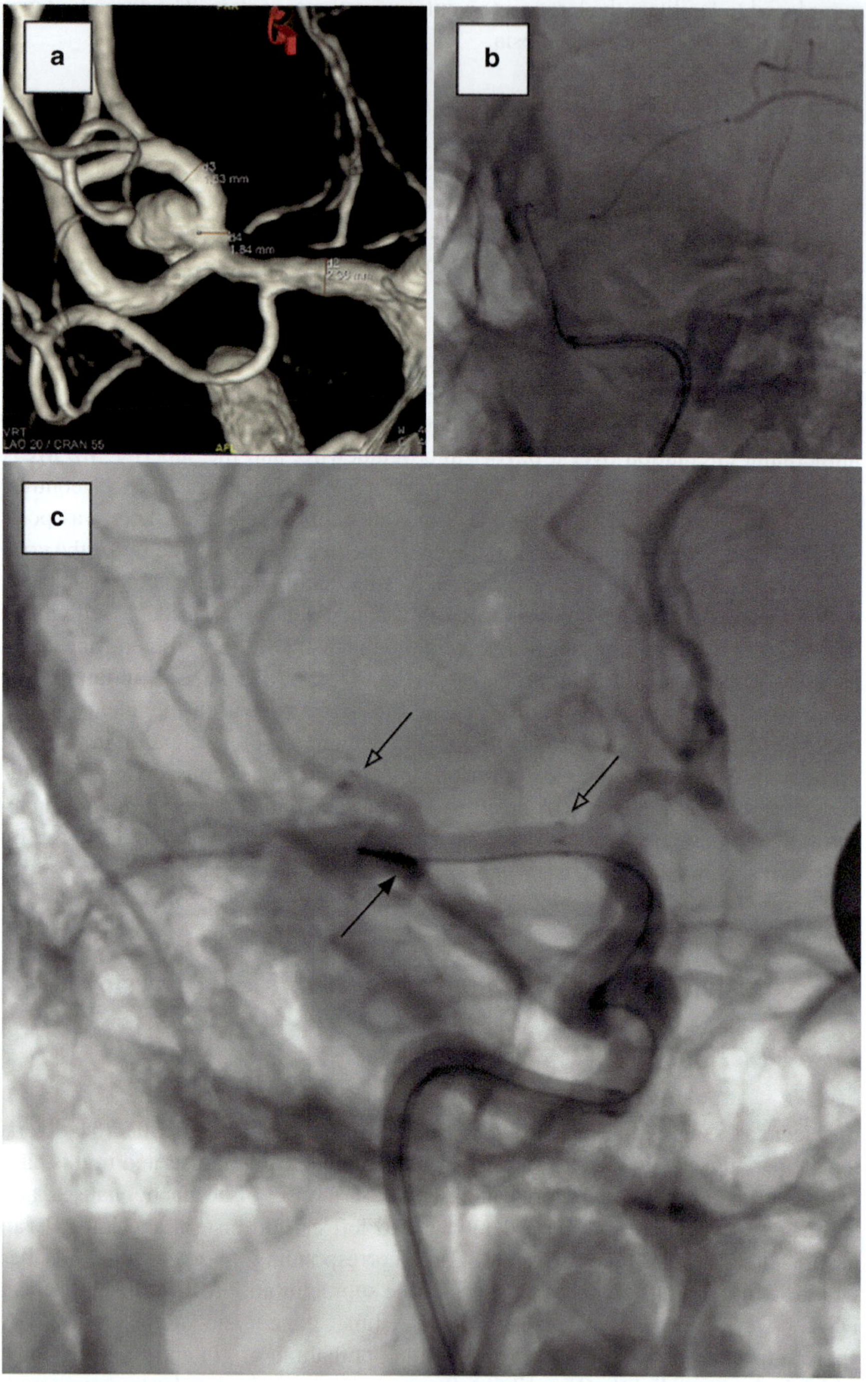
a
b
c
VRT
LAO 20 / CRAN 55

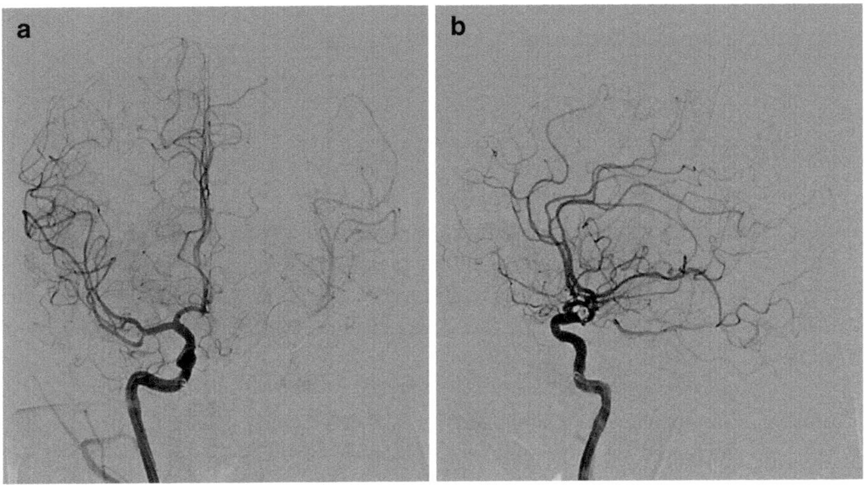

Fig. 17.4 Final arterial phase DSA, right ICA injection following intervention demonstrates a modified Raymond-Roy Class IIIa result. (**a**) PA view. (**b**) Lateral view

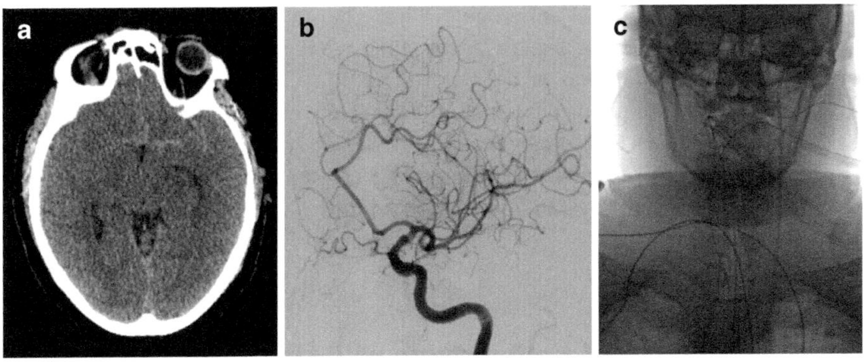

Fig. 17.5 (**a**) CT head demonstrates SAH in left carotid and sylvian cisterns (open arrow). (**b**) Arterial phase DSA, left ICA injection, lateral view shows a subtle ICA blister aneurysm of the dorsal ICA. (**c**) Unsubtracted radiograph, PA view shows the course of radial catheter from right subclavian to left ICA. (Figure reproduced with permission of Dr. Justin Singer, MD)

Fig. 17.3 (**a**) 3D rotational angiography, right ICA injection. (**b**) Unsubracted superselective M2 angiogram, lateral view. A guide catheter is positioned in the distal petrous ICA. (**c**) Unsubracted angiogram, right ICA injection, PA view demonstrates successful jailing of the coil delivery catheter by the stent (distal and proximal markers indicated by open arrows). A single loop of coil is placed within the aneurysm prior to stenting (closed arrow) placement of a flow diverting stent, utilizing the same equipment for access, planning, and closure as described in "Case Description".

Procedure

Access Prior to the start of the procedure, the patient received a loading dose of aspirin and clopidogrel. Standard monitoring, prep, and TR access of the right radial artery was performed following the technique described in "Case Description", and a 5/6F slender glide sheath was placed. The procedure was performed under general anesthesia.

Planning The sheath was exchanged for a 0.088″ guide sheath (100 cm long), which was navigated into the left distal ICA over a 5-Fr Simmons 2 (Fig. 17.5c). Routine projections and 3D rotation angiogram were obtained. Stent sizing and magnified working views were derived from 3D acquisition.

Intervention A distal access catheter was navigated into the left MCA over an offset catheter and a 0.014″ microguidewire. The guide sheath was then further advanced to the vertical petrous ICA for stability (Fig. 17.6a), and 6000 units of heparin was administered as an IV bolus. The flow diverting stent was deployed using standard technique as described in Fig. 17.6b, ensuring bridging of the diseased ICA segment. Post-deployment runs demonstrated good wall apposition (Fig. 17.6c) and stasis (not shown) within the aneurysmal sac. Six-month follow-up angiogram (Fig. 17.6d) showed appropriate vascular reconstruction and vessel wall remodeling.

Right Occipital AVM Embolization with Onyx

Case Description

The current case demonstrates safe navigation of a radial artery loop, as well as an instance in which TR access was utilized to mitigate the risks associated with femoral artery catheterization. A 58-year-old female with past medical history of morbid obesity (BMI 48), HTN, and DM presented with a right occipital parenchymal ICH. Subsequent femoral DSA confirmed a right occipital Spetzler-Martin grade III arteriovenous malformation (AVM), and complicated by a large right retroperitoneal hematoma requiring NSICU admission and resuscitation secondary to high femoral access and closure device malfunction. She presented for her first session of staged embolization of the AVM. Basic equipment for the procedure includes:

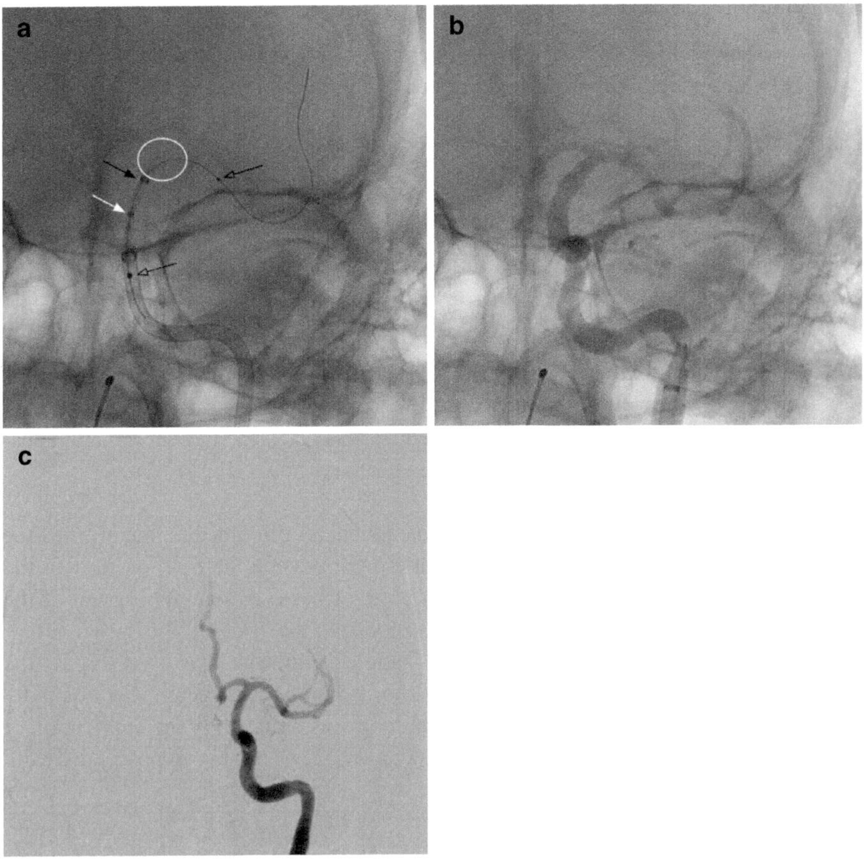

Fig. 17.6 (**a**) Unsubtracted radiograph, working view shows stent deployment. The intermediate catheter (closed black arrow) is advanced beyond the aneurysm. Markers (open arrows) signify the proximal and distal ends of the sent pusher. The stent is deployed from its delivery microcatheter (white arrow) within the intermediate catheter, which is then pulled back for final deployment of the stent into the vessel (white circle). (**b**) Post-deployment angiogram, working view shows good wall opposition. (**c**) Arterial phase DSA, right ICA injection, PA view at 6-month follow-up shows no evidence of stenosis or dissection. (Figure reproduced with permission of Dr. Justin Singer, MD)

- Access
  - Micropuncture access set and a 5/6-Fr slender sheath
  - 0.070″ or 0.071″ navigable guiding catheter
- Planning
  - >125 cm 5-Fr selecting catheter (e.g., Simmons or Berenstein select)
  - 150 cm Bentson guidewire
  - 0.035″ or 0.038″ stiff guidewire

- Intervention
  - Dimethyl sulfoxide (DMSO)–compatible microcatheter with detachable tip
  - Ethylene vinyl alcohol embolic system
- Closure
  - Radial puncture compression device

Procedure

Access Standard monitoring, prep, and TR access of the right radial artery was performed following the technique described in "Case Description", and a 5/6F slender glide sheath was placed. The procedure was performed under general anesthesia. Initial radial angiogram through the sheath is shown (Fig. 17.7a).

Planning As the Simmons 2 catheter was advanced through the sheath into the radial artery, resistance was encountered at a point beyond the field of view of the initial radial angiogram. The catheter was brought back, and an angiogram of the brachial bifurcation showed a 360-degree loop at the root of the radial artery (Fig. 17.7b). Under roadmapping, a 0.018″ angled glidewire was used to pass the loop into the brachial artery, over which the Simmons 2 catheter was coaxially passed into the subclavian artery. The radial loop was reduced by the application of gentle traction to the Simmons 2 catheter (Fig. 17.7c, d). Planning proceeded with

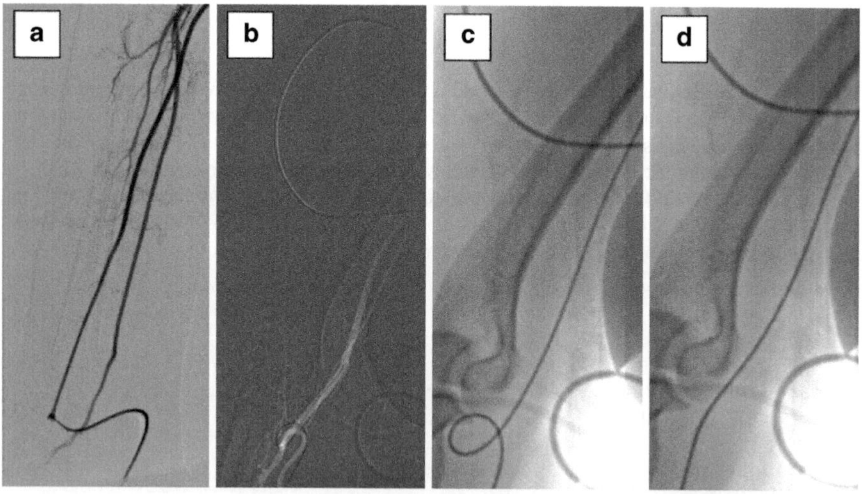

Fig. 17.7 Access through looped origin of the radial artery. (**a**) Initial radial angiogram demonstrates no abnormalities. (**b**) Radial roadmap including the bifurcation point demonstrates a loop at the radial artery origin. (**c**) The Simmons 2 catheter navigated through the loop over an angled guidewire. (**d**) After gentle traction on the catheter and guidewire, the loop is straightened

a full diagnostic cerebral angiogram performed using standard technique (Fig. 17.8a, b).

Intervention The diagnostic catheter was exchanged for a 0.071″ guide sheath over a 260 cm exchange wire. The guide was then advanced into the right vertebral artery over a 5-Fr Berenstein select catheter and glidewire. The selecting catheter and wire were removed, and a DSA was obtained in magnified working views. Intervention proceeded with embolization of selected posterior cerebral artery (PCA) feeders using Onyx 18 liquid embolic system through a DMSO–compatible microcatheter with detachable tip. The catheters were removed and the radial access

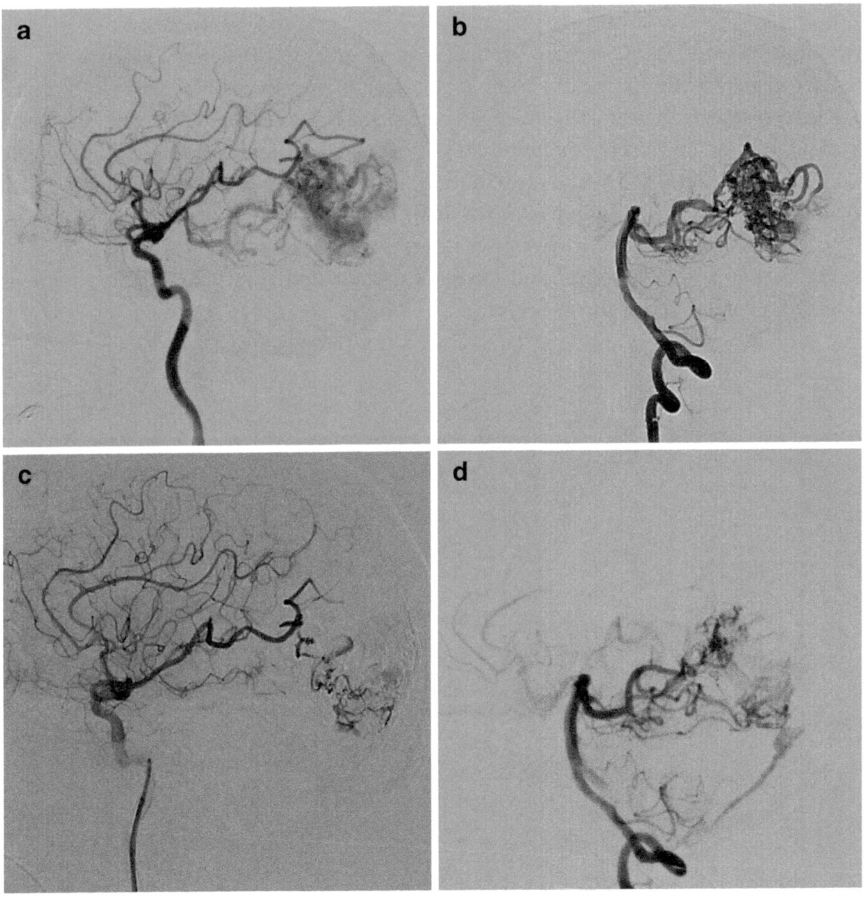

Fig. 17.8 Arterial phase DSA, lateral views, pre- and post-embolization. (**a**) Pre-embolization right ICA injection shows two small feeders via the right MCA angular branch supplying a right occipital AVM with superficial drainage. (**b**) Pre-embolization right vertebral injection demonstrates the main AVM supply arising from the PCA circulation. The AVM measures approximately 4 cm along its longest axis. (**c-d**) Follow-up DSAs after four sessions of staged embolization show a marked reduction of AVM volume and AV shunting, amenable to transvenous closure

site was closed with a compressive band. The patient was transferred to the NSICU in stable condition at their neurologic baseline. The patient returned for three subsequent staged embolizations of additional right PCA, right MCA, and bilateral middle meningeal artery feeders (Fig. 17.8c, d), and at the time of writing is scheduled to undergo final transvenous closure of the AVM.

Direct Aspiration Thrombectomy of Distal Basilar Occlusion

Case Description

In some cases of large vessel occlusion involving the posterior circulation, TR access may provide the fastest route to the lesion. A 57-year-old male with a past medical history of cardiac valve repair and prior right cerebellar infarct presented via EMS for acute-onset right hemiparesis, facial droop, and dysarthria. He was last seen normal 2.5 hours prior to presentation, and NIH Stroke scale on arrival was 13. At baseline, the patient is independent in all activities of daily living.

CTH showed chronic R cerebellar infarct without hemorrhage, and CTA head/neck showed a left vertebral and basilar tip occlusion (Fig. 17.9). The patient is deemed a candidate for thrombectomy.

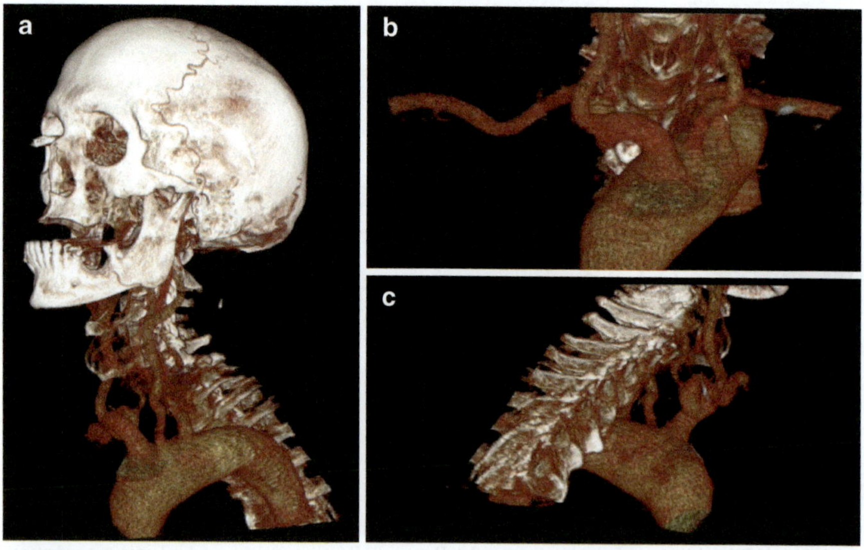

Fig. 17.9 Preprocedural CTA, 3D reconstruction in three views demonstrates an unfolded aorta and severe right proximal subclavian tortuosity. (**a**) The right vertebral artery originates from the posterior aspect of the subclavian loop. (**b**) The course of the distal subclavian artery is relatively straightforward. (**c**) View from right side more clearly demonstrates subclavian loop

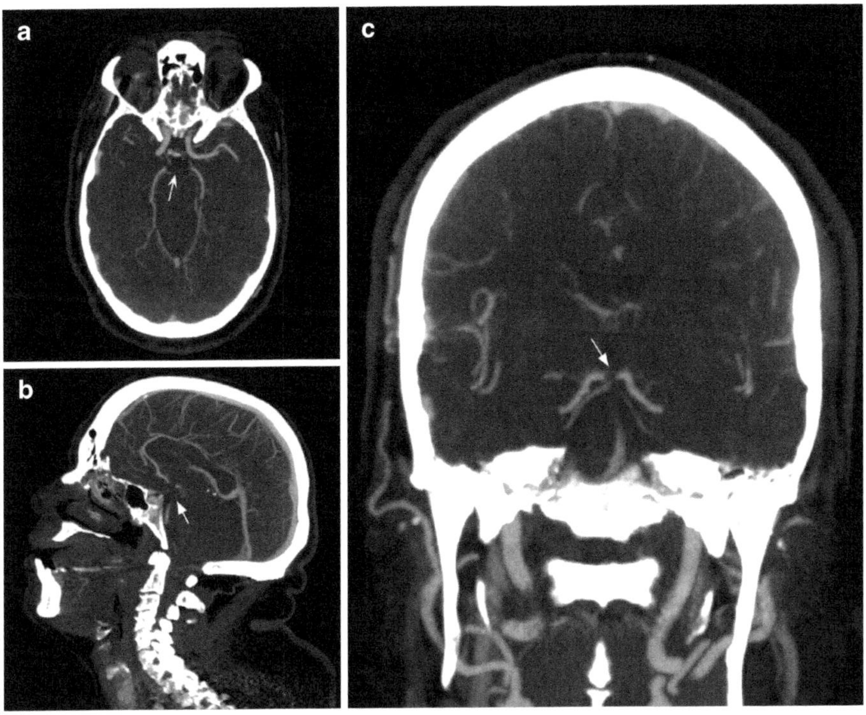

Fig. 17.10 Preprocedural CTA, maximum intensity projections demonstrate filling defect at the basilar apex (white arrow), with good collateralization. (**a**) Axial view. (**b**) Sagittal view. (**c**) Coronal view

Prior to the procedure, careful review of the patient's CTA head/neck (3D reconstruction in Fig. 17.10) revealed an unfolded aorta and severe right proximal subclavian tortuosity, leading to a right vertebral artery origin that emanated from the posterior aspect of a subclavian loop. This contrasted the relatively straightforward course of the distal subclavian artery, prompting the decision to pursue right vertebral catheterization via transradial approach. A basic equipment list for this procedure includes:

- Access
  - Micropuncture access set and a 5/6-Fr slender sheath
  - 0.088″ navigable guide sheath
- Planning
  - 150 cm Bentson guidewire
  - 180 cm 0.038″ stiff guidewire
- Intervention
  - Stent retriever and/or intermediate catheter with aspiration tubing
  - 2.7-Fr microcatheter
  - 0.016 microguidewire

- Closure
  - Radial puncture compression device

Procedure

Access Standard monitoring, prep, and TR access of the right radial artery was performed following the technique described in "Case Description", and a 5/6F slender glide sheath was placed. In order to mitigate the risk hypotension, a nitroglycerin was not included in the radial cocktail. The procedure was performed under monitored anesthesia care.

Planning The sheath was exchanged over a Bentson wire for a 0.088″ guide catheter, which was advanced into the right subclavian artery. Using roadmapping and guidewire, the guide was brought up into the right vertebral artery. DSA performed 5 minutes after radial puncture demonstrated a filling defect at the basilar tip without opacification of the right PCA or superior cerebellar artery (SCA) (Fig. 17.11a, b). Based on this finding, the decision was made to proceed with stroke intervention.

Intervention A coaxial system consisting of an intermediate catheter, microcatheter, and microwire was advanced into the intracranial circulation. The intermediate catheter was brought to the face of the clot, and direct aspiration was initiated. Three minutes later, with aspiration still running, the intermediate catheter was retrieved under secondary aspiration through the guide catheter. Follow-up angiogram through the guide catheter performed 12 minutes after radial puncture demonstrated full recanalization of the previously occluded basilar bifurcation (Fig. 17.11c, d). The guide catheter was removed and the radial access site was closed with a compressive band. The patient's immediate post-procedure exam improved to NIHSS 6, and they were transferred to the NSICU in stable condition.

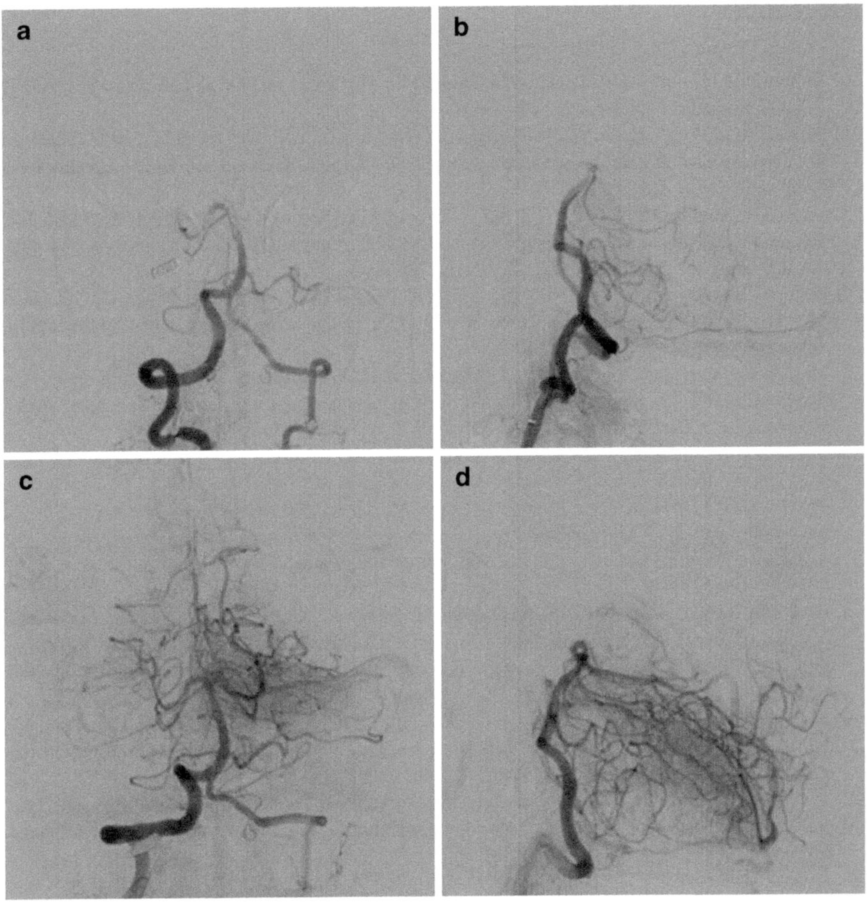

Fig. 17.11 Arterial phase DSA, right vertebral injection, PA and lateral views pre- and post-thrombectomy. (**a** and **b**) Pre-thrombectomy DSA reveals occlusive thrombus at the basilar tip. (**c** and **d**) Post-thrombectomy DSA demonstrated full recanalization of the previously occluded basilar bifurcation. There is hyperperfusion in the left SCA territory in keeping with established infarct

References

1. Nohara AM, Kallmes DF. Transradial cerebral angiography: technique and outcomes. AJNR Am J Neuroradiol. 2003;24(6):1247–50.
2. Brunet MC, Chen SH, Sur S, McCarthy DJ, Snelling B, Yavagal DR, Starke RM, Peterson EC. Distal transradial access in the anatomical snuffbox for diagnostic cerebral angiography. J Neurointerv Surg. 2019;1(7):710–3.
3. Chen SH, Snelling BM, Shah SS, Sur S, Brunet MC, Starke RM, Yavagal DR, Osbun JW, Peterson EC. Transradial approach for flow diversion treatment of cerebral aneurysms: a multicenter study. J NeuroInterv Surg. 2019b;11:796–800.
4. Levy EI, Boulos AS, Fessler RD, Bendok BR, Ringer AJ, Kim SH, Qureshi AI, Guterman LR, Hopkins LN. Transradial cerebral angiography: an alternative route. Neurosurgery. 2002;51(2):335–40; discussion 340-2.
5. Matsumoto Y, Hongo K, Toriyama T, Nagashima H, Kobayashi S. Transradial approach for diagnostic selective cerebral angiography: results of a consecutive series of 166 cases. Am J Neuroradiol. 2001;22(4):704–8.
6. Snelling BM, Sur S, Shah SS, Marlow MM, Cohen MG, Peterson EC. Transradial access: lessons learned from cardiology. J NeuroInterv Surg. 2018;10(5):487–92.
7. Zussman BM, Tonetti DA, Stone J, Brown M, Desai SM, Gross BA, Jadhav A, Jovin TG, Jankowitz BT. Maturing institutional experience with the transradial approach for diagnostic cerebral arteriography: overcoming the learning curve. J NeuroInterv Surg. 2019;11(12):1235–8.
8. Chalouhi N, Sweid A, Saiegh F, Mahtabfar A, Ghosh R, Mouchtouris N, Khanna O, Romo V, Tjoumakaris S, Gooch R, Rosenwasser RH, Jabbour P. Initial experience with transradial intraoperative angiography in aneurysm clipping: technique, feasibility, and case series. Chalouhi et al: World Neurosurgery. 2020;134:e554–e58.
9. Osbun JW, Patel B, Levitt MR, Yahanda AT, Shah A, Dlouhy KM, Thatcher JP, Chicoine MR, Kim LJ, Zipfel GJ. Transradial intraoperative cerebral angiography: a multicenter case series and technical report. J NeuroInterv Surg. 2019;12(2):170–5.
10. Chen SH, Brunet M-C, Sur S, Yavagal DR, Starke RM, Peterson EC. Feasibility of repeat transradial access for neuroendovascular procedures. J Chen et al: Neurointerv Surg. 2020;12(4):431–34.
11. Goland J, Doroszuk G. Transradial approach for endovascular diagnosis and treatment of ruptured cerebral aneurysms: a descriptive study. Surg Neurol Int. 2019;10:87.
12. Goland J, Doroszuk G, Garbugino S, Ypa M. Transradial approach to treating endovascular cerebral aneurysms: case series and technical note. Surg Neurol Int. 2017;8:73.
13. Lawson MF, Velat GJ, Fargen KM, Hoh BL, Mocco J. Direct radial artery access with the 070 neuron guide catheter for aneurysm coiling: a novel application of the neuron catheter for cerebral interventions. Neurosurgery. 2012;71(2 Suppl Operative):onsE329–34.
14. Sajnani N, Bogart DB. Retroperitoneal hemorrhage as a complication of percutaneous intervention: report of 2 cases and review of the literature. Open Cardiovasc Med J. 2013;7:16–22. https://doi.org/10.2174/1874192401307010016.
15. Chen SH, Snelling BM, Sur S, Shah SS, McCarthy DJ, Luther E, Yavagal DR, Peterson EC, Starke RM. Transradial versus transfemoral access for anterior circulation mechanical thrombectomy: comparison of technical and clinical outcomes. J NeuroInterv Surg. 2019c;11(9):874–8.
16. Haussen DIC, Nogueira RG, DeSousa KG, Pafford RN, Janjua N, Ramdas KN, Peterson EC, Elhammady MS, Yavagal DIR. Transradial access in acute ischemic stroke intervention. J NeuroInterv Surg. 2016;8(3):247–50.
17. Khanna O, Sweid A, Mouchtouris N, Shivashankar K, Xu V, Velagapudi L, Stricsek G, Amllay A, Pavlos T, Reid Gooch M, Tjoumakaris S, Rosenwasser RH, Jabbour PM. Radial artery catheterization for neuroendovascular procedures. Stroke. 2019;50(9):2587–90.

Chapter 18
Acute Hemorrhage and Trauma

David Kestenbaum and Robert Blue

General Considerations

To CTA or not to CTA

A CT angiogram is almost always recommended prior to intervention for bleeding. A CTA is more sensitive in the detection of active hemorrhage as compared to conventional angiography (0.25 ml/min vs. 0.5 ml/min, respectively) [1]. In some cases, bleeding is successfully controlled by empiric embolization of a particular vessel or territory identified on preoperative CTA despite a negative invasive angiogram [2]. Particularly in the case of GI hemorrhage, CTA is indispensable in its ability to accurately identify the offending vessel/vascular territory among the entirety of the mesenteric vasculature, saving valuable procedure time and improving outcomes.

Although the primary utility of a preoperative CTA is to localize a bleeding vessel or identify active hemorrhage, there are a number of additional reasons a preoperative scan is useful. In cases of trauma, more than one site of active bleeding can be present and may be missed on invasive imaging. Additionally, alternative pathology may be identified which may be more appropriately treated by open surgery, as in the case of bowel ischemia that has progressed to infarction. Being able to identify the patient's anatomy and any anatomic variants can help cut down the time required to control the hemorrhage and reduce the risks.

D. Kestenbaum · R. Blue (✉)
Department of Diagnostic, Molecular and Interventional Radiology,
Icahn School of Medicine at Mount Sinai, New York, NY, USA

A. M. Fischman et al. (eds.), *Transradial Access in Interventional Radiology*,
https://doi.org/10.1007/978-3-030-81678-0_18

In specific cases, such as hemorrhage due to pelvic fracture and postpartum hemorrhage, it is reasonable to forgo preoperative imaging. Post-partum hemorrhage is often rapid and difficult to control. As a rule of thumb, if an obstetric surgeon is calling you for help with post-partum hemorrhage, the bleeding is likely to be quite severe, and you should usually proceed directly to pelvic angiography. It should be noted though that when possible, preoperative scanning in these patients can still be beneficial in identifying multiple bleeding vessels, gynecologic surgical complications, and in the case of pelvic trauma, occult fractures.

Radial Access and Impaired Blood Clotting

Assessing a patient's CBC and INR is always part of the pre-operative workup for IR procedures for hemorrhage. At many institutions, a platelet count >40,000/microliter and an INR <1.7 are generally recommended for arterial interventions. These standards, however, were developed in part to avoid access site hemorrhage and pseudoaneurysm formation at the common femoral artery. In patients with cirrhosis and severe liver dysfunction, it is often difficult to fully correct the platelet count and INR, and infusions of platelets and fresh frozen plasma can also paradoxically exacerbate hemorrhage by increasing preload.

The radial artery is quite easily identifiable a few millimeters below the surface of the skin, and for this reason, compression of the artery access site post procedure is dramatically simpler than compression of a common femoral artery access site. At our institution, hemostasis is achieved using the TR Band (Terumo, Shibuya City, Tokyo), which is placed over the access site for 1–2 hours post procedure. Manual palpation is used to confirm the presence of a distal radial pulse after inflation of the band over the access site. Because the Barbeau test is performed before the procedure to assess for adequate collateral palmar circulation, and because the distal radial pulse is assessed after band placement, it is possible to leave the band in place for more than 2 hours if bleeding persists, which can be of especial utility in unstable ICU patients. Moreover, a recent study demonstrated that transradial access in patients with INR >1.5 appears to be safe [3]. At our institution patients are not routinely advised to hold their antiplatelet or anticoagulant medications prior to noncoronary transradial procedures.

The "Radial Cocktail" in the Setting of Hemorrhage

In general, immediately after placing a sheath in the left radial artery, "radial cocktail" is administered, consisting of 3000 units heparin, 200 micrograms nitroglycerin, and 2.5 mg verapamil. The goal of this regimen is to reduce the risk of radial artery thrombosis post-procedure. In hemorrhagic patients, however, the addition of any of these medications may exacerbate hemorrhage. It is recommended, therefore, that in the case of hemodynamic instability, the radial cocktail be avoided completely. In cases in which the patient has a stable blood pressure and heart rate, it is reasonable to give verapamil and nitroglycerin without heparin. A pre-procedure Barbeau examination is always performed prior to radial artery access, and an A, B, or C result is necessary to confirm adequate collateral blood flow to the hand.

n-Butyl Cyanoacrylate for Hemorrhage

n-Butyl cyanoacrylate (nBCA) glue can be used as a permanent embolic for the treatment of hemorrhage in many settings, and is especially helpful in cases of acute hemorrhage in which a patient's platelets and/or clotting cascade are not fully functional [4, 5]. However, several specific concerns must be addressed when using glue due to its particular mechanism of action. TRUFILL n-BCA Liquid Embolic System (Johnson and Johnson, New Brunswick, NJ, USA) is an nBCA manufactured for intravascular use and is FDA approved for intracranial arteriovenous malformations, but it has been used off-label in many non-neurologic interventions. Histoacryl (B. Braun, Bethlehem, PA, USA) is a skin adhesive consisting of nBCA and is similarly used off-label for embolization. nBCA is not radio-opaque and must be mixed with either tantalum powder or lipiodol prior to administration in order to be seen fluoroscopically. Care must be taken to mix the glue in a glass container, as lipiodol will warp and destroy standard polypropylene syringes and basins. At our institution, most nBCA arterial embolizations are achieved with a 3:1 solution of lipiodol/nBCA, though some applications will call for a thicker or thinner solutions depending on the size of the target vessels and the desired degree of penetration. The larger the ratio of lipiodol to nBCA, the "thinner" the solution will be, and the further it will penetrate before polymerizing.

nBCA should only be administered through a microcatheter, ideally 2.4F or smaller. The catheter must be flushed with 5% dextrose solution at least 3 times prior to administration of the nBCA solution to prevent premature polymerization within the catheter. If the nBCA comes in contact with blood, saline, or contrast, it will polymerize. The nBCA solution should be administered in 0.2–0.4 ml aliquots using a polycarbonate syringe (Medalion; Merit Medical, South Jordan, UT, USA) and should be followed immediately by 5% dextrose flushes to fully eject it from the microcatheter. This should be done slowly under fluoroscopic guidance. If it appears that the full volume of the glue aliquot cannot be completely administered without causing reflux and/or nontarget embolization, the microcatheter should be quickly removed to prevent adherence of the catheter to the target vessel. For this reason, the base catheter should always be positioned carefully, such that any adherent glue sheared off during withdrawal of the microcatheter will not cause nontarget embolization of a critical vessel. Power injection should not be performed through the microcatheter after glue embolization has been performed; the microcatheter must be replaced.

Thorax

Arteries originating from the aorta at or above the level of T8 can be difficult to cannulate from a radial approach due to the limited maneuverability of the catheter within the aorta near the aortic arch. Especially if the patient is older, and has a tortuous aorta, these cases can be incredibly frustrating from the radial artery.

When preoperative imaging reveals that the origin of a bleeding intercostal or bronchial artery emerges at or below the level of the T8 vertebral body, a transradial approach is ideal. Approach is initiated with a 5F Sarah radial catheter and a 260 cm Bentson wire to access the descending aorta. Once the Bentson wire is deep in the descending aorta, the Sarah is exchanged for a 100 cm 4–5 F pigtail catheter, and a flush aortogram is performed at or above the suspected vessel origin. Of note, the Sarah has side holes and may be used for flush angiography runs, though the pigtail catheters result in superior aortograms. After identifying the target vessel, the 5F Sarah radial catheter may be replaced over a Bentson wire. After positioning the Sarah, a 2.8F microcatheter (Progreat, Terumo) is recommended for bronchial arteries, and a 2.4F catheter (Progreat, Terumo) is recommended for intercostal arteries.

Bronchial Artery Embolization

A 2.8F microcatheter is preferred for bronchial arteries because large particles used in bronchial artery embolization are less likely to become clogged in the larger microcatheter. A 0.018-inch Fathom microwire (Boston Scientific, Marlborough, MA, USA) is useful for vessel selection. Selective angiography is performed within the target bronchial artery, and special care must be taken to identify any vascular supply to the spinal cord or other nontarget vessels. Once the bronchial artery is selectively catheterized, and the microcatheter is positioned sufficiently beyond its origin, embolization may be performed with large particles, ideally 300–700 micron, such as Embospheres (Merit). After embolization, follow-up angiography should be performed from the microcatheter to assess vessel occlusion.

Sample Setup

- 110 cm 5F Sarah radial catheter
- 280 cm and 150 cm Bentson wires
- 4-5F 100 cm pigtail flush catheter
- 150 cm 2.8F Progreat microcatheter
- 180 cm 0.018-inch Fathom microwire
- 300–700 micron particles

Intercostal Artery Embolization

The same general technique as above is utilized, though in the case of an intercostal artery bleed, subselection with a 2.4F 150 cm microcatheter such as a Progreat is recommended. The smaller 2.4F microcatheter is recommended because liquid embolics or coils will likely be used. At our institution, 3:1 lipiodol/nBCA glue is the most frequently utilized embolic for intercostal artery bleeds. If this is planned, special care must be taken to optimize both base catheter and microcatheter positioning in order to minimize the risk of glue embolization into the abdominal aorta. Of the available microcoils, detachable coils are preferred, such as Concerto (Medtronic, Minneapolis, MN, USA). A glue-embolization of an intercostal artery bleed is seen in Fig. 18.1.

Sample Setup

- 110 cm 5F Sarah radial catheter
- 280 cm and 150 cm Bentson wires
- 4-5F 100 cm pigtail flush catheter
- 150 cm 2.4F Progreat microcatheter
- 180 cm 0.018-inch Fathom microwire
- n-Butyl cyanoacrylate glue/lipiodol
- Concerto detachable coils

When in Doubt

Do not be afraid to prep the groin and plan for common femoral artery access when attempting embolization of a thoracic artery, especially in cases in which the thoracic aorta is tortuous. A CTA in these cases is very helpful to localize the bleed or

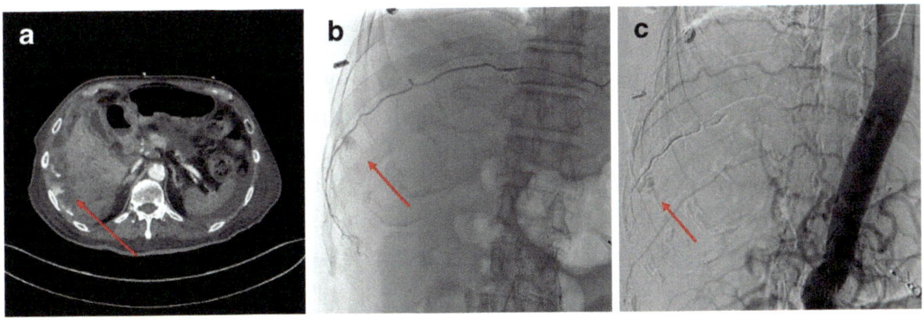

Fig. 18.1 70-year-old male with bleeding after percutaneous biliary drain removal. (**a**) CTA demonstrated arterial extravasation in right upper quadrant, suspected intercostal artery source. (**b**) Selective catheterization and angiography of the right tenth intercostal artery demonstrates active extravasation of contrast. Embolization was performed using 3:1 lipiodol/nBCA glue. (**c**) Post-embolization angiogram performed from the base catheter demonstrates a glue cast in the distal portion of the right tenth intercostal artery and absence of extravasation

at least a suspicious hypertrophied bronchial artery. Interestingly, a 5F Sarah radial catheter is also quite useful when introduced via femoral approach and is often the first choice for cannulating intercostal and bronchial arteries at our institution.

Abdomen

As with thoracic hemorrhage, there is a common transradial setup used for most forms of arterial hemorrhage in the abdomen. Most vessels in the abdomen can be easily reached with a Sarah radial base catheter and a 150 cm microcatheter. This combination is employed for bleeding vessels in the liver, spleen, kidney, and gastrointestinal (GI) tract, similar to the way in which the same reverse curve catheter may be used to for each of these regions when approaching from the groin. Hemorrhagic masses (most frequently ruptured HCC) can be treated from a transradial approach with the same general technique employed in hepatic oncologic embolizations, exchanging the chemo–/radio-therapeutic agent for a conventional embolic such as particles or nBCA. As with thoracic arterial interventions, abdominal embolizations performed from the radial artery vary in difficulty according to the tortuosity of the aorta, and pre-procedure imaging of the chest should always be reviewed if available.

Gastrointestinal Tract Hemorrhage

GI bleeding is one of the most frequently encountered indications for emergent embolization. Only arterial sources of GI hemorrhage may be selectively embolized in IR. For this reason, pre-procedure CTA is essential to confirm an arterial source, determine the offending vascular territory, and potentially discover the underlying etiology. Of special concern is bleeding from a fresh surgical anastomosis, as embolization of these already hypovascular regions appears to increase the risk of anastomotic failure [6]. If a patient with anastomotic bleeding is too unstable for conventional surgery, the patient and surgical team must be briefed on the increased risk of perianastomotic necrosis and anastomotic failure after an embolization.

The celiac artery and both the superior and inferior mesenteric arteries (SMA and IMA) are all easily accessible from a transradial approach using a 110 cm 5F Sarah radial catheter and 150 cm Bentson wire. In tall patients, the SMA and IMA may be cannulated using a 125 cm catheter such as the 4F Tempo Aqua VER (Cordis, Santa Clara, CA, USA). A 125 cm FH3 catheter (Merit) is helpful for cannulation of the left gastric artery (LGA) or the inferior phrenic arteries because of its sharp distal turn. If LGA access is required and a catheter with an abrupt 90-degree distal turn is not available, a transfemoral approach using a reverse curve catheter should be considered as the LGA can otherwise be difficult to cannulate from above.

In most cases, the abdominal aorta is accessed using a Sarah radial catheter and a 150 cm Bentson wire as usual, and digital subtraction angiography (DSA) is performed from the proximal celiac artery or SMA. The same injection rate for DSA may be used in the celiac and the SMA, 5 ml/s for a 25 ml total volume. Special care must be taken to include the entire vascular territory in the angiogram whenever possible. Keep in mind: review of raw angiographic images (without digital subtraction) can be useful to identify bleeding vessels in the presence of bowel peristalsis. Subselective catheterization may then be performed using a 2.4F 150 cm microcatheter such as a Progreat along with an 0.018-inch 180 cm microwire such as the Fathom. Successive runs of DSA are then performed through the microcatheter in order to identify and cannulate a target hemorrhagic vessel.

In forming a plan for embolization, consider the collateral vascular supply to the area in question. For example, if bleeding into the duodenum is identified in a branch of the gastroduodenal artery (GDA), it is reasonable to perform coil embolization of the GDA, as there is generally robust collateral supply to ensure perfusion of the duodenum even without the GDA. Conversely, if a tertiary branch of the right colic artery is found to be bleeding, special care must be taken to embolize from the most distal position possible and with a minimum of embolic, so as to preserve the colon's tenuous collateral blood supply [7].

At our institution, nBCA glue is the generally preferred embolic, and the above-described method is recommended using 0.2 ml or smaller aliquots. Detachable or pushable microcoils such as Concerto may also be used with precision, but should be avoided in patients without a functional clotting cascade. Gelfoam is discouraged, as there is often less accuracy in its administration, and recanalization is possible. A sample coil embolization of a cecal arterial bleed is shown in Fig. 18.2.

Sample Setup

- 110 cm 5F Sarah radial catheter
- 150 cm Bentson wire
- 150 cm 2.4F Progreat microcatheter
- 180 cm 0.018-inch Fathom microwire

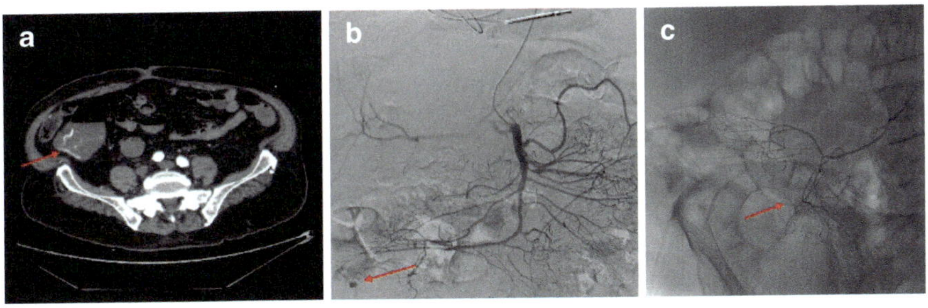

Fig. 18.2 85-year-old male with GI tract hemorrhage. (**a**) CTA demonstrated an arterial bleed in the cecum. (**b**) SMA angiogram performed from left radial approach revealed a small bleeding pseudoaneurysm in the cecum. (**c**) Hemostasis was achieved after superselective angiogram, vessel selection, and deployment of a single 4 × 3.7 mm pushable coil

- n-Butyl cyanoacrylate glue/lipiodol
- Concerto detachable coils

Stent-Assisted Embolization

In patients with bleeding from a truncated short vessel, such as in the case of a GDA stump rupture after a Whipple procedure, without a stent to provide a backwall for coil placement, embolization of such a very short vessel can be quite difficult. In this situation, stent-assisted coiling can be performed from a transradial approach (Fig. 18.3). A 6F system will be used in order to deliver the stent. A 6F radial sheath is used (Terumo), followed by a 6F guide catheter such as a 6F 100 cm JR-4 runway

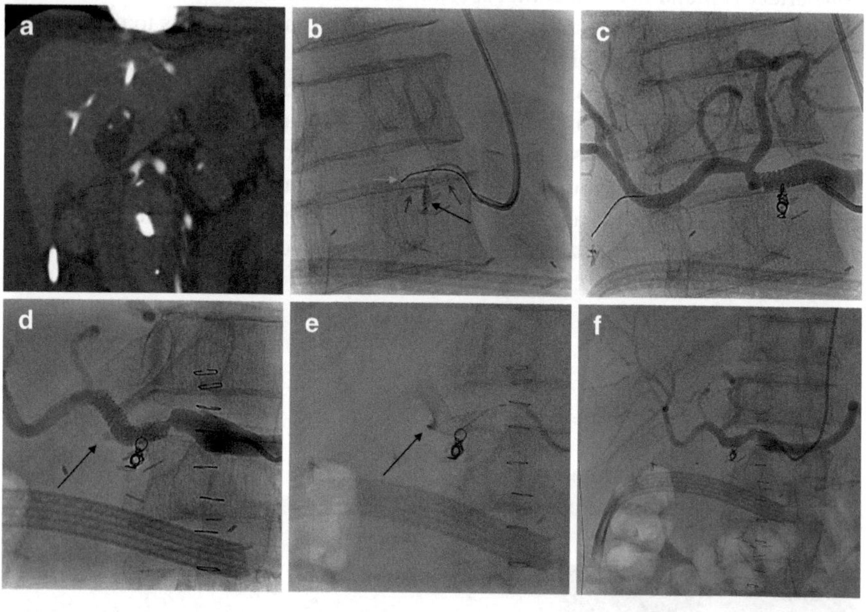

Fig. 18.3 72-year-old male post op day 6 after Whipple surgery for cholangiocarcinoma presenting with abdominal pain and clinical concern for bleeding. (**a**) CT angiogram demonstrated active bleeding (not shown) from the GDA. (**b**) A bare metal stent (blue arrows) was deployed across the GDA origin. A microcatheter (black arrow) was inserted between the interstices of the stent, while a safety microwire (green arrow) was left within the stent lumen. (**c**) After coil deployment into the GDA stump, an angiogram was performed from the common hepatic artery revealing patency of the proper hepatic artery and stent and occlusion of the GDA stump. (**d**) After 24 hours, the patient continued to bleed, and angiography was repeated demonstrating a small blister pseudoaneurysm originating from the stented portion of the common hepatic artery (black arrow). (**e**) A 0.1 ml aliquot of 3:1 lipiodol/nBCA glue was used for stent-assisted glue embolization (black arrow) using the same approach as previously utilized. (**f**) Final angiogram demonstrated occlusion of the blister pseudoaneurysm with radiopaque glue/lipiodol mixture. No further bleeding was seen in this patient

(Boston Scientific). Because a 6F catheter may approximate the diameter of the radial artery, a 3-way hemostasis valve such as the Guardian II (Teleflex, Wayne, PA, USA) and a pressure bag containing saline (with or without added heparin depending on the severity of the patient's hemorrhage) should be attached to ensure adequate flow through the catheter as it is advanced over a Bentson wire and up the radial artery. This same Bentson wire and 6F guide catheter may be used to cannulate the abdominal aorta and subsequently the Celiac artery. An atraumatic 0.014-inch microwire sufficient for delivery of a stent such as a 180 cm Balanced Middleweight Wire (BMW, Abbott, Chicago, IL, USA) or Stabilizer wire (Cordis) can then be used to target the vessel for stent deployment.

Herculink balloon-expandable bare-metal stents are most commonly used in our institution (Abbott), and range from 4 to 7 mm in diameter, though slightly larger diameters are achievable with balloon dilatation. After the stent is positioned across the target vessel, angiography may be performed as needed through the 3-way hemostatic valve to achieve ideal deployment. After deployment across the target vessel, such as the GDA, a 2.4F or smaller microcatheter is then placed in the stent lumen, and a microwire such as a Fathom may be used to advance the microcatheter through the interstices of the stent and into the hemorrhagic vessel. Detachable coils such as Concertos may then be used to completely occlude the vessel, using the stent as a backwall.

Sample Setup

- 6F radial sheath
- 100 cm 6F JR-4 runway guide catheter
- Guardian II hemostatic valve with pressure bag
- 150 cm Bentson wire
- 180 cm BMW 0.014-inch microwire
- Herculink balloon-expandable stent
- 150 cm 2.4 or 2.0F Progreat microcatheter
- 180 cm 0.018-inch Fathom microwire
- Concerto detachable coils

Splenic Hemorrhage

Splenic laceration is a feared complication of abdominal trauma and occurs frequently as a result of automotive accidents involving both drivers and pedestrians. Interventional radiologists are frequently involved in the treatment of splenic lacerations, specifically in patients in whom bleeding is identified from the spleen on the initial CT scan, but who are otherwise hemodynamically stable without need for emergent exploratory laparotomy.

The splenic artery is easily accessed using a Sarah radial catheter from the radial artery using the previously described techniques. It should be noted, however, that it is often helpful to perform selective angiography within the splenic artery, rather than celiac artery, when evaluating splenic hemorrhage. Rates for ideal DSA in this setting are 5 ml/s for 15–20 ml volume. The results of the angiogram will dictate the plan for embolization, and can be stratified into the following two categories:

- *Diffuse hemorrhage from multiple sites.* In this setting, a proximal embolization is necessary. The goal of a proximal splenic embolization is to decrease the overall blood flow to the spleen, while allowing it to remain perfused via collaterals from the short gastric arteries and other collateral pathways. To perform a proximal splenic embolization, first identify the branches of the splenic artery that directly supply the pancreas, such as the greater pancreatic artery and the various short perforators. A 2.4F microcatheter, such as a Progreat, is then placed into the splenic artery distal to the dorsal pancreatic artery but proximal to the hilar bifurcation and the greater pancreatic artery in order to preserve collateral flow. Detachable coils such as Concertos may then be deployed to form a scaffold in this location. Pushable coils may then be deployed into the scaffold to completely occlude the vessel. A completion angiogram should be performed within the splenic artery to confirm vessel occlusion, to assess for residual bleeding, and to confirm collateral perfusion of the splenic parenchyma.
- *Hemorrhage from 1 to 3 sites.* In this setting, a distal embolization is preferred, specifically targeting the distal bleeding vessels. The same approach is utilized to catheterize the splenic artery as mentioned previously. Next, a 150 cm 2.4F microcatheter such as a Progreat should be positioned using a 180 cm 0.018-inch microwire (Fathom) into the most distal position possible with respect to the bleeding branch vessel. Glue is frequently used in this setting to achieve permanent embolization of a tertiary bleeding vessel (3:1 lipiodol/nBCA, 0.2 ml aliquots), though detachable or pushable coils may also be used. A gelfoam slurry may be utilized, though this provides a less durable embolic effect. If gelfoam is to be used, a 2.8F microcatheter is recommended to reduce chance of clogging. As above, a completion angiogram is recommended from the base catheter in the splenic artery to confirm successful embolization.

Sample Setup

- 110 cm 5F Sarah radial catheter
- 150 cm Bentson wire
- 150 cm 2.4F Progreat microcatheter
- 180 cm 0.018-inch Fathom microwire
- Pushable or detachable coils (for proximal or distal embolization)
- n-Butyl cyanoacrylate glue/lipiodol (for distal embolization)

Renal Hemorrhage

Renal lacerations are common following trauma and are effectively treated from the left radial artery. To simplify, the same approach utilized for distal splenic artery embolization may be applied for renal parenchymal hemorrhage. The renal arteries are easily catheterized from above using a Sarah radial catheter. A highly specific distal embolization must be performed in the setting of a renal laceration to avoid damaging healthy renal parenchyma. For this reason, the most common embolics at our institution are detachable coils and glue. A sample renal bleed embolization is shown in Fig. 18.4.

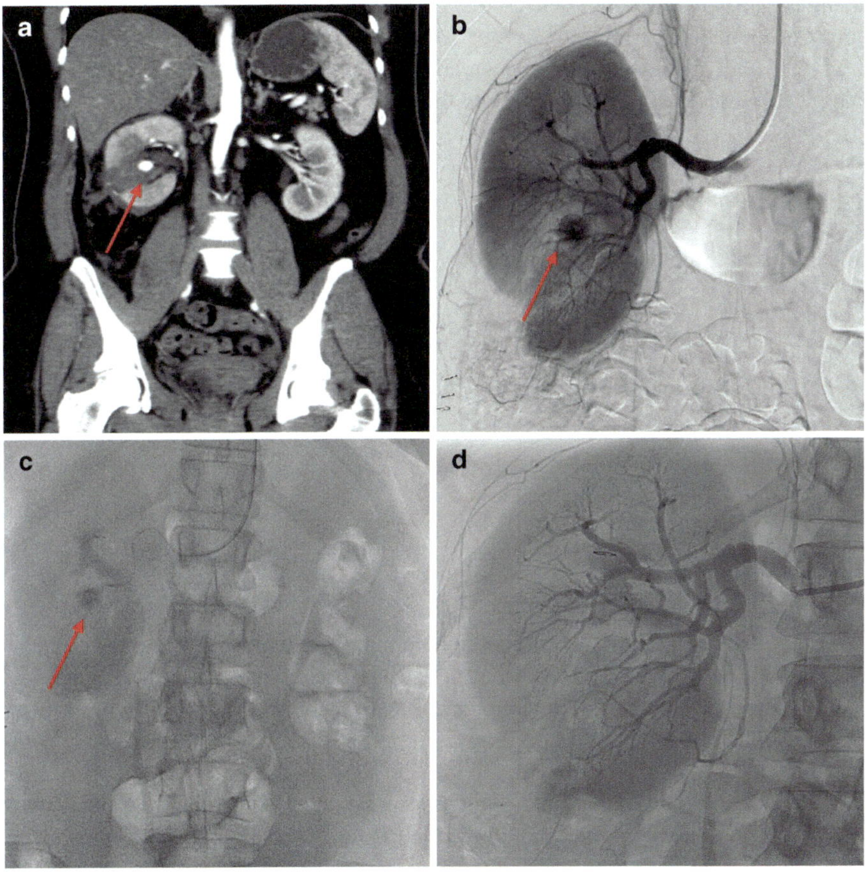

Fig. 18.4 46-year-old female with right flank pain and concern for bleeding after undergoing a partial nephrectomy for a renal cell carcinoma. (**a**) CTA demonstrated a 1 cm pseudoaneurysm in the resection bed. (**b**) Right renal angiogram from a transradial approach demonstrated the pseudoaneurysm. (**c**) The right renal artery branch supplying the pseudoaneurysm was selected, and a nBCA glue embolization was performed using 0.2-ml aliquots of 3:1 lipiodol/nBCA until the pseudoaneurysm was filled. (**d**) Postembolization angiogram from the base catheter confirms absence of flow in the pseudoaneurysm with preserved flow to the remainder of the kidney

A ruptured angiomyolipoma (AML) represents a specific cause of renal hemorrhage related to the rupture of a benign fatty tumor. For ruptured AMLs, renal angiography is performed from the Sarah radial catheter positioned just within the renal artery. Care is taken to identify all of the arteries feeding the AML, as incomplete embolization may result in recurrence. Selective catheterization is then performed using a 150 cm 2.4F microcatheter (Progreat) and a 0.018-inch microwire (Fathom). The catheter should be positioned in the feeding vessels such that nontarget embolization of the healthy renal parenchyma is avoided as much as possible. After a suitable position has been achieved, embolization is performed using 100–500 micron particles (Embospheres) or a liquid embolic such as nBCA. The goal of either liquid or particle embolization is the embolization of distal vessels; therefore a thinner nBCA solution such as 4:1 or 5:1 lipiodol/nBCA may be utilized to improve penetration into the tumor. After embolization, the microcatheter is removed, and an angiogram is performed from the base catheter to assess for residual bleeding/perfusion of the mass and the kidney.

Sample Setup

- 110 cm 5F Sarah radial catheter
- 150 cm Bentson wire
- 150 cm 2.4F Progreat microcatheter (or 2.8F in the case of particle embolization)
- 180 cm 0.018-inch Fathom microwire
- n-Butyl cyanoacrylate glue/lipiodol
- 100–500 micron particles

Pelvis

Of all the sites of hemorrhage discussed herein, transradial treatment of pelvic hemorrhage offers the most advantages over transfemoral. As discussed in the chapters on prostate and uterine embolizations, the cannulation of the iliac arteries from above is much easier from above than from below. Using a simple curved-tip catheter such as the Aqua Tempo VER, the left and right iliac arteries may be alternately catheterized in a matter of seconds from transradial approach, rather than necessitating a lengthy repositioning when performed from either the left or right common femoral artery.

Additionally, pelvic binders, placed in the setting of open-book fractures of the pelvis, can complicate access of the femoral arteries during intervention. The binder must be removed for common femoral artery access, and this can cause further hemorrhage and destabilization of the patient's fracture. Worse, it's often a bloody mess under there depending on the mechanism of injury. In these cases in particular, left radial artery access provides a route for embolization without the need to compromise the patient, and also has a lower risk of post-procedure access-site hemorrhage.

Traumatic Pelvic Hemorrhage

The left radial artery is accessed as usual, and a 5F radial sheath is placed. A 125 cm 4F catheter with a curved tip, such as an Aqua Tempo VER, may be used in concert with a 150 cm Bentson wire to advance the catheter all the way from the radial artery to the common iliac arteries. When performing the initial angiogram in the pelvis, the most thorough option is to exchange the catheter over a 260 cm Bentson wire for a 100 cm 4 or 5F pigtail catheter and perform a flush aortogram just above the bifurcation. This will provide the most comprehensive visualization of any pelvic bleeder. Alternatively, if a specific site of hemorrhage is already suggested based on CT, angiography may be performed from the common or internal iliac arteries via the VER catheter. This is generally sufficient, as almost all sources of pelvic hemorrhage in the setting of trauma will arise from an internal iliac artery branch.

When possible, a specific distal bleeding branch should be catheterized using a 150 cm microcatheter, and embolization should be performed with coils, glue, or Gelfoam. If Gelfoam will be used, a 2.8F microcatheter should be employed. Otherwise, a 2.4F microcatheter is ideal for deployment of glue and coils. In the case of a patient with multiple site of hemorrhage arising from the internal iliac artery, or in a hemodynamically unstable patient, embolization of the anterior division of the internal iliac artery with gelfoam may be performed from the base catheter without the use of a microcatheter.

Sample Setup

- 125 cm 4F Aqua Tempo VER catheter
- 150 cm Bentson wire
- 150 cm 2.4F Progreat microcatheter (or 2.8F if gelfoam will be used)
- 180 cm 0.018-inch Fathom microwire
- n-Butyl cyanoacrylate glue, gelfoam slurry, detachable or pushable microcoils

Post-partum Hemorrhage

Post-partum uterine hemorrhage can be readily treated from a left transradial approach using a 4F 125cm catheter such as the Tempo Aqua VER using the same general technique as uterine artery embolization in the treatment of uterine fibroids. Similar to the cases of pelvic trauma discussed above, multiple sites of hemorrhage may be identified, and gelfoam embolization of the anterior division of one or both internal iliac arteries may be helpful to achieve hemostasis quickly. Often, however, a specific distal bleeding vessel will be identified, and in this case the vessel should be selectively catheterized and embolized with a 2.4F microcatheter using the same method above.

Hematuria

Hematuria from a bleeding prostate or bladder can be treated in a similar fashion to a prostate artery embolization for BPH. In both procedures, the 125 cm VER catheter is advanced down the descending aorta, and an angiogram is performed in the internal iliac arteries. Ideally, a site of bleeding is identified on a pre-procedure CTA. If a specific bleed is identified, a 150 cm 2.4 microcatheter (Progreat) is advanced in concert with an 0.018-inch microwire (Fathom) into the target vessel as distally as possible, and selective embolization is performed using nBCA or coils. More frequently, however, as in the setting of hemorrhagic cystitis following radiation therapy or prostate hemorrhage following transurethral resection of the prostate (TURP), the feeding vessels should be empirically embolized with large particles from the superior and inferior vesicles arteries (hemorrhagic cystitis) or prostatic arteries (post-TURP hemorrhage), respectively, taking care to avoid nontarget embolization. In the setting of hemorrhagic cystitis, a 2.8F microcatheter should be used, along with large particles (500–700 micro Embospheres). Reduction in flow, rather than complete vessel occlusion, is desired. The same techniques used for transradial embolization of BPH may be utilized to treat prostate artery hemorrhage.

Sample Setup

- 125 cm 4F Aqua Tempo VER catheter
- 150 cm Bentson wire
- 150 cm 2.4F Progreat microcatheter (or 2.8F if gelfoam will be used)
- 180 cm 0.018-inch Fathom microwire
- n-Butyl cyanoacrylate glue, particles, or detachable microcoils

Tips

1. Review chest imaging pre-procedure to evaluate aortic tortuosity.
2. CTA is always helpful, but is specifically NOT required for post-partum hemorrhage or pelvic fractures with hemorrhage on conventional CT.
3. Consider using a permanent liquid embolic in coagulopathic patients (cirrhosis, DIC, etc.).
4. Transradial approach is generally safe even for coagulopathic patients.
5. In pelvic trauma patients in a pelvic binder, transradial access is almost always superior to transfemoral.

References

1. Wortman JR, Landman W, Fulwadhva UP, Viscomi SG, Sodickson AD. CT angiography for acute gastrointestinal bleeding: what the radiologist needs to know. Br J Radiol. 2017;90(1075):20170076. https://doi.org/10.1259/bjr.20170076.
2. Muhammad A, Awais M, Sayani R, et al. Empiric Transcatheter Arterial Embolization for Massive or Recurrent Gastrointestinal Bleeding: Ten-year Experience from a Single Tertiary Care Center. Cureus. 2019;11(3):e4228. Published 2019 Mar 11. https://doi.org/10.7759/cureus.4228.
3. Titano JJ, Biederman DM, Zech J, et al. Safety and Outcomes of Transradial Access in Patients with International Normalized Ratio 1.5 or above. J Vasc Interv Radiol. 2018;29(3):383–88. https://doi.org/10.1016/j.jvir.2017.11.010.
4. Yata S, Ohuchi Y, Adachi A, Endo M, Takasugi S, Tsukamoto K, Matsumoto K, Kodani M, Makishima J, Fujii S. Is glue embolization safe and effective for gastrointestinal bleeding?. Int J Gastrointest Interv 2018;7:158–61. https://doi.org/10.18528/gii180030.
5. Encarnacion CE, Kadir S, Beam CA, Payne CS. Gastrointestinal bleeding: treatment with gastrointestinal arterial embolization. Radiology. 1992;183(2):505–08. https://doi.org/10.1148/radiology.183.2.1561358.
6. Fernández de Sevilla Gómez E, Vallribera Valls F, Espin Basany E, et al. Postoperative small bowel and colonic anastomotic bleeding. Therapeutic management and complications. Cir Esp. 2014;92(7):463–67. https://doi.org/10.1016/j.ciresp.2014.03.002.
7. Pham T, Tran BA, Ooi K, et al. Super-Selective Mesenteric Embolization Provides Effective Control of Lower GI Bleeding. Radiol Res Pract. 2017;2017:1074804. https://doi.org/10.1155/2017/1074804.

Chapter 19
Transulnar Arterial Access

Daryl Goldman, Jun Yeop Lee, and Mona Ranade

Abbreviations

RA	Radial artery
TFA	Transfemoral arterial access
TRA	Transradial arterial access
TUA	Transulnar arterial access
UA	Ulnar artery

Introduction/Background

While the radial artery is increasingly becoming a more preferred access site for coronary and peripheral interventions, there are several relative contraindications including radial artery anatomical variations, tortuosity, and small radial artery caliber [1]. Ulnar artery access is a favorable alternative technique for percutaneous image-guided procedures when radial access is contraindicated, or the radial artery must be preserved. Transulnar approach for percutaneous coronary procedures was first performed by Terashima et al. on patients originally determined to have inadequate ulnar blood supply to perform transradial access (TRA) [2]. Since then, several studies have utilized transulnar access (TUA) as an alternative to both

D. Goldman (✉) · J. Y. Lee
Department of Diagnostic, Molecular and Interventional Radiology, Icahn School of Medicine at Mount Sinai, New York, NY, USA
e-mail: daryl.goldman2@mountsinai.org; junyeop.lee@icahn.mssm.edu

M. Ranade
Department of Radiology, University of California, Los Angeles, Los Angeles, CA, USA
e-mail: mranade@mednet.UCLA.edu

A. M. Fischman et al. (eds.), *Transradial Access in Interventional Radiology*,
https://doi.org/10.1007/978-3-030-81678-0_19

transfemoral access (TFA) and TRA reporting similar safety and efficacy of TUA and TRA [1–15].

The safety and efficacy of TUA has primarily been reported for coronary interventions. Multiple randomized controlled trials and single-center studies have shown that interventions via TUA achieves similar rates of success when compared to TRA, and with comparable rates of complications. When performed by the experienced operator, rates of complications of TUA, including major adverse cardiac events, such as MI, vessel revascularizations, stroke and mortality, and access site complications, such as hematoma, arterial stenosis or occlusion, pseudoaneurysm, and ulnar nerve injury, were similar to those of TRA, if not better [3, 5, 7, 11]. Additionally, TRA and TUA have similar operation-related parameters, including total procedure time and fluoroscopy time [7]. While limited, various studies have also utilized TUA for peripheral and visceral interventions and have reported similar success rates [12, 13]. Despite data suggesting feasibility and safety of TUA as a possible alternative to TRA, TUA is still rarely performed for coronary, peripheral, and visceral interventions.

Patient Selection

Patient selection is an important consideration for TUA (Table 19.1). In general selection criteria are often similar for TUA and TRA [6]. Ulnar access is often performed when patients are contraindicated for radial access; such conditions include small radial artery size, excessive tortuosity of the radial artery, variant radial artery anatomy including radial loop, past radial artery occlusion, and type D Barbeau test result. While presence of a type D Barbeau waveform indicates suboptimal anatomy, several studies suggest that TUA is still safe and feasible [8]. Prior to selecting patients for TUA, collateral flow to the hand and patency of ulnopalmar arch should be tested via both Barbeau and reverse Barbeau test, and sonographic evaluation of the anatomy and sizes of the forearm arteries must be performed.

Table 19.1 Relative indications and contraindications to TUA

Indications for TUA consideration	Relative contraindications
Barbeau D waveform	Ulnar artery <2 mm
Radial artery loop/tortuosity/anatomical variations	Aortic arch atherothrombosis/calcification
ESRD and potential for future HD access, functional upper extremity HD access involving the radial artery, potential for future CABG	Radial artery occlusion
Radial artery <2 mm	Ulnar artery vasospasm
Severe radial artery vasospasm	Operator inexperience
Past radial artery occlusion	Ulnar artery anatomical variations (rare)

The ulnar artery is often reported to be similar in size to the radial artery, although it is located relatively deeper and is less compressible than the radial artery. Additionally, the ulnar nerve and ulnar vein lie adjacent to the ulnar artery, and trauma to these structures during arterial access should be avoided [9]. Given the ulnar artery's deeper course in the wrist and proximity of the ulnar nerve, transulnar access may be technically more difficult. Various studies have reported higher crossover rates to TFA during TUA than TRA, primarily when operators were inexperienced with ulnar access [7]. Likewise, rates of vasospasm, time to access the artery, and total procedure time were all increased for TUA when performed under inexperienced operators [10, 11]. However, these same studies reported that such differences disappear once the operator is familiarized with the ulnar artery, with as little as 50 attempts sufficient to bring down the rate of complications to that of TRA [7].

The most significant complication of ulnar access is access site bleeding. In our experience, access site related bleeding can be occult and if not noticed early, can lead to compartment syndrome. The ulnar artery is deeper in the wrist and may not be positioned directly on top of the underlying bone; the artery thus frequently rolls when gaining access. Positioning the artery in its most stable position, typically pinning it against the ulna, is important to achieve post procedure hemostasis. Accessing the artery closer to the wrist is advised as compared to radial artery access where it can be safely accessed further up the forearm if necessary. If there is concern for hematoma and other access site bleeding at the end of the procedure, two TR bands should be placed – one directly over the ulnar access site, and the other proximal to it with half the amount of air (Fig. 19.3). This applies non-occlusive pressure on the access site and allows for reduced blood flow through the artery. The ipsilateral radial artery may also be compressed to enhance the ulnar flow [8]. Upon removal of the TR band(s), patients must be thoroughly evaluated for access site complications and presence of pulses [12].

Ulnar Artery Access Technique (Figs. 19.1 and 19.2)

1. Evaluate the ulnar artery patency using ultrasound.
2. Perform a reversed Allen test (Barbeau test) with ulnar compression to confirm patency of the ulnopalmar arch using pulse oximetry.

Table 19.2 Ulnar access sheaths

Device name	Manufacturer
Flexor Radial Introducer	Cook Medical, Inc (Bloomington, IN)
RadialSource, Avanti	Cordis (Bridgewater Township, NJ)
PreludeEASE	Merit Medical Systems, Inc (South Jordan, UT)
Adelante Radial	Oscor, Inc (Palm Harbor, FL)
Engage TR	St Jude Medical, Inc (St Paul, MN)
Glidesheath, Glidesheath Slender	Terumo Interventional Systems (Vaughan, Ontario)
VSI Radial	Vascular Solutions, Inc (Minneapolis, MD)

3. Position the left wrist to the side of the patient, supinated and dorsiflexed. Place a rolled towel underneath the wrist for support. Secure the hand in this position to the arm board with tape (Fig. 19.1).
4. Prep and drape in the normal sterile fashion.
5. Identify the access site with ultrasound visualization. The ulnar artery should be accessed over the ulnar styloid (Fig. 19.2).
6. Perform single-wall ulnar artery micropuncture under real-time ultrasound visualization.
7. Perform Seldinger technique with a 21-gauge micropuncture needle and 0.018 wire.
8. NOTE: Be mindful of adjacent ulnar nerve (lateral to medial approach).
9. Exchange needle for a micropuncture sheath.
10. 5F hydrophilic Glidesheath over a 0.035 wire without creating a skin incision.
11. Administer the "anti-spasmodic cocktail" through the sheath.
    (a) 3000 U heparin, 200mcg nitroglycerin, 2.5 mg of verapamil.
12. NOTE: Hemodilute the cocktail and inject slowly to reduce burning sensation.

Ulnar Artery Closure Technique: (Fig. 19.3)

1. Perform ulnar artery closure while maintaining patent hemostasis in order to reduce the rate of ulnar artery occlusion.
2. Insufflate the TR Band with 15-18 cc of air (versus <15 cc for TRA).
3. Continue patent hemostasis for a longer time period (120–180 minutes vs. 90 minutes for TRA access).

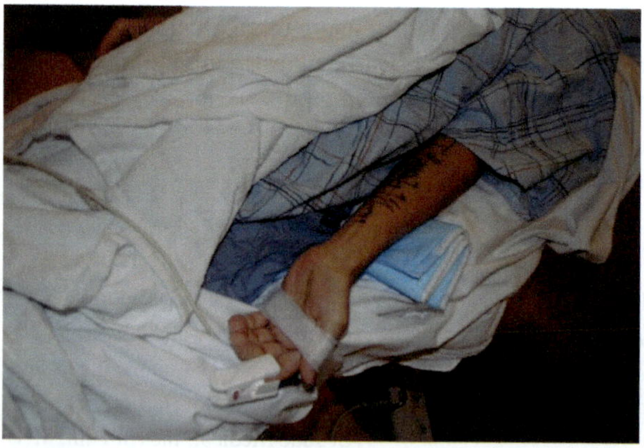

Fig. 19.1 Ulnar artery access patient positioning

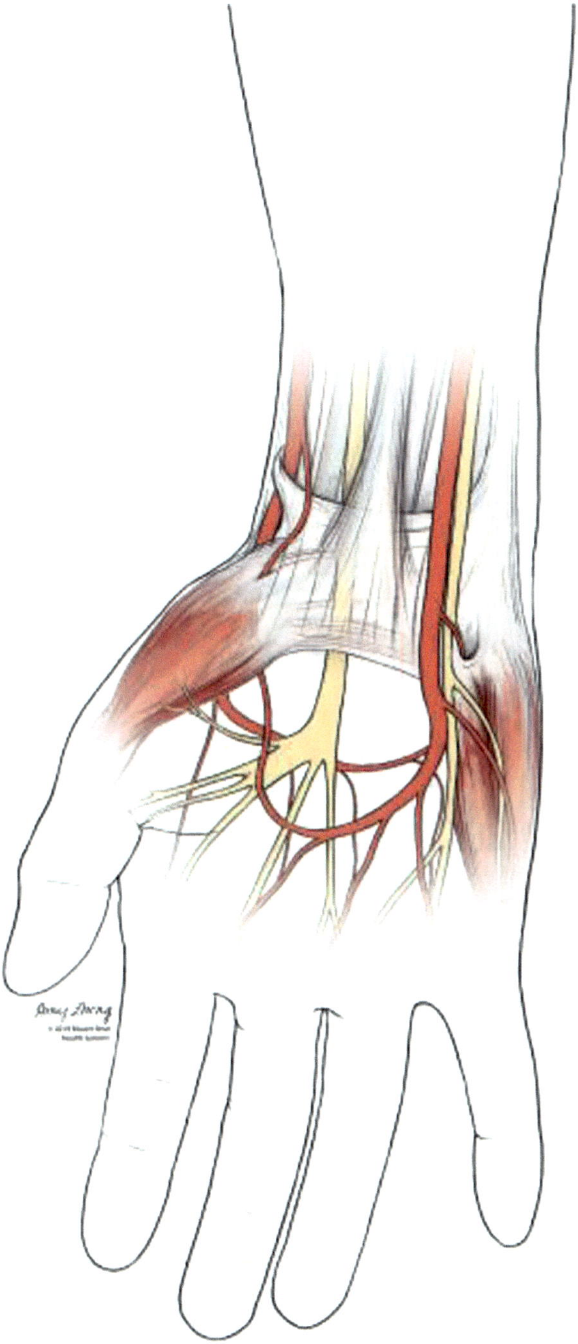

Fig. 19.2 Arterial anatomy of the forearm

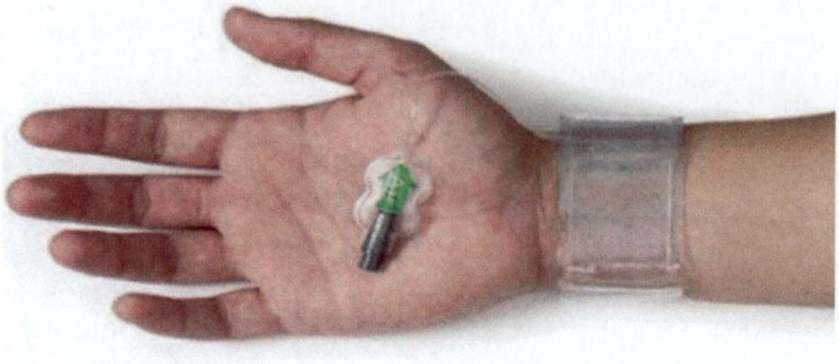

Fig. 19.3 Ulnar artery access closure

Table 19.3 Arterial compression devices

Device name	Manufacturer
HemoBand	Hemoband Corporation (Portland, OR)
TR Band	Terumo Interventional Systems (Vaughan, Ontario)
Zephyr-Dual Model 9200 Vascular Compression Device	Advanced Vascular Dynamics (Latham, NY)
Zephyr-Dual Vascular Compression Device	Advanced Vascular Dynamics (Latham, NY)

Authors Equipment List (Tables 19.2 and 19.3)

Transulnar Arterial Cases

Case 1

Renal Arteriovenous Fistula Embolization with n-BCA Liquid Embolic Agent
60 M with history of end-stage-renal-disease status post renal transplant, presenting 1-week post biopsy of renal transplant with elevating creatinine and Doppler ultrasound demonstrating evidence of renal transplant arteriovenous fistula (AVF). Patient had a left radiocephalic dialysis fistula and the decision was made to access the left ulnar artery.

Procedure

1. Obtain ulnar artery access as described earlier in this chapter (21-guage/4Fr Micropuncture Introducer Set, 4Fr 10-cm Glidesheath Slender (Terumo)) (Fig. A and B).
2. Administer the antispasmodic cocktail as described earlier in this chapter.
3. Navigate through the arm and into the right external iliac artery with a 0.035 × 150 cm Bentson Guidewire (AngioDynamics) and a 4Fr × 125 cm Tempo Aqua Vert Diagnostic Catheter (Cordis). Perform a diagnostic angiogram. Findings: Patent right main transplant renal artery arising from the right external iliac artery (Fig. C).
4. Select and catheterize the right main transplant renal artery and perform a DSA angiogram (Fig. D). Findings:

   (a) Transplant renal angiogram demonstrates focal irregularity of the renal arterial branch at the interpolar region near the hilum. There is early filling of a draining renal vein in this region and global decreased perfusion of the transplant kidney parenchyma. Findings are compatible with patient's known history of renal AVF.

5. Advance a 2.4Fr × 130 cm Progreat Microcatheter (Terumo) over a 0.16in × 180 cm, 25 cm tip Fathom Guidewire (Boston Scientific), and perform selective catheterization of the renal transplant distal hilar arterial branch supplying the fistula.
6. Perform embolization: Inject 0.8 cc of n-BCA liquid embolic agent slowly until near stasis is achieved (Fig. E).
7. Remove the microcatheter and retract the diagnostic catheter to the main renal artery, and perform completion angiography (Fig. F and G). Findings:

   (a) Successful occlusion of the AVF and increased perfusion throughout the transplant kidney.

8. Remove the catheter, guidewire, and sheath from the arm, and apply the TR Band Radial Artery Compression Device (Terumo) as described earlier in this chapter for 120–180 minutes.

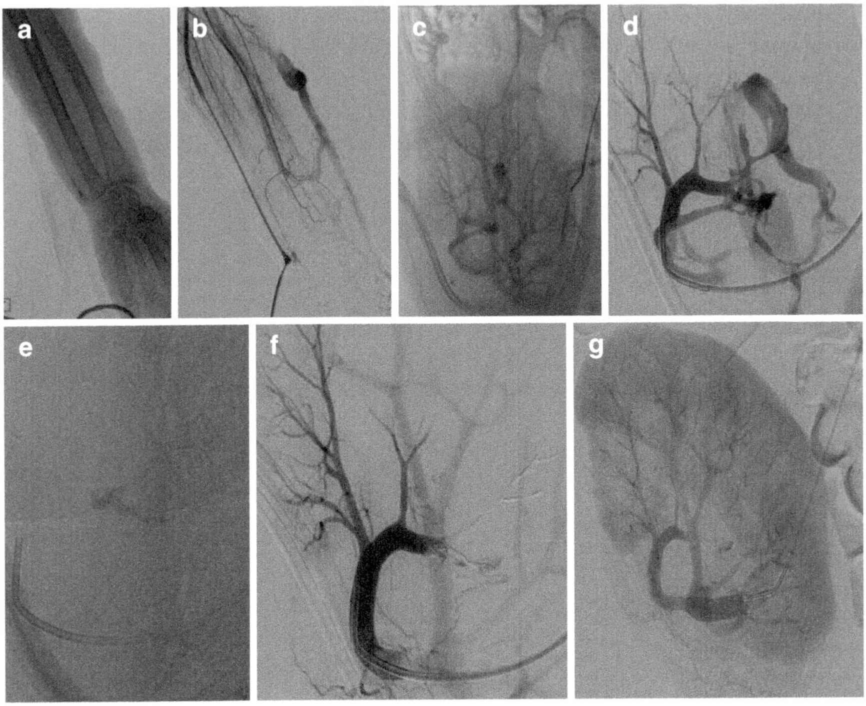

Case 2

Hepatic Chemoembolization

63-year-old with hepatocellular carcinoma. Barbeau waveform D.

Procedure

1. Obtain ulnar artery access as described earlier in this chapter (21-guage/5Fr Micropuncture Introducer Set, 5Fr 10-cm Glidesheath Slender (Terumo) (Fig. A).
2. Administer the antispasmodic cocktail as described earlier in this chapter.
3. Navigate through the arm and into the descending aorta with a 0.035 × 150 cm Bentson Guidewire (AngioDynamics) and a 5Fr × 110 cm Sarah Radial Diagnostic Catheter (Terumo).
4. Select the common hepatic artery and perform angiography, which demonstrates conventional hepatic anatomy and multiple areas of tumor blush within the right hepatic lobe (Fig. B).
5. Advance a 3Fr × 135 cm Renegade Hi-Flo Microcatheter (Boston Scientific) over a 0.16in × 180 cm, 25 cm tip Fathom Guidewire (Boston Scientific), and selectively catheterize the vessels feeding the tumors (Fig. C).
6. Perform embolization with 150 mg Adriamycin mixed with 10 mL of Lipiodol followed by 1 vial of 100 LC Bead Embolization Particles (BTG). Diagnostic angiogram shows adequate staining of the tumors (Fig. D).
7. Completion angiography from the right hepatic artery (Fig. E) demonstrates successful embolization of the target lesions.
8. Remove the catheter, guidewire, and sheath from the arm, and apply the TR Band Radial Artery Compression Device (Terumo) for 120–180 minutes.

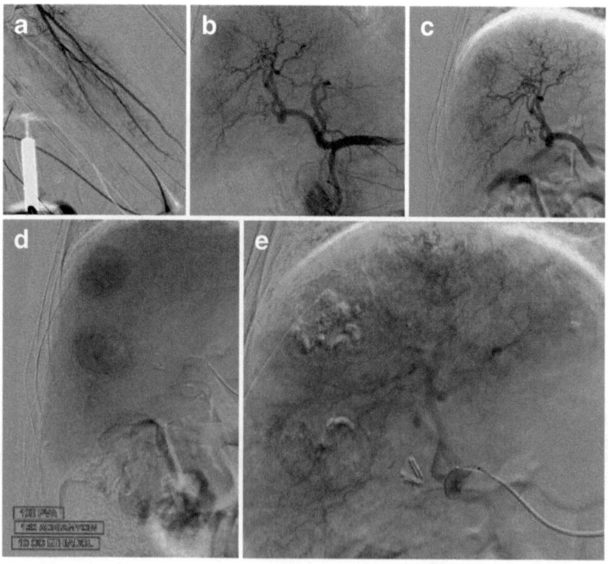

References

1. Mason PJ, Shah B, Tamis-Holland JE, et al. An update on radial artery access and best practices for transradial coronary angiography and intervention in acute coronary syndrome: a scientific statement from the American Heart Association. Circ Cardiovasc Interv. 2018;11:e000035.
2. Terashima M, Meguro T, Takeda H, et al. Percutaneous ulnar artery approach for coronary angiography: a preliminary report in nine patients. Catheter Cardiovasc Interv. 2001;53:410–4.
3. Gokhroo R, Bisht D, Padmanabhan D, Gupta S, Kishor K, Ranwa B. Feasibility of ulnar artery for cardiac catheterization: AJmer ULnar ARtery (AJULAR) catheterization study. Catheter Cardiovasc Interv. 2015;86:42–8.
4. Ruzsa Z, Toth K, Nemes B, et al. Transradial and transulnar access for iliac artery interventions using sheathless guiding systems: a feasibility study. Catheter Cardiovasc Interv. 2016;88:923–31.
5. Roghani-Dehkordi F, Mansouri R, Khosravi A, Mahaki B, Akbarzadeh M, Kermani-Alghoraishi M. Transulnar versus transradial approach for coronary angiography and angioplasty: considering their complications. ARYA Atheroscler. 2018;14:128–31.
6. de Andrade PB, Tebet MA, Nogueira EF, et al. Transulnar approach as an alternative access site for coronary invasive procedures after transradial approach failure. Am Heart J. 2012;164:462–7.
7. Gokhroo R, Kishor K, Ranwa B, et al. Ulnar artery interventions non-inferior to radial approach: AJmer Ulnar ARtery (AJULAR) intervention working group study results. J Invasive Cardiol. 2016;28:1–8.
8. Sattur S, Singh M, Kaluski E. Trans-ulnar catheterization and coronary interventions: from technique to outcomes. Cardiovasc Revasc Med. 2017;18:299–303.
9. Kar S. Systematic review of alternative access for cardiac catheterization and percutaneous coronary intervention: dorsal distal radial and ulnar artery catheterization. Catheter Cardiovasc Interv. 2019;94(5):706–13.
10. Hahalis G, Tsigkas G, Xanthopoulou I, et al. Transulnar compared with transradial artery approach as a default strategy for coronary procedures: a randomized trial. The Transulnar or Transradial Instead of Coronary Transfemoral Angiographies Study (the AURA of ARTEMIS Study). Circ Cardiovasc Interv. 2013;6:252–61.
11. Dahal K, Rijal J, Lee J, Korr KS, Azrin M. Transulnar versus transradial access for coronary angiography or percutaneous coronary intervention: a meta-analysis of randomized controlled trials. Catheter Cardiovasc Interv. 2016;87:857–65.
12. Zybulewski A, Edwards M, Kim E, et al. Transulnar approach as an alternative to transradial approach in non-coronary intervention: safety, feasibility and technical factors. J Vasc Access. 2017;18:250–4.
13. Gatzopoulos D, Rigatou A, Kontopodis E, et al. Alternative access site choice after initial radial access site failure for coronary angiography and intervention. J Geriatr Cardiol. 2018;15:585–90.
14. Kuo F, Park J, Chow K, Chen A, Walsworth MK. Avoiding peripheral nerve injury in arterial interventions. Diagn Interv Radiol. 2019;25:380–91.
15. Seto AH, Kern MJ. Transulnar catheterization: the road less traveled. Catheter Cardiovasc Interv. 2016;87:866–7.

Chapter 20
Distal Transradial Arterial Access

Daryl Goldman, Raghuram Posham, and Mona Ranade

Abbreviations

dTRA	Distal transradial arterial access
RA	Radial artery
TFA	Transfemoral arterial access
TRA	Transradial arterial access

Introduction/Background

Distal transradial artery access (dTRA) in the anatomical snuffbox is a safe and feasible alternative for percutaneous image-guided procedures [1–5]. Distal radial artery access is performed by accessing the deep radial artery just distal to the branch of the superficial palmer arch and just proximal to the artery to the princeps pollicis [2, 3]. The radial artery size at the anatomical snuffbox is not significantly different than at the wrist, allowing for safe and feasible access at both locations [3]. The distal aspect of the radial artery is located superficially and runs along the trapezium and scaphoid bones, theoretically allowing for easier post-procedure hemostatic control [1, 3, 5] (Fig. 20.1). Due to the superficial location of the distal radial artery, dTRA has advantages including fewer puncture site complications, faster post-procedural hemostasis, and may be a preferred method for patients as it allows for movement at the wrist during post-procedural hemostasis [1–3, 5]. Additionally, dTRA may be preferred for patients who are unable to supinate the arm allowing for increased intraprocedural comfort for these patients. Importantly, accessing the

D. Goldman (✉) · R. Posham
Department of Diagnostic, Molecular and Interventional Radiology, Icahn School of Medicine at Mount Sinai, New York, NY, USA
e-mail: daryl.goldman2@mountsinai.org

M. Ranade
Department of Radiology, University of California, Los Angeles, Los Angeles, CA, USA
e-mail: mranade@mednet.UCLA.edu

A. M. Fischman et al. (eds.), *Transradial Access in Interventional Radiology*,
https://doi.org/10.1007/978-3-030-81678-0_20

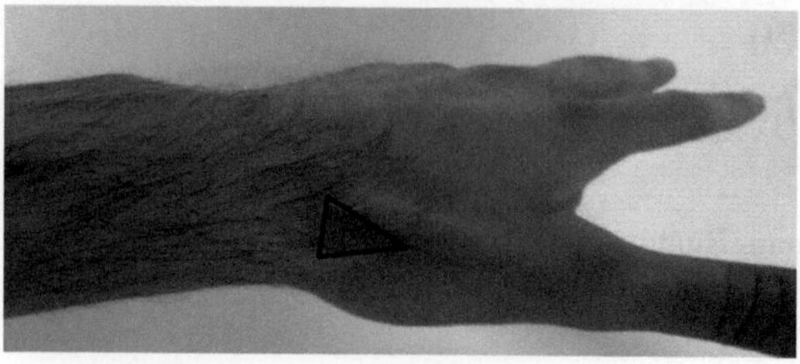

Fig. 20.1 Anatomic snuffbox

radial artery distally at the anatomic snuffbox allows for preserved antegrade flow to the hand via the superficial palmar arch and has been shown to reduce the incidence of radial artery occlusion and subsequent hand ischemia [1–5].

Patient Selection

As is the case in any traditional radial access procedure, patient selection for dTRA is an important consideration. In most cases, patients that are good candidates for TRA are also good candidates for dTRA. In certain cases, dTRA may be preferred over TRA; these include patients who are coagulopathic or are unable to discontinue anticoagulation, and patients with limited supination of the arm, as positioning for dTRA may be preferable [1–5] (Table 20.1).

Importantly, the anatomical snuffbox contains other important anatomic structures, including the cephalic vein and superficial branches of radial nerve. As damage to unintended structures can lead to complications, including hematoma, tendon damage, irritation of the underlying periosteum, and/or radial nerve injury, care must be taken not to damage these structures when accessing the artery. Ultrasound guidance should be used to identify landmarks and accurately access the vessel. In addition, the Barbeau test is recommended to evaluate for ulnopalmar patency, although some studies have doubted the usefulness of the Barbeau test for radial procedures [3]. Importantly, Patients with systemic or vascular disease can present with unreliably weak radial pulses, and proximal radial artery occlusions can present with a distal pulse due to robust palmar collaterals [3].

Distal Transradial Arterial Access Step-by-Step Technique

1. Identify the anatomical snuffbox (Fig. 20.1).
2. Evaluate the distal radial artery patency using ultrasound.
3. Perform an Allen test (Barbeau test) with distal radial compression to confirm patency of the radial palmer arch using pulse oximetry.

Table 20.1 Relative indications and contraindications to dTRA

Indication for dTRA consideration	Relative contraindications
Coagulopathy/unable to discontinue anticoagulation	Radial artery <2 mm
Patient preference	Aortic arch atherothrombosis/calcification
Inability to supinate arm	Radial artery occlusion
	Radial artery loop
	Barbeau D waveform
	ESRD and potential for future HD access, functional upper extremity HD access

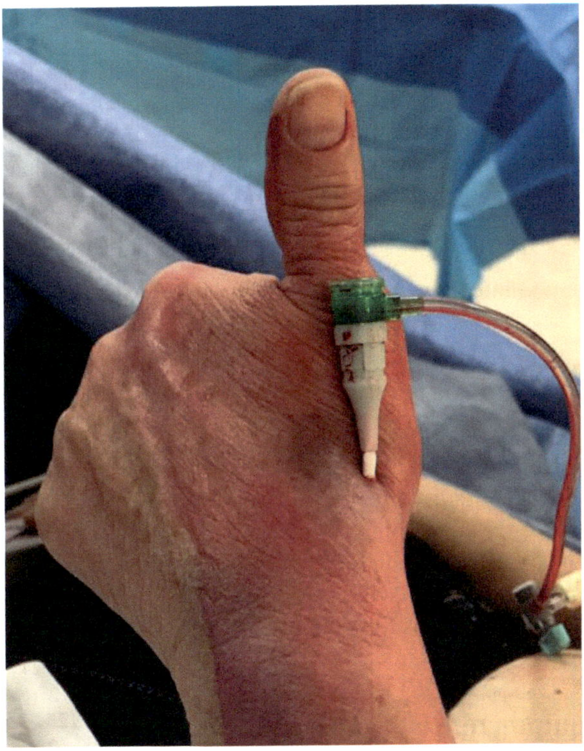

Fig. 20.2 Anatomic snuffbox; distal transradial arterial access site

4. Position the patient with the arm by their side at 90° of abduction (thumbs up position, Fig. 20.2) or across the body toward the contralateral groin. Secure the hand in this position to the arm board with tape.
5. Prep and drape in the normal sterile fashion.
6. Identify the access site with ultrasound visualization; identify the metacarpal of the thumb and index finger, and then adjust the ultrasound probe, so first the trapezium and then the scaphoid is visualized under the artery. Then pick any area along the radial artery between the scaphoid and the trapezium, while staying distal to the superficial branch of the radial artery (Fig. 20.3).

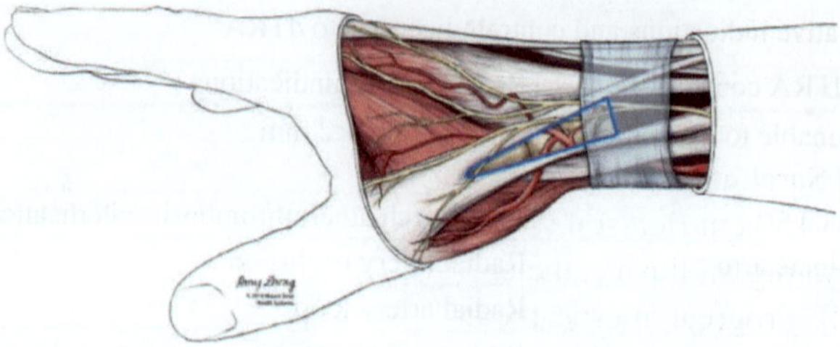

Fig. 20.3 Arterial anatomy of the anatomic snuffbox. (Printed with permission from ©Mount Sinai Health System)

7. Perform single-wall distal radial artery micropuncture under real-time ultrasound visualization.
8. Perform Seldinger technique with a 21-gauge micropuncture needle and 0.018 wire.
9. Exchange needle for a micropuncture sheath.
10. 5F hydrophilic Glidesheath over a 0.035 wire without creating a skin incision.
11. Administer the "anti-spasmodic cocktail" through the sheath.
    (a) 3000 U heparin, 200mcg nitroglycerin, 2.5 mg of verapamil.
12. NOTE: Hemodilute the cocktail and inject slowly to reduce burning sensation.

Distal Transradial Arterial Closure Technique: (Fig. 20.4)

1. Perform distal radial artery closure while maintaining patent hemostasis in order to reduce the rate of radial artery occlusion.
2. Apply a Safeguard Radial Compression Device (Merit Medical) to the access site.
3. Insufflate the Safeguard Radial Compression device until patent hemostasis is achieved (approximately 3 cc of air).
4. Continue patent hemostasis for a minimum of 90 minutes.

Authors Equipment List (Tables 20.2 and 20.3)

Distal Transradial Arterial Cases

Case 1

Left Shoulder Mass Pre-operative Embolization

79 M with metastatic renal cell carcinoma to the left shoulder with plan to undergo surgical resection, requiring presurgical embolization. Barbeau waveform type B.

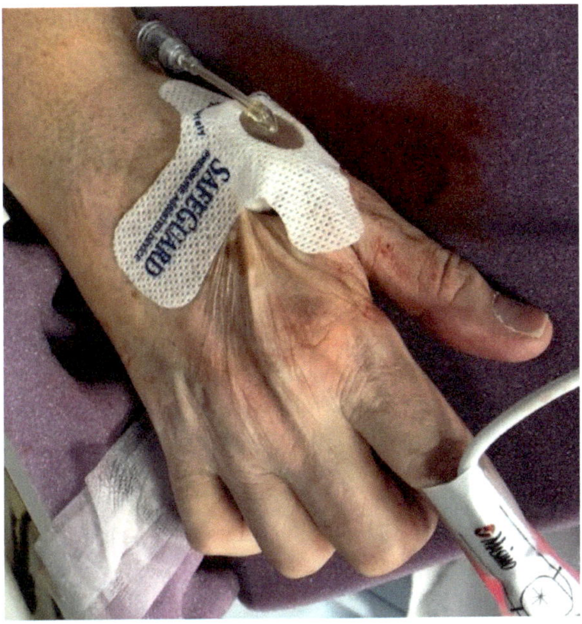

Fig. 20.4 Distal transradial arterial closure

Table 20.2 Distal radial access sheaths

Device name	Manufacturer
Flexor Radial Introducer	Cook Medical, Inc (Bloomington, IN)
RadialSource, Avanti	Cordis (Bridgewater Township, NJ)
PreludeEASE	Merit Medical Systems, Inc (South Jordan, UT)
Adelante Radial	Oscor, Inc (Palm Harbor, FL)
Engage TR	St Jude Medical, Inc (St Paul, MN)
Glidesheath, Glidesheath Slender	Terumo Interventional Systems (Vaughan, Ontario)
VSI Radial	Vascular Solutions, Inc (Minneapolis, MD)

Table 20.3 Radial arterial compression devices

Device name	Manufacturer
VasoStat	Forge Medical (Philadelphia, PA)
PreludeSYNC DISTAL	Merit Medical Systems, Inc (South Jordan, UT)

Procedure

1. Obtain distal radial access as described earlier in this chapter (21-guage/5Fr Micropuncture Introducer Set, 5Fr 10-cm Glidesheath Slender (Terumo)).
2. Administer the antispasmodic cocktail as described earlier in this chapter.

3. Navigate to the proximal axillary artery with a 0.035 × 130 cm Bentson Guidewire (AngioDynamics) and a 4Fr × 65 cm Berenstein Diagnostic Catheter (Cordis).
4. Perform left upper extremity angiography. Findings:
   (a) Large left shoulder mass with multiple supplying feeders from the left axillary artery, circumflex humeral artery, and circumflex scapular artery.
5. Exchange the Berenstein catheter for a 4Fr × 65 cm Soft-Vu Diagnostic Cather (AngioDynamics), and select the left posterior circumflex artery which is noted to supply the anterior aspect of the mass (Fig. A).
6. Advance a 2.4Fr × 130 cm Progreat Microcatheter (Terumo) over a 0.16in × 180 cm, 25 cm tip Fathom Guidewire (Boston Scientific) to the distal left posterior circumflex, and perform superselective angiography, with findings confirming tumor blush of the superior aspect of the mass, with collateral supply from circumflex, scapular, acromial, and clavicular artery branches (Fig. B).
7. Perform embolization with 500 um Embozene Microspheres (Boston Scientific). Angiographic endpoint: near-stasis (not static, contrast visible for at least 5 heartbeats). Post embolization angiography confirms significantly decreased tumor blush.
8. Retract the microcatheter and subselect the left circumflex scapular artery, and advance the system to the distal aspect of the vessel. Perform superselective angiography, demonstrating tumor blush of the inferior aspect of the mass with branches from the clavicular and acromial artery (Fig. C).
9. Perform embolization with 500 um Embozene Microspheres (Boston Scientific). Angiographic endpoint: near-stasis (not static, contrast visible for at least 5 heartbeats). Post embolization angiography confirms significantly decreased tumor blush.
10. Perform completion angiography from the axillary artery. Findings:
    (a) Significantly decreased vascular flow to the left shoulder mass with small residual enhancement (Fig. D and E).
11. Remove the catheter, guidewire, and sheath from the arm, and apply the VasoStat hemostatis device (Forge Medical) for 90.. minutes.

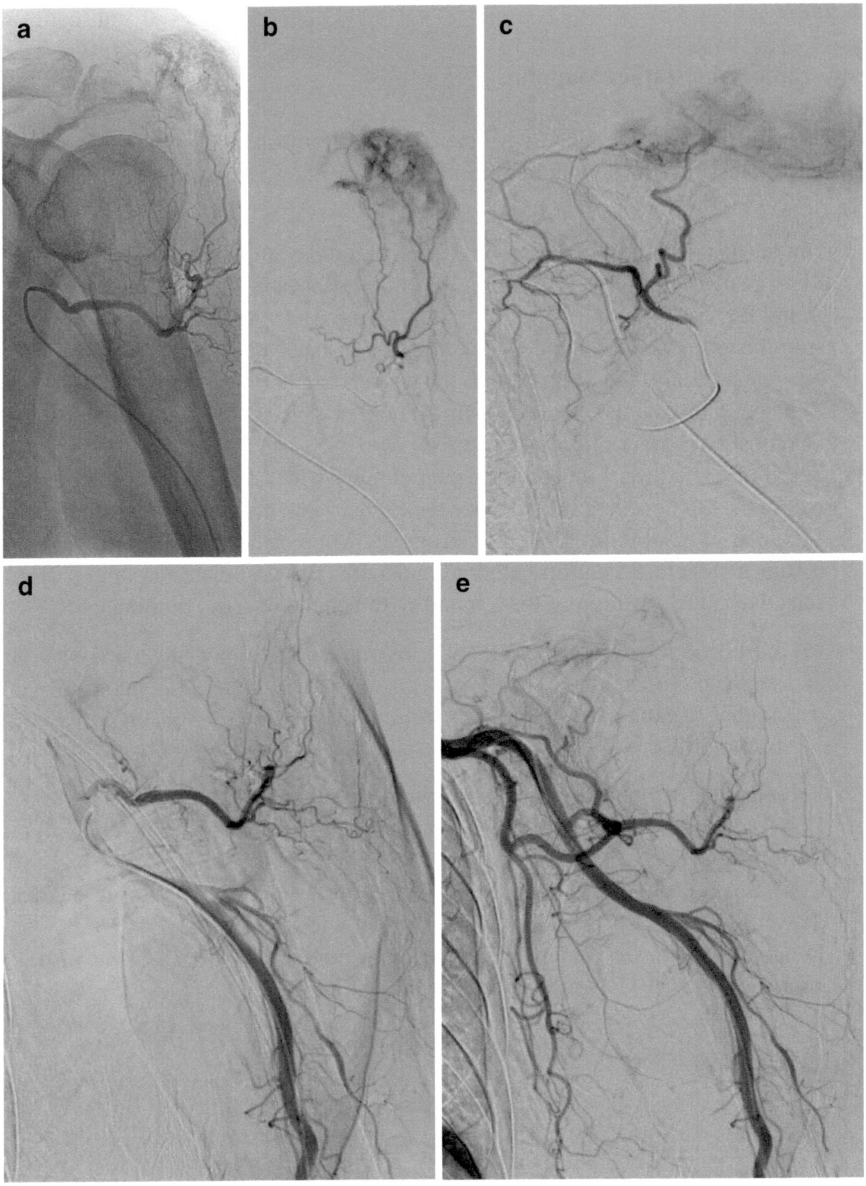
a
b
c
d
e

Case 2

Pre-radioembolization Mapping

76 M with unresectable HCC with portal vein thrombus, right lobe atrophy, and elevated total bilirubin and alpha-fetoprotein. Barbeau waveform type C.

Procedure

1. Obtain distal radial access as described earlier in this chapter (21-guage/5Fr Micropuncture Introducer Set, 5Fr 10-cm Glidesheath Slender (Terumo)) (Fig. A and B).
2. Administer the antispasmodic cocktail as described earlier in this chapter.
3. Navigate through the arm and into the descending aorta with a 0.035 × 130 cm Bentson Guidewire (AngioDynamics) and a 5Fr × 110 cm Sarah Radial Diagnostic Catheter (Terumo).
4. Select the celiac artery and perform angiography, which demonstrates tumor blush within the left hepatic lobe. Advance the catheter into the common hepatic artery.
5. Advance a 2.4Fr × 130 cm Progreat Microcatheter (Terumo) over a 0.16in × 180 cm, 25 cm tip Fathom Guidewire (Boston Scientific), and perform selective catheterization of the left and right hepatic arteries. Findings:
   (a) Left hepatic artery catheterization: hypervascular tumor blush arising from segment 4 branch.
   (b) Right hepatic artery catheterization: no evidence of hypervascular tumor blush.
6. Subselect the segment 4 branch supplying the tumor (Fig. D).
7. Deliver TC-99 MAA into the segment 4 hepatic artery branch supplying the tumor.
8. Cone Beam CT (CBCT) was performed intraprocedurally to confirm adequate delivery of the MAA to the intended segment 4 lesion (Fig. E).
9. Remove the catheter, guidewire, and sheath from the arm, and apply the VasoStat hemostatis device (Forge Medical) for 90.. minutes.

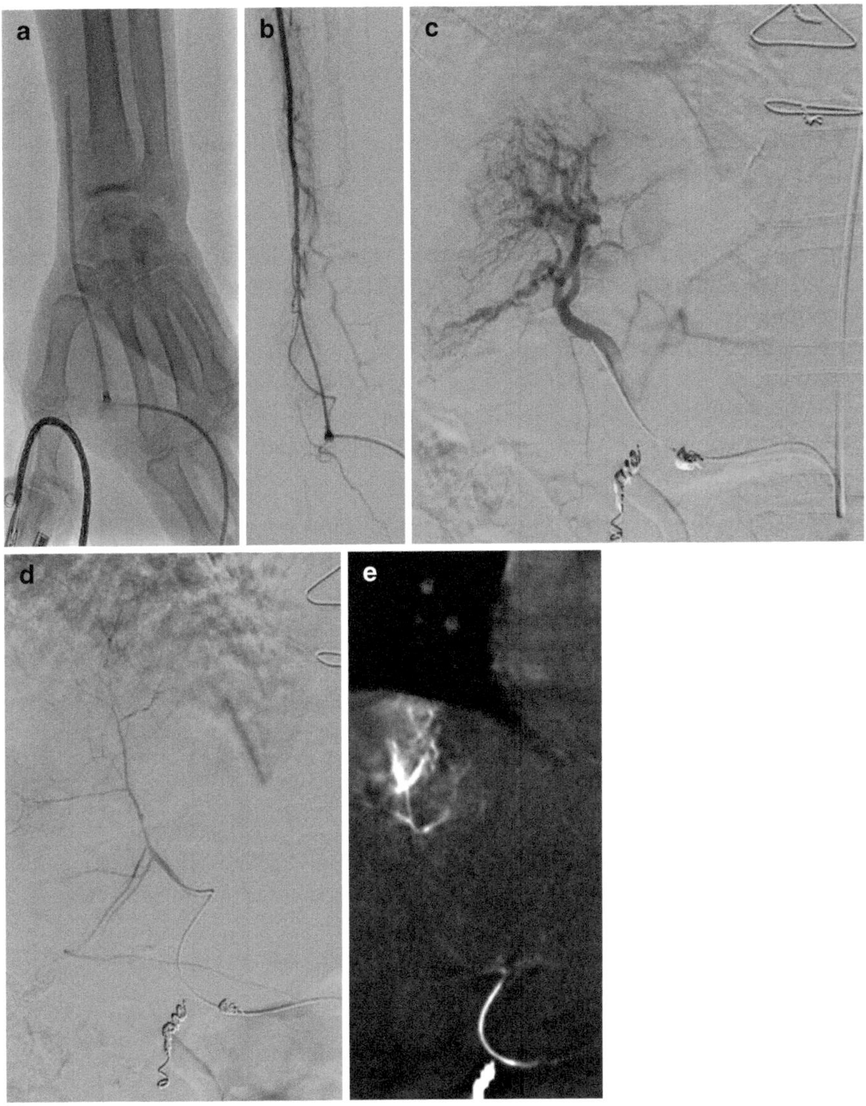
a
b
c
d
e

Case 3

Embolization of Left Humerus Metastatic Hepatocellular Carcinoma Mass

68 M with metastatic hepatocellular carcinoma to the left humerus causes pathologic fracture. Barbeau waveform type B.

Procedure

1. Obtain distal radial access as described earlier in this chapter (21-guage/5Fr Micropuncture Introducer Set, 5Fr 10-cm Glidesheath Slender (Terumo)).
2. Administer the antispasmodic cocktail as described earlier in this chapter.
3. Navigate to the proximal axillary artery with a 0.038in × 180 cm Angled Tip Glidewire (Terumo) and 5Fr × 65 cm Soft-Vu Diagnostic Catheter (AngioDynamics).
4. Perform left upper extremity angiography from the left axillary artery (Figs. A and B). Findings:

   (a) Tumor blush overlying the proximal left humerus at the site of pathologic fracture.

5. Advance a 2.4Fr × 130 cm Progreat Microcatheter (Terumo) over a 0.16in × 180 cm, 25 cm tip Fathom Guidewire (Boston Scientific) into the left circumflex humeral artery.
6. Perform selective angiography from the left circumflex humeral artery (Fig. C). Findings:

   (a) Approximately 70% of the tumor vasculature supplied by the left circumflex humeral artery.

7. Perform embolization with 500 um Embozene Microspheres (Boston Scientific). Angiographic endpoint: near-stasis (not static, contrast visible for at least 5 heartbeats) (Fig. D).
8. Perform completion angiography from the axillary artery (Fig. E). Findings:

   (a) Significantly decreased tumor blush.

9. Remove the catheter, guidewire, and sheath from the arm, and apply the VasoStat hemostatis device (Forge Medical) for 90.. minutes.

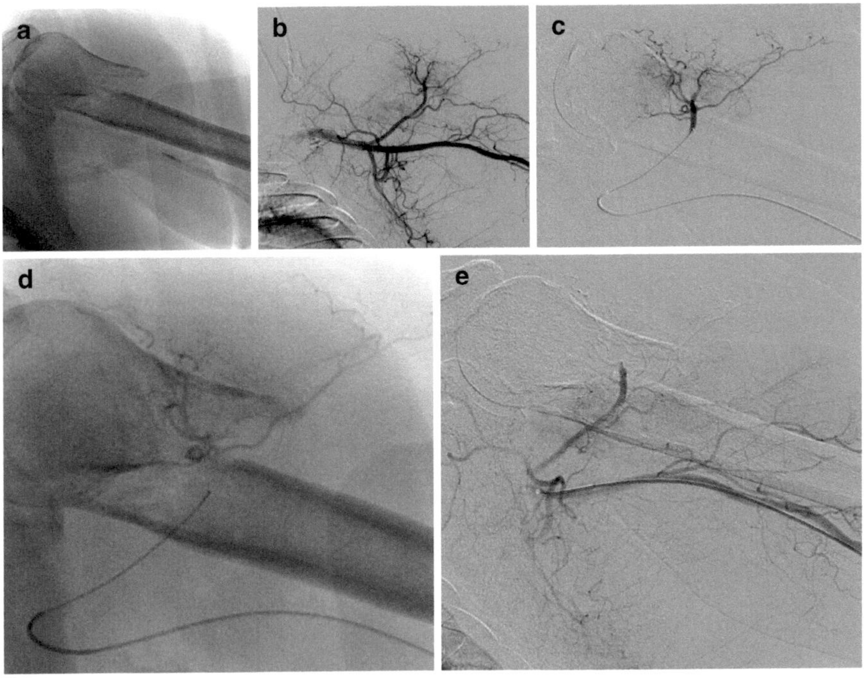

References

1. van Dam L, Geeraedts T, Bijdevaate D, van Doormaal PJ, The A, Moelker A. Distal radial artery access for noncoronary endovascular treatment is a safe and feasible technique. J Vasc Interv Radiol. 2019;30(8):1281–5.
2. Kiemeneij F. Left distal transradial access in the anatomical snuffbox for coronary angiography (ldTRA) and interventions (ldTRI). EuroIntervention. 2017;13(7):851–7.
3. Hadjivassiliou A, Kiemeneij F, Nathan S, Klass D. Ultrasound-guided access of the distal radial artery at the anatomical snuffbox for catheter-based vascular interventions: a technical guide. EuroIntervention. 2021;16(16):1342–8.
4. Hadjivassiliou A, Chung J, Liu D, Klass D. 4:12 PM abstract no. 159 technical feasibility and safety of left distal transradial access for percutaneous image-guided procedures. J Vasc Interv Radiol. 2018;29(4):S71.
5. Pua U, Sim JZT, Quek LHH, Kwan J, Lim GHT, Huang IKH. Feasibility study of "snuffbox" radial access for visceral interventions. J Vasc Interv Radiol. 2018;29(9):1276–80.

Chapter 21
Transradial Access for Bariatric Embolization

Mario A. Cedillo, Kirema Garcia-Reyes, and Aaron M. Fischman

Abbreviations

BAE	Bariatric arterial embolization
CBCT	Cone-beam computed tomography
CHA	Common hepatic artery
DSA	Digital subtraction angiography
GEA	Gastroepiploic artery
IDE	Investigational device exemption
LGA	Left gastric artery
SA	Splenic artery

Introduction

Obesity is a major public health concern in the United States with significant morbidity and mortality [1]. In patients who don't respond to traditional treatments (such as diet modification, exercise, behavioral therapy, medications), surgery can be considered to treat obesity. Bariatric surgeries such as Roux-en-Y gastric bypass and sleeve gastrectomy have proven effective in producing large and sustained weight loss but pose significant risks of morbidity and mortality [2]. The weight loss from bariatric surgery has been attributed to a decrease in an appetite mediating hormone called ghrelin, a 28-amino acid peptide that is produced primarily in the gastric fundus [3]. The gastric fundus is supplied predominantly by the left gastric artery (LGA) [4]. Bariatric arterial embolization (BAE) is an image-guided therapy that delivers targeted embolics to the gastric arteries (usually the LGA) to induce localized ischemia and downregulation of the appetite mediated hormone ghrelin

M. A. Cedillo · K. Garcia-Reyes · A. M. Fischman (✉)
Department of Diagnostic, Molecular and Interventional Radiology,
Icahn School of Medicine at Mount Sinai, New York, NY, USA
e-mail: aaron.fischman@mountsinai.org

A. M. Fischman et al. (eds.), *Transradial Access in Interventional Radiology*,
https://doi.org/10.1007/978-3-030-81678-0_21

[5]. The benefits of BAE have been reported in multiple clinical trials which report a favorable safety profile and potential efficacy in treating obesity by suppressing ghrelin production, resulting in early weight loss and abdominal fat loss [6–8]. Radial access is of particular interest in treating severely obese patients where femoral access may be more technically challenging. Additionally, radial access in morbidly obese patients (BMI > 40) may have less bleeding and less access site complications when compared to femoral access [9]. Although the short-term weight loss benefit of BAE appears promising, the long-term benefit remains unclear, and continued investigation should be performed in the context of an investigational device exemption (IDE). This chapter will discuss conventional and variant gastric vascular anatomy as well as key technical considerations for successful transradial BAE.

Anatomical Considerations

Visceral Anatomy of the Stomach

The stomach is a muscular and hollow organ made up of five anatomical/histological sections: the cardia, fundus, body, antrum, and pylorus. Located to the left and superior to the cardia just below the diaphragm is a dome-shaped fundus. The fundus harbors most of the gastric neuroregulatory pathways involved with appetite stimulation and satiety. Within the fundus are X/A cells responsible for producing 75–90% of the body's ghrelin, the primary appetite stimulating hormone of the body [5].

Conventional Gastric Arterial Anatomy

The celiac trunk arises from the aorta at the level of T12 and gives off three major branches including the LGA, splenic artery (SA), and common hepatic artery (CHA) (Figs. 21.1 and 21.2). The LGA is the smallest of the three branches and typically branches first, supplying the lesser curvature of the stomach (Figs. 21.1 and 21.2). The LGA provides the majority of arterial supply to the gastric fundus, with the gastroepiploic artery (GEA) providing additional supply in some patients. The right gastric artery arises from the CHA and, like the LGA, supplies the lesser curvature of the stomach (Figs. 21.1 and 21.2). The left GEA and short gastric arteries branch from the SA and supply the greater curvature of the stomach. The right GEA branches from the gastroduodenal artery and also supplies the greater curvature of the stomach (Figs. 21.1 and 21.2).

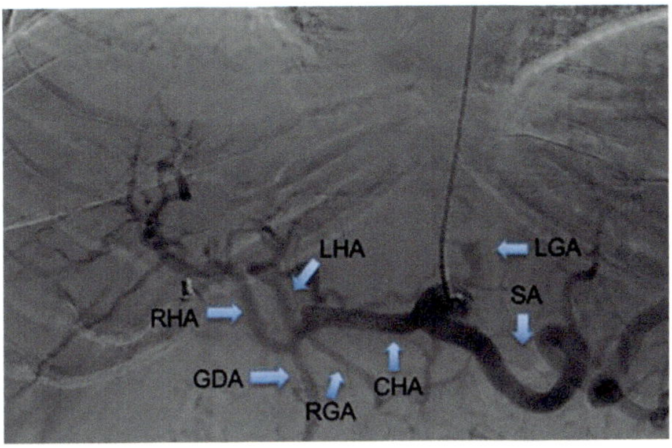

Fig. 21.1 Conventional celiac trunk anatomy. Diagnostic angiogram via a 5 F Sarah radial catheter with the tip at the origin of the celiac axis. The three main branches arising from the celiac artery are the left gastric artery (LGA), splenic artery (SA), and common hepatic artery (CHA). Additional arteries are the gastroduodenal artery (GDA), right gastric artery (RGA), right hepatic artery (RHA), and left hepatic artery (LHA)

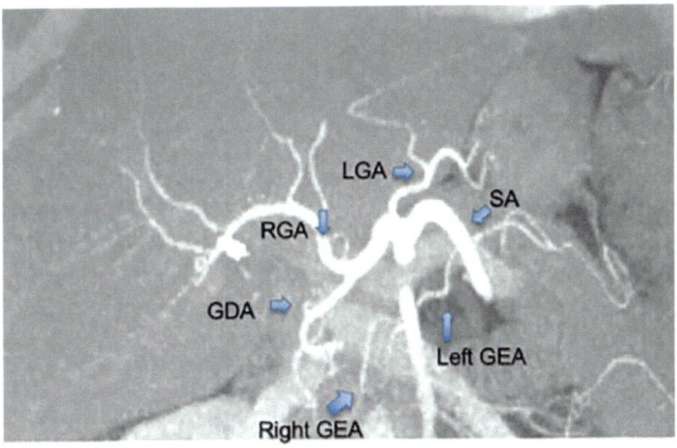

Fig. 21.2 Conventional gastric arterial anatomy. Maximum-intensity projection coronal CBCT angiogram demonstrates the left gastric artery (LGA) arising from the celiac artery, and the right gastric artery (RGA) arising from the common hepatic artery (CHA). The left gastroepiploic artery (GEA) arises from the splenic artery (SA), while the right GEA arises from the gastroduodenal artery (GDA)

Variant Gastric Arterial Vascular Anatomy

Recognition of anatomical variants is critical to avoid complications such as undertreatment and nontarget embolization, which may result in gastric mucosal ulceration, erosion, or gastritis. The morphological variations of the celiac trunk are

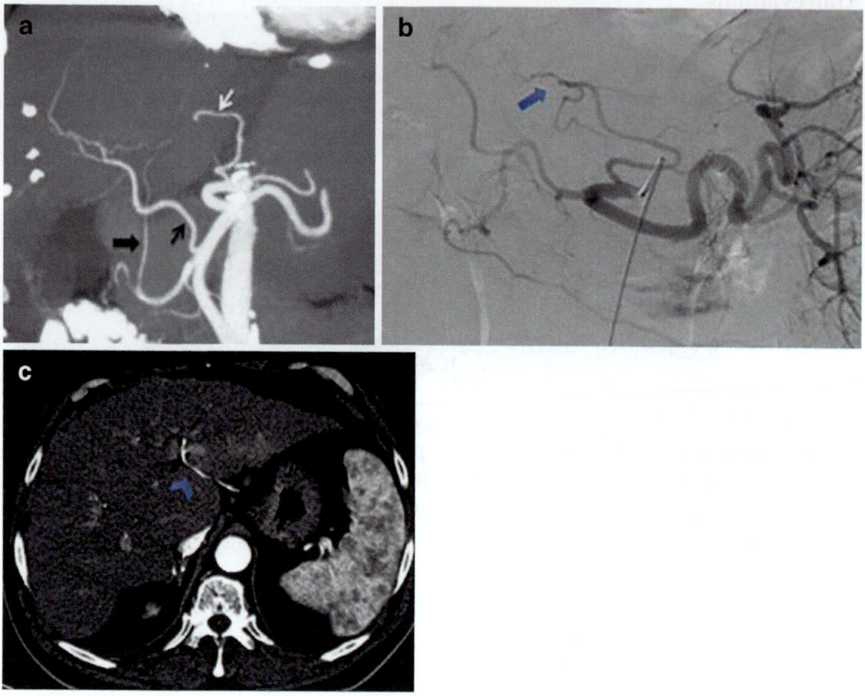

Fig. 21.3 Variant gastric arterial anatomy. (**a**) Maximum-intensity projection coronal CT angiogram image demonstrates a replaced left hepatic artery (LHA) arising from LGA (white arrow). Additional replaced right hepatic arteries are (RHAs) seen originating from the superior mesenteric artery (black arrows). (**b**) Conventional angiogram reveals an accessory LHA arising from LGA (blue arrow), which can be seen coursing along the ligamentum venosum (**c**) on contrast-enhanced axial abdominal CT images (blue arrowhead)

frequent and can be seen 25–75% of patients [10]. Variant examples include a replaced or accessory left hepatic artery arising from LGA, which poses risk of non-target embolization to the liver (Fig. 21.3). A variant esophageal artery can arise from the proximal LGA and would require more distal embolization to avoid esophageal artery embolization. Additional variations include a replaced LGA from a right inferior phrenic artery (Fig. 21.4) or LGA arising directly from the aorta (Fig. 21.5).

Benefits of Transradial Approach in BAE

Although BAE is feasible both from a transradial or transfemoral approach, data from coronary intervention literature suggests that a transradial approach results in less bleeding and access site complications in morbidly obese patients (BMI > 40) [9]. Additionally, transradial approach BAE has been shown to be safe and efficacious for visceral interventions in morbidly obese patients with a 100% technical success rate and no major complications [11].

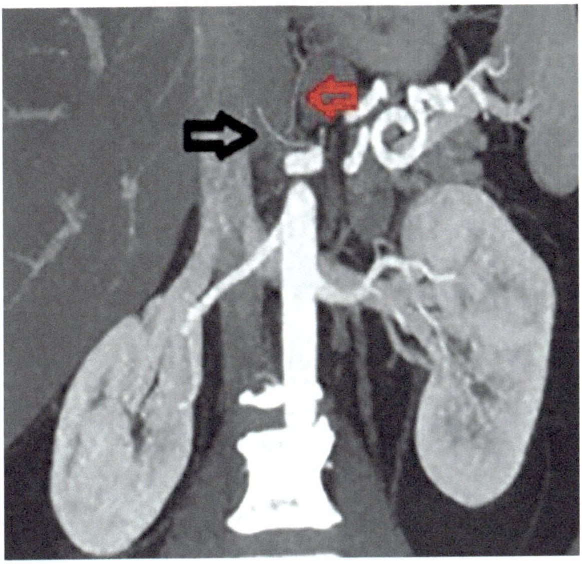

Fig. 21.4 Coronal CT angiogram demonstrates a replaced LGA (red arrow) arising from the right phrenic artery (black arrow)

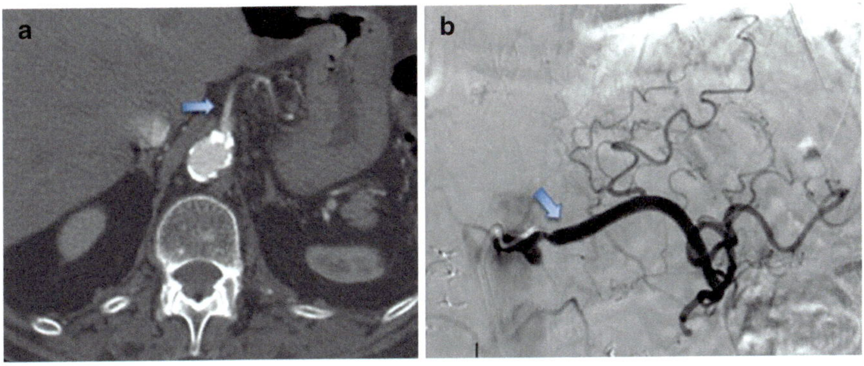

Fig. 21.5 Axial CT (**a**) and conventional angiography (**b**) demonstrate a replaced LGA arising directly from the aorta (blue arrow)

Technical Considerations

General Transradial BAE Technique

While there is no standardized transradial BAE technique to date, multiple clinical trials have reported successful transradial BAE techniques [6, 7, 12, 13], as detailed in Table 21.1. The basic steps of the procedure include radial access, cannulation of the celiac trunk, angiographic imaging of downstream branches, cannulation of the

Table 21.1 Transradial BAE techniques used in obesity clinical trials

Author (reference)	Weiss [6, 7]	Syed [12]	Pirlet [13]
Celiac artery access	100 or 110 cm length 5 F ultimate radial (merit medical) or 5 F Sarah (Terumo medical, Tokyo, Japan) catheter	4-F or 5-F Simmons 1 catheter (length not reported)	125 cm 5-F right Judkins catheter (Boston Scientific, USA)
Celiac artery DSA	Yes	Yes	Yes
LGA access	2.9 F high-flow microcatheter (maestro; merit medical)	Coaxial microcatheter (size or brand not reported)	Same 5F right Judkins catheter
Bead size	300–500-μm Embosphere microspheres (merit medical)	Bead block microspheres 300–500 μm (biocompatibles, Farnham, United Kingdom)	300–500 μm polyvinyl alcohol (PVA) particles (cook medical, Ireland)
Confirmation of stasis	Yes	Yes	Yes
Intraarterial vasodilating agents	200 mg of nitroglycerin, 2.5 mg of verapamil, and 3000 units injected slowly through LGA over 3–5 min	None reported	None reported
Additional technique	CBCT after celiac artery DSA and after LGA embolization		

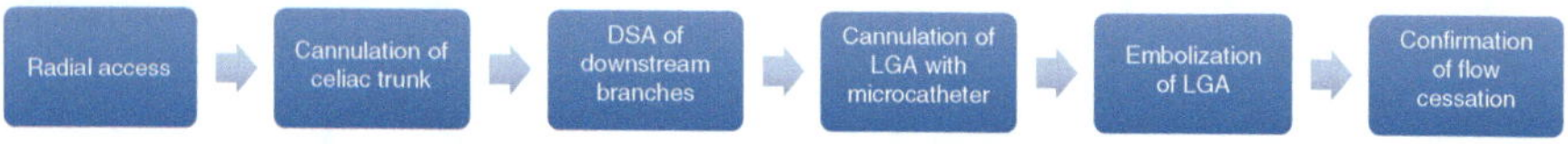

Fig. 21.6 Basic step-by-step diagram of transradial BAE procedure

LGA with a microcatheter, embolization of LGA, and confirmation of flow cessation (Fig. 21.6).

Catheter Selection

After obtaining radial access via Seldinger technique, a 5 F Sarah radial catheter (Merit Medical) or Ultimate radial catheter (Terumo Medical, Tokyo, Japan) may be used to select the celiac artery. Careful attention should be made to the acute angle of the origin of LGA when using the radial guide catheter. Newer diagnostic catheters, such as the 5 F FH-3 catheter (Merit Medical), have been developed to more readily catheterize LGA from a transradial approach. A high-flow microcatheter is then used to select more distal vasculature followed by injection of embolic particles. Targeted embolization of the GEA can also be considered based on its perceived contribution to the fundal blood supply. In the Bariatric Embolization of Arteries for the Treatment of Obesity trial, only 20% of patients had just LGA embolized while 80% had both LGA and GEA embolized [6, 7]. In cases where there is high concern for reflux and concern for nontarget embolization, an antireflux microcatheter such as a Surefire Infusion system (Surefire Medical, Westminster, Colo) can be considered.

Intra-arterial Vasodilation

In order to prevent spasm and achieve more distal penetration prior to LGA embolization, a vasodilating cocktail can be administered in the LGA, such as 200 mg of nitroglycerin, 2.5 mg of verapamil, and 3000 units of heparin. This injection should be performed slowly over the course of 3–5 minutes.

Bead Size

The optimal bead size for BAE remains unknown. Theoretically, smaller bead sides can penetrate more distally but may also have a higher risk of gastric ischemia and ulceration. Early animal studies have demonstrated success with smaller distally penetrating embolic agents such as sclerosants and 40-um particles [14]. In contrast, multiple human clinical trials have used larger 300–500 um size beads with encouraging results and a favorable safety profile [6, 7, 12, 13]. Further studies are necessary to determine the ideal bead size for BAE.

Particle Embolization

To prevent nontarget embolization, careful attention should be made to identify the arterial supply to the gastric fundus and potential anatomic variants, which can be obtained with celiac digital subtraction angiography (DSA) and cone-beam computed tomography (CBCT) (Artis Zeego; Siemens, Forchheim, Germany). Once anatomy is delineated and the LGA or GEA is subselected, delivery of embolic particles should be made as distally into the vessel as possible. Injecting the particles too proximally can lead to nontarget embolization to the stomach antrum. Embolization of the chosen vessel should be performed to stasis with a dilute particle solution, such as a 2 mL vial of embolic particles diluted in 20 cc of contrast and 20 cc of normal saline. Repeat CBCT can then be performed to confirm distribution of embolics and to assess for nontarget embolization.

Post-procedural Considerations

After the procedure, patients should be closely monitored for complications such as nausea, vomiting, and epigastric discomfort. Patients should also be informed of potential risk of gastric ulcers which may manifest as transient or postprandial abdominal pain. For prevention and treatment of gastric ulcers, a proton pump inhibitor such as omeprazole in combination with sucralfate should be given up to 6 weeks post-procedure. In some cases, upper endoscopy can be considered to monitor ulcers in patients who are at higher risk or severely symptomatic.

Conclusion

Bariatric artery embolization may serve as a technically feasible and safe option for treating obesity, although long-term benefits remain investigational. A transradial approach should be considered for morbidly obese patients to reduce the risk of bleeding and access site complications. A clear understanding of gastric vascular anatomy and potential variants is critical in preventing nontarget embolization and undertreatment. Mapping of the vasculature supplying the gastric fundus is critical and can be achieved from the left gastric artery with the use of digital subtraction angiography or cone-beam computed tomography.

References

1. Meldrum DR, Morris MA, Gambone JC. Obesity pandemic: causes, consequences, and solutions—but do we have the will? Fertil Steril. 2017;107(4):833–9.
2. O'Rourke RW, Andrus J, Diggs BS, Scholz M, McConnell DB, Deveney CW. Perioperative morbidity associated with bariatric surgery: an academic center experience. Arch Surg. 2006;141(3):262–8.
3. Cummings DE, Weigle DS, Frayo RS, et al. Plasma ghrelin levels after diet-induced weight loss or gastric bypass surgery. N Engl J Med. 2002;346(21):1623–30.
4. Arepally A, Barnett BP, Montgomery E, et al. Catheter-directed gastric artery chemical embolization for modulation of systemic ghrelin levels in a porcine model: initial experience. Radiology. 2007;244:138–43.
5. Zhong BYB-Y, Ba GA, Weiss CR. An overview of what we currently know about weight loss expectations associated with bariatric embolization. Endovasc Today. 2012;7:85–90.
6. Weiss CR, Akinwande O, Paudel K, et al. Clinical safety of bariatric arterial embolization: preliminary results of the BEAT obesity trial. Radiology. 2017;283:598–608.
7. Weiss CR, Abiola GO, Fischman AM, et al. Bariatric embolization of arteries for the treatment of obesity (BEAT obesity) trial: results at 1year. Radiology. 2019;291:792–800.
8. Bai ZB, Qin YL, Deng G, et al. Bariatric embolization of the left gastric arteries for the treatment of obesity: 9-month data in 5 patients. Obes Surg. 2018;28:907–15.
9. Hibbert B, Simard T, Wilson KR, et al. Transradial versus transfemoral artery approach for coronary angiography and percutaneous coronary intervention in the extremely obese. JACC Cardiovasc Interv. 2012;5:819–26.

10. Pirlet C, Ruzsa Z, Costerousse O, Nemes B, Merkely B, Poirier P, et al. Transradial left gastric artery embolization to treat severe obesity: a pilot study. Catheter Cardiovasc Interv. 2019;93:365–70. https://doi.org/10.1002/ccd.27846.
11. Biederman DM, Marinelli B, O'Connor PJ, et al. Transradial access for visceral endovascular interventions in morbidly obese patients: safety and feasibility. J Vasc Access. 2016;17:256–60.
12. Syed MI, Morar K, Shaikh A, et al. Gastric artery embolization trial for the lessening of appetite nonsurgically (GET LEAN): six-month preliminary data. J Vasc Interv Radiol. 2016;27:1502–8.
13. Zagyapan R, Kürkçüoğlu A, Bayraktar A, Pelin C, Aytekin C. Anatomic variations of the celiac trunk and hepatic arterial system with digital subtraction angiography. Turk J Gastroenterol. 2014;25(Suppl 1):104–9.
14. Paxton BE, Kim CY, Alley CL, et al. Bariatric embolization for suppression of the hunger hormone ghrelin in a porcine model. Radiology. 2013;266(2):471–9.

Index

A
Abdomen
  GI bleeding, 200, 201
  renal hemorrhage, 205, 206
  splenic hemorrhage, 203, 204
  stent-assisted embolization, 202, 203
  transradial setup, 200
Abdominal aortic aneurysm (AAA)
  infrarenal, 87
  juxtarenal, 87
  repair of, 87
  suprarenal, 87
Access-site hematoma, 41
  incidence, 38
Active clotting time (ACT), 67, 79
Acute circuit thrombosis, 148, 149, 158
Acute hemorrhage and trauma
  abdomen
    GI bleeding, 200, 201
    renal hemorrhage, 205, 206
    splenic hemorrhage, 203, 204
    stent-assisted embolization, 202, 203
    transradial setup, 200
  CT angiogram, 195, 196
  n-butyl cyanoacrylate (nBCA) glue, 197
  pelvis
    hematuria, 208
    post-partum uterine hemorrhage, 207
    traumatic pelvic hemorrhage, 207
  radial access and impaired blood clotting, 196
  radial cocktail, 196, 197
  thorax
    bronchial artery embolization, 198
    intercostal artery embolization, 199
    preoperative imaging, 198
Allen test, 22, 222
Anatomic success, 148
Aneurysm sac, 87
Angiography suite setup
  Barbeau test, 25
  equipment/medication list, 26
  left *vs.* right radial approach, 26
  patient positioning, 26–28
  physical exam of the wrist, 25
  radial access, 28
  relative contraindications, 25
Angiomyolipoma (AML), 206
Anticoagulation/antiplatelet therapy, 5
Anti-thrombotic therapy, 98
Aortic aneurysm, 87
Aortic arch, asymmetry of, 165
Aortic endoleak
  algorithm, 94
  anti-thrombotic therapy, 98
  complex endograft endoleak management, 99
  diagnosis/post-evar surveillance, 93
  prevention, 99–100
  radial access, 100
  risks, 87
  TEVAR endoleak management, 98
  type I
    classification, 88–90
    management and approach, 94, 95
  type II
    classification, 88–91
    management and approach, 95, 96
  type III
    classification, 88, 89, 91, 92
    management and approach, 97
  type IV

A. M. Fischman et al. (eds.), *Transradial Access in Interventional Radiology*,
https://doi.org/10.1007/978-3-030-81678-0

Aortic endoleak (*cont.*)
classification, 88, 89, 92
management and approach, 97
type V
classification, 88, 89, 93
management and approach, 97
Aortoiliac arterial disease
aortic arch and monitoring, 66
catheter and sheath systems, 66
covered stents, 65
descending aorta navigation, 66
interventions, 65
preprocedural patient selection, 66
radial artery access, 66
secondary access site, 65
sheaths and guiding catheters, 67
stent grafts, 65, 66
techniques and specific tools, 66
Arch navigation, 166
Arterial compression devices, 213, 216
Atherectomy, 77
AV fistulas, 44
incidence, 38

B
Balloon maceration, 149
Barbeau test, 15, 16, 25, 213, 222
Bariatric arterial embolization (BAE)
anatomical considerations
conventional celiac trunk anatomy, 235
conventional gastric arterial anatomy, 234, 235
variant gastric arterial vascular anatomy, 235–237
visceral anatomy of stomach, 234
benefits of, 234, 236
post-procedural considerations, 240
procedural steps, 238
technical considerations
bead size, 239
catheter selection, 238, 239
intra-arterial vasodilation, 239
particle embolization, 239
standardized transradial technique, 237, 238
Bariatric surgery, 233
Brachial artery
anatomy, 11
loop, 12
variants and frequency, 12
Bronchial artery embolization, 198

C
Carnevale system, 138
Carotid and vertebral intervention
arch navigation, 166
equipment list, 165, 166
left ICA primary stenting, 171–173
left vertebral artery origin angioplasty and stent, 173, 174
right ICA angioplasty and stenting, 169–171
right vertebral artery stenting, 167–169
Simmons 2 shape formation, 167
transradial CAS, 164
Carotid artery stenting (CAS), 163
Catheter and sheath systems, 66
Catheter granuloma, 47
incidence, 38
Catheter/sheath entrapment
incidence, 38
Chimney or snorkel technique, 99
Co-axial guide catheter approach, 52
Compartment syndrome
forearm, 43
hand, 43
Compartment syndrome/hand ischemia, 38
Complex endograft endoleak management, 99
Conventional celiac trunk anatomy, 235
Conventional gastric arterial anatomy, 234, 235
Coronary angiography, 4, 5
Coronary arterial bypass graft (CABG) surgery, 5
Coronary arterial disease (CAD), 5

D
Device-related complications
catheter granuloma, 47
sheath entrapment, 46
Dialysis interventions, 148
Distal basilar occlusion, 190–193
Distal radial arteriotomy, 1
Distal radial artery access (dTRA)
advantages, 221
anatomic snuffbox, 222, 223
arterial anatomy, 223
closure technique, 224
distal radial access sheaths, 225
left humerus metastatic hepatocellular carcinoma mass, 230
left shoulder mass pre-operative embolization, 224, 226

patient selection, 222
post-procedure hemostatic control, 221
pre-radioembolization mapping, 228
radial arterial compression devices, 225
relative indications and contraindications, 223
Dotter's aortic root injection method, 4

E
Embolization
persistent left circumflex humeral artery bleed, 120
right brachial artery branches, 117
Endovascular aortic repair (EVAR), 87

F
Forearm compartment syndrome, 43

G
Gastric neuroregulatory pathways, 234

H
Hand compartment syndrome, 43
Hematoma
access-site, 41
compartment syndrome, 43
with extensive ecchymosis, 43
radial artery perforation, 42
Hematuria, 208
Hemodialysis access intervention
access, 150
access approach, 147
acute circuit thrombosis, 148, 149, 158
adjunctive medication, 150
balloon maceration/mechanical thrombectomy, 149
circuit evaluation, 147
closure, 150
dialysis, 148
disadvantages, 148
dysfunction, 148, 153
elective and urgent basis, 147
fistula or graft, 147
limitation, 148
non-maturation, 148, 155, 156
occluded anastomosis, 150
percutaneous access, 149
primary evidence, 151–153
radiocephalic fistula, 149
reflux angiography with outflow compression, 147
standard approach, 147
Hemostasis
equipment list, 33
inflatable wrist bands, 31, 32
non-occlusive patent hemostasis, 31
physical examination, 32
post-procedure care and complications, 33, 34
pulse oximeter waveform, 31
Hepatic chemoembolization, 218
Hepatocellular carcinoma (HCC), 58
Herculink balloon-expandable bare-metal stents, 203
Hypervascular malignancies, 58

I
Inferior mesenteric artery (IMA) aneurysm, 52, 54
Infrainguinal disease, 77
aortoiliac and infrainguinal lesions, 79
descending aorta navigation, 78
drug-coated balloons and drug eluting stent options, 77
5Fr self-expandable sinus-superflex-518, 77
limiting factor, 77
over-the-write (OTW) devices, 78
radial artery access, 78
with second access site, 78
6Fr 119 and 149cm destination slender sheath, 77
subintimal paths, 77
techniques and specific tools, 78
vessel perforation, 78
Infrainguinal lower extremity interventions, 76
Intercostal artery embolization, 199
Interventional oncology (IO) procedures
hepatocellular carcinoma, 58
intra-arterial treatments, 58
liver metastasis, 58
methodology, 58, 59
transradial access, 59, 60
Intra-arterial IO treatments, 58
Intra-arterial vasodilation, 239
Intraoperative angiography, 178
Intravascular access, history of, 2

L

Left arteriovenous fistula, thrombosis of, 118, 119
Left ICA primary stenting, 171–173
Left subclavian arteriovenous malformation, 114
Left subclavian artery embolization, with persistent endoleak, 115, 116
Left vertebral artery origin angioplasty and stent, 173, 174
LICA blister aneurysm embolization with flow diversion, 183, 186
Liver metastasis, 58

M

Macroaggregated albumin (MAA) mapping, 58
Mechanical thrombectomy, 149
Modified Allen test, 15

N

Neuroangiography, 179–181
Neurologic complications, 45
Neurologic deficits, incidence, 38
Neuromuscular complications, 45, 46
Nonhealing foot wound, 84–86
Non-occlusive patent hemostasis, 31
Nonselective coronary angiography, 2
Nursing assessment
  history, 21, 22
  informed consent, 20, 21
  medications, 22
  patient education and orientation, 20
  physical exam, 21

O

Obesity, 233
Occluded popliteal artery and posterior tibial artery, 82–84
Occlusive aortography method, 4
Over-the-write (OTW) devices, 78

P

Pain control methods, 125
Pelvis
  hematuria, 208
  post-partum uterine hemorrhage, 207
  traumatic pelvic hemorrhage, 207
Percutaneous arterial catheterization, 3
Percutaneous coronary angiography, 5
Percutaneous coronary interventions (PCIs), 5
Percutaneous thoracic aortography, 3
Percutaneous transluminal coronary angioplasty (PTCA), 5
Percutaneous transradial access, 2
Percutaneous transradial coronary angiography, 2
Percutaneous transradial coronary balloon angioplasty, 2
Peripheral arterial disease (PAD)
  aortoiliac arterial disease
    aortic arch and monitoring, 66
    catheter and sheath systems, 66
    covered stents, 65
    descending aorta navigation, 66
    interventions, 65
    preprocedural patient selection, 66
    radial artery access, 66
    secondary access site, 65
    sheaths and guiding catheters, 67
    stent grafts, 65, 66
    techniques and specific tools, 66
  behavioral changes, 64
  endovascular or surgical intervention, 64
  factors, 64
  infrainguinal disease, 77
    aortoiliac and infrainguinal lesions, 79
    descending aorta navigation, 78
    drug-coated balloons and drug eluting stent options, 77
    5Fr self-expandable sinus-superflex-518, 77
    limiting factor, 77
    over-the-write (OTW) devices, 78
    radial artery access, 78
    with second access site, 78
    6Fr 119 and 149cm destination slender sheath, 77
    subintimal paths, 77
    techniques and specific tools, 78
    vessel perforation, 78
    with second access site, 78
  interventions, 65
  lower extremity arterial anatomy, 76
  lower extremity interventions, 64
  medical and behavior management, 64
  nonhealing foot wound, 84–86
  occluded popliteal artery and posterior tibial artery, 82–84
  pharmaceutical interventions, 64
  prevalence, 63
  relative indications and contraindications, 64

- right common iliac and external iliac stenosis, 67, 69, 71, 72
  - superficial femoral artery in-stent neointimal hyperplasia, 79, 81, 84
  - symptomatic and asymptomatic individuals, 64
- Persistent left circumflex humeral artery bleed, 120
- Postoperative coronary arteriography, 5
- Post-partum hemorrhage, 196
- Post-partum uterine hemorrhage, 207
- Pre/intraoperative embolization, 97
- Prophylactic ipsilateral ulnar artery compression, 33, 40
- Prostate artery embolization (PAE)
  - advantages of, TRA, 134
  - with alternative BPH treatments, 133
  - alternative diagnoses, 135
  - angiography, 139
  - Carnevale system, 138
  - clinical cases, 141, 142
  - clinical workup, 135
  - closure and post-procedure care, 141
  - 90-degree abduction position, 139
  - disadvantages of, 135
  - embolization, 140
  - equipment list, 135
  - 5F diagnostic catheter, 139
  - history, 133
  - left arm adduction position, 139
  - left internal iliac artery, 140
  - pre-procedure setup, 136, 137
  - radial access considerations, 136–138
  - radial artery access, 134
  - transradial/ransulnar access *vs.* transfemoral access, 134
  - tube angulation, 139
  - variable anatomy, 138
- Prostatectomy, 133
- Pseudoaneurysms, 44
  - incidence, 38

R

- Radial arterial compression devices, 225
- Radial arteritis, 44
  - anatomy, 12, 13
  - blood supply, hand, 14
  - gray scale visualization, 16
  - loop, 13
  - sonographic assessment, 16
  - triphasic waveform, 16
  - variants and frequency, 13
- Radial artery dissection, incidence, 38
- Radial artery occlusion (RAO)
  - adequate systemic anticoagulation, 40
  - consequences, 41
  - due to the protective effects, 40
  - incidence, 38, 40
  - IR practices, 40
  - patent hemostasis, 40
  - prophylactic ipsilateral ulnar artery compression, 40
  - risk factors, 40
  - treatment, 41
  - unfractionated heparin, 40
- Radial artery perforation, 42
  - incidence, 38
- Radial artery spasm (RAS)
  - effective prophylactic method, 38
  - incidence, 38
  - manifestation, 38
  - multifocal, 38
  - procedural management, 39
  - transradial procedure with initial puncture and sheath placement, 38
- Radial endarterectomy procedure, 46
- Radiocephalic fistula, 149
- Renal and mesenteric artery disease
  - balloon expandable stent placement, 52, 53
  - co-axial guide catheter approach, 52
  - complete occlusion, 52, 54
  - with flow improvement, 52, 53
  - large angiomyolipoma, 53, 55
  - large inferior mesenteric artery aneurysm, 52, 54
  - mass vascularity, 53, 55
  - no touch technique, 52
  - Onyx cast, 54
  - severe ostial stenosis, 52, 53
  - wire stabilization, 52
- Renal arteriovenous fistula embolization with n-BCA liquid embolic agent, 216, 217
- Renal hemorrhage, 205, 206
- Right ICA angioplasty and stenting, 169–171
- Right occipital AVM embolization with Onyx, 186, 188
- Right vertebral artery stenting, 167–169

S

- Seldinger technique, 3
- Sheathless Eaucath systems, 66
- Simmons 2 shape formation, 167
- Single-wall puncture technique, 28
- Smallest-diameter hydrophilic sheath, 28
- Sones' early coronary angiographic studies, 5

Sones' selective method, 4
Splenic hemorrhage, 203, 204
Subclavian and upper arm interventions
  embolization
    persistent left circumflex humeral artery bleed, 120
    right brachial artery branches, 117
  immediate ambulation, 113
  left arteriovenous fistula, thrombosis of, 118, 119
  left subclavian arteriovenous malformation, 114
  left subclavian artery embolization, with persistent endoleak, 115, 116
Supra-aortic neuro-interventions, 164

T
Thoracic aortic aneurysm (TAA), 87
TR Band®, 32
Traditional transvenous approach, 148
Transarterial embolization, 96
Transcaval and ventral approaches, 96
Transfemoral coronary artery stent placement, 5
Translumbar embolization, 96
Transradial access, 2
Transradial approach
  ACCESS study, 6
  in interventional cardiology, 5, 6
  interventional radiology, 6–8
  MORTAL, RIVAL, RIFLE STEACS, and MATRIX studies, 6
  origins, 2–5
  radial artery
    surgical exposure, 3
Transradial artery catheterization, 1
Transradial endovascular advanced therapies (TREAT), 2
Transradial endovascular arterial intervention, 131
Transradial interventions, 2
Transradial noncoronary, 2
Transulnar arterial access (TUA)
  arterial compression devices, 213, 216
  closure technique, 214, 216
  coronary and peripheral interventions, 211
  forearm, arterial anatomy of, 215
  hepatic chemoembolization, 218
  patient positioning, 214
  patient selection, 212, 213
  percutaneous coronary procedures, 211
  relative indications and contraindications, 212
  renal arteriovenous fistula embolization with n-BCA liquid embolic agent, 216, 217
  safety and efficacy, 212
  technique, 213
  vs. TRA, 212
  ulnar access sheaths, 213
TRA-related pseudoaneurysms, 44
Traumatic pelvic hemorrhage, 207

U
Ulnar access sheaths, 213
Ulnar artery access, 211
Ulnopalmar arch patency, 25
Ulnopalmar patency, 222
Unruptured right MCA wide-neck bifurcation aneurysm, stent-assisted coiling of, 178, 182, 183, 185
Uterine artery embolization (UAE)
  advantages, 124
  conventional catheter/guidewire combinations, 124
  microcatheter, 126, 127
  pain management, 125
  patient satisfaction, 125
  safety, 124, 125
  symptomatic uterine fibroids, 125–127
  technical considerations, 130, 131
  tools, 124
  unstable patient with postpartum bleeding, 128

V
Variant gastric arterial vascular anatomy, 235–237
Vascular complications
  AV fistulas, 44
  dissection, 43
  radial arteritis, 44
  TRA-related pseudoaneurysms, 44

W
Whipple procedure, 202

Y
Yttrium-90 microspheres, 58

GPSR Compliance

The European Union's (EU) General Product Safety Regulation (GPSR) is a set of rules that requires consumer products to be safe and our obligations to ensure this.

If you have any concerns about our products, you can contact us on ProductSafety@springernature.com

In case Publisher is established outside the EU, the EU authorized representative is:

Springer Nature Customer Service Center GmbH
Europaplatz 3
69115 Heidelberg, Germany

Batch number: 10732090

Printed by Printforce, the Netherlands